P9-DEM-510

Foldable Intraocular Lenses

Evolution, Clinicopathologic Correlations, and Complications

Foldable Intraocular Lenses

Evolution, Clinicopathologic Correlations, and Complications

DAVID J. APPLE, MD

Center for Research on Ocular Therapeutics and Biodevices, Albert Florens Storm Eye Institute, Department of Ophthalmology, Medical University of South Carolina, Charleston, South Carolina

GERD U. AUFFARTH, MD

Department of Ophthalmology, University of Heidelberg, Germany

QUN PENG, MD

Center for Research on Ocular Therapeutics and Biodevices, Albert Florens Storm Eye Institute, Department of Ophthalmology, Medical University of South Carolina, Charleston, South Carolina

NITHI VISESSOOK, MD

Center for Research on Ocular Therapeutics and Biodevices, Albert Florens Storm Eye Institute, Department of Ophthalmology, Medical University of South Carolina, Charleston, South Carolina

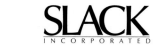

SLACK
INCORPORATED

6900 Grove Rd. • Thorofare, NJ 08086

Publisher: John H. Bond
Editorial Director: Amy E. Drummond
Design Editor: Lauren Biddle Plummer

Copyright © 2000 by SLACK Incorporated

All rights reserved. No part of this book may be reproduced, stored in a retrieval system or transmitted in any form or by any means, electronic, mechanical, photocopying, recording or otherwise, without written permission from the publisher, except for brief quotations embodied in critical articles and reviews.

The procedures and practices described in this book should be implemented in a manner consistent with the professional standards set for the circumstances that apply in each specific situation. Every effort has been made to confirm the accuracy of the information presented and to correctly relate generally accepted practices. The author, editor, and publisher cannot accept responsibility for errors or exclusions or for the outcome of the application of the material presented herein. There is no expressed or implied warranty of this book or information imparted by it.

Care has been taken to ensure that drug selection and dosages are in accordance with currently accepted/recommended practice. Due to continuing research, changes in government policy and regulations, and various effects of drug reactions and interactions, it is recommended that the reader review all materials and literature provided for each drug, especially those that are new or not frequently used.

Any review or mention of specific companies or products is not intended as an endorsement by the author or the publisher.

Foldable intraocular lenses: evolution, clinicopathologic correlations, and complications/ David J. Apple...[et al.].
    p. ; cm.
   Includes bibliographical references and index.
   ISBN 1-55642-435-3 (alk. paper)
   1. Intraocular lenses, I. Apple, David J., 1941-
   [DNLM: 1. Lenses, Intraocular. WW 358 F6635 2000]
   RE988 .F654 2000
   617.7'4206--dc21   00-029134

Printed in Canada

Published by: SLACK Incorporated
                     6900 Grove Road
                     Thorofare, NJ 08086 USA
                     Telephone: 856-848-1000
                     Fax: 856-853-5991
                     World Wide Web: www.slackbooks.com

Contact SLACK Incorporated for more information about other books in this field or about the availability of our books from distributors outside the United States.

Authorization to photocopy items for internal or personal use, or the internal or personal use of specific clients, is granted by SLACK Incorporated, provided that the appropriate fee is paid directly to Copyright Clearance Center, 222 Rosewood Drive, Danvers, MA 01923 USA, 978-750-8400. Prior to photocopying items for educational classroom use, please contact the CCC at the address above. Please reference Account Number 9106324 for SLACK Incorporated's Professional Book Division.

For further information on CCC, check CCC Online at the following address: http://www.copyright.com.

Last digit is print number: 10 9 8 7 6 5 4 3 2 1

DEDICATION

To Sir Harold Ridley, MA, MD, Cantab., FRCS, England, Fellow of the Royal Society, London—the inventor of the intraocular lens.

"An invasion of armies can be resisted, but not an idea whose time has come."

—Victor Hugo

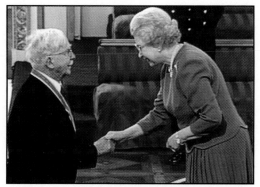

Investiture of Knighthood on Harold Ridley by Queen Elizabeth II, February 9, 2000. (Courtesy of David J. Apple, MD, Charleston, SC, and Ian Collins and Donald Munro, Rayner, Ltd., United Kingdom.)

CONTENTS

ABOUT THE AUTHORS

David J. Apple, MD
Center for Research on Ocular Therapeutics and Biodevices, Storm Eye Institute, Department of Ophthalmology, Medical University of South Carolina, Charleston
Professor of Ophthalmology and and Pathology

Formerly, Professor and Chairman, Department of Ophthalmology
Pawek-Vallotton Chair of Biomedical Engineering
Director, Ocular Pathology Laboratory and Center for Research on Ocular Therapeutics and Biodevices
Albert Florens Storm Eye Institute, Medical University of South Carolina, Charleston, South Carolina
Director, World Health Organization (WHO) Collaborating Centre for Prevention of Blindness
Distinguished Senior U.S. Scientist Awardee, Alexander von Humbolt Foundation
Formerly: Professor of Ophthalmology and Pathology, University of Utah Health Sciences Center, Salt Lake City, Utah

Priv.-Doz. Dr. Med. Gerd U. Auffarth, MD
Department of Ophthalmology, University of Heidelberg, Germany

Associate Professor of Ophthalmology
Department of Ophthalmology
Ruprecht-Karls-University of Heidelberg, Germany

Qun Peng, MD
Center for Research on Ocular Therapeutics and Biodevices, Storm Eye Institute, Department of Ophthalmology, Medical University of South Carolina, Charleston

Assistant Professor of Ophthalmology
Assistant Director, Ocular Pathology Laboratory and Center for Research on Ocular Therapeutics and Biodevices
Albert Florens Storm Eye Institute, Medical University of South Carolina, Charleston, South Carolina

Nithi Visessook, MD
Center for Research on Ocular Therapeutics and Biodevices, Storm Eye Institute, Department of Ophthalmology, Medical University of South Carolina, Charleston

Senior Research Fellow, Ocular Pathology and Center for Research on Ocular Therapeutics and Biodevices
Albert Florens Storm Eye Institute, Medical University of South Carolina, Charleston, South Carolina

CONTRIBUTING AUTHORS

Roberto Bianchi, MD
Center for Research on Ocular Therapeutics and Biodevices,
Charleston, South Carolina

Marcela Escobar-Gomez, MD
Center for Research on Ocular Therapeutics and Biodevices,
Charleston, South Carolina

Suresh K. Pandey, MD
Center for Research on Ocular Therapeutics and Biodevices,
Charleston, South Carolina

Edgar L. Ready, M.S
Center for Research on Ocular Therapeutics and Biodevices,
Charleston, South Carolina

Enrique Roig, MD
Center for Research on Ocular Therapeutics and Biodevices,
Charleston, South Carolina

Robert J. Schoderbek, Jr, MD
Center for Research on Ocular Therapeutics and Biodevices,
Charleston, South Carolina

Kerry Solomon, MD
Center for Research on Ocular Therapeutics and Biodevices,
Charleston, South Carolina

Kaidi Tourort, MD
Center for Research on Ocular Therapeutics and Biodevices,
Charleston, South Carolina

Liliana Werner, MD, PhD
Center for Research on Ocular Therapeutics and Biodevices,
Charleston, South Carolina

ACKNOWLEDGMENTS

We would like to thank Joyce B. Edmonds, HT; Beau Evans; Rose Hayes; Daphne Hoddinott; Maddie Manuel; Lucia McClendon; Sebastian Ober; Krista Ramonas; and Theodora R. Redmon.

We thank all Eyebanks nationwide that have provided invaluable support to the research analyses provided in this text.

PREFACE

The evolution of the cataract surgery–intraocular lens (IOL) operation since Harold Ridley's (now Sir Harold Ridley, as of February 9, 2000, see Dedication and Figure P-1) invention of the IOL 50 years ago has been one of the most stellar achievements of modern medicine. Benefits provided to patients with cataracts have increased dramatically, especially in the industrialized world. The mediocre visual rehabilitation provided by aphakic spectacles—often associated with moderate to severe complications of the surgery—has been replaced by precise pseudophakic optical rehabilitation with fewer complications. The advent of small-incision surgery made possible by phacoemulsification and foldable IOLs represents a major milestone in this evolutionary process.

Today's foldable IOLs are generally very good, but not perfect. Specific differences among today's designs exist. We are currently in a period of fine-tuning the technology. The goal of this text is to provide clinically relevant information that bridges the gap between purely clinical considerations regarding modern IOL surgery and basic scientific investigations regarding this surgical subspecialty.

Surgeons today choose IOLs primarily according to clinical experience; as a result of information gained from IOL manufacturers' research, development, and marketing; and after evaluation of service and financial issues. In this text we share a large database of information and illustrative material that we have accumulated on foldable IOLs over the last two decades—material that will further assist surgeons in the IOL selection process.

We present a viewpoint that heretofore has rarely been readily available to clinicians; namely, clinicopathologic correlation. Pathologic analyses on a large number of specimens have enabled us to determine subtle differences among various modern foldable IOL designs, especially in relation to variations in postoperative tissue reactions within capsular bags of eyes implanted with various IOL designs and biomaterials. We have chosen not to provide specific opinions or recommendations regarding which may be the "best" foldable IOL(s). Rather, a careful reading of the text and tables, as well as the illustrations and their legends—almost all of which contain new and previously unpublished material—should speak for itself. The information presented should provide new insights for the surgeon that will assist him or her in choosing a preferred foldable IOL.

This is not a book on surgical techniques. Excellent discussions of operative techniques, such as phacoemulsification and sutureless cataract surgery, as well as details regarding anesthesia, incision size and location, and IOL insertion techniques with or without injectors, and other important topics, have been presented in numerous previous publications, with input from the masters in these fields. Several have been published by SLACK Incorporated (referenced in Chapter 1). These need not be repeated here. Clinical investigations (including Food and Drug Administration–mandated studies) are ongoing on many foldable IOL designs. Because in many cases the results are not final, details regarding clinical results and outcomes are best reserved for future publications.

Many publications detailing basic scientific investigations on foldable IOLs are now readily available to the reader and therefore need not be covered here. Such studies include comprehensive listings of manufacturers' specifications, physical properties, and chemical formulations of IOL biomaterials, and details regarding design and manufacture of foldable IOLs and physiologic optics of IOLs, including multifocals.

Bridging the gap between the clinician and the basic scientist is accomplished by focusing directly on clinicopathologic analysis and correlation of tissue specimens containing foldable IOLs. The main source of information is the large database of human eyes obtained postmortem with posterior chamber IOLs accumulated in our research center between 1982 and the present. With few exceptions, the main sources of specimens and data are physicians and Eyebanks in the continental United States.

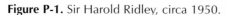

Figure P-1. Sir Harold Ridley, circa 1950.

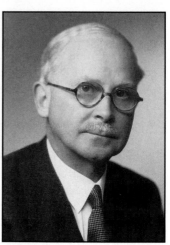

We cannot cover all parameters regarding foldable IOLs, we limit our observations to findings gleaned from direct analysis of specimens in our Center. We have attempted to avoid speculation of purely clinical themes. For example, we refrain from discussion on such topics as possible IOL–induced visual aberrations and glare—topics that are important but not well addressed in a laboratory setting. However, we can comment with confidence on basic tissue reactions, such as anterior and posterior capsular opacification, centration, and overall safety and tolerance of the IOL in the eye.

Detailed presentations, illustrations, and, of course, conclusions can only be made on foldable IOLs that are available for implantation in the United States (and therefore available to our database). We provide a comparative listing and catalogue of selected foldable IOLs not available in our USA autopsy database. However, we are unable to offer nearly as much clinically relevant clinicopathologic correlation as is possible with the IOLs available to us in the United States. Various positive or negative observations we make regarding each individual IOL design are based on our clinicopathologic studies. Many clinical observations and conclusions regarding outcomes in the literature are anecdotal. Therefore, we minimize referral to these both in the pathologic evaluations and reference material.

In a computer-assisted literature search, we found a total of 7284 citations of IOL–related articles between 1966 and the present! Detailed referencing of these is far outside the scope of this text. The reader interested in further detail can search the Internet rather than have us provide a huge bibliography. We have attempted to confine the selected references in the text to those most relevant to the stated focus; namely, clinicopathologic correlation of foldable IOLs.

The origin of the above mentioned database stems from the 1983 founding of the Center for Intraocular Lens Research, co-founded by Randall Olson, MD, and the senior author, David J. Apple, MD, in Salt Lake City, Utah. This center was transferred to Charleston, SC in 1988. Because of evolving research in other fields related to biomedical engineering, including refractive surgical procedures and devices, we have changed the name to the Center for Research on Ocular Therapeutics and Biodevices. The growth of the database of IOL–related material, beginning with IOL number 1 in late 1982 and moving to IOL number 16,000 and beyond by 2000, reflects the rapid growth of the specialty of cataract surgery–IOL implantation and attests to the success of the Center.

The database consists largely of two major subgroups. The first subgroup consists of IOLs explanted from patients' eyes that had IOL–related complications. The second subgroup—most important to this text—consists of the large and unique database of human eyes obtained post-mortem containing IOLs. By the year 2000, this collection of eyes numbered over 7000. We are grateful to the eye banks nationwide that have provided us with these specimens. Most important for purposes of this text is the fact that the number of foldable IOLs being accessioned is growing rapidly. This publication provides us an opportunity, for the first time, to present data and illustrations from this unique collection of research tissue.

Except for a very few selected illustrations and tables provided by professional colleagues and industry, the overwhelming majority of materials in this book, both textual and visual, are original from our Center. All lens manufacturers were notified of the preparation of this book and invited to submit up-to-date information and illustration material of their choice. The information provided here is unbiased and not influenced by manufacturers. It represents solely the opinions of the authors and staff of the Center for Research on Ocular Therapeutics and Biodevices. Preparation of this book was funded by our general laboratory fund and not by specific manufacturers. Therefore, what is presented is unbiased.

We originally intended to limit our focus and discussion to the most current information available to us regarding modern foldable lenses. However, at the suggestion of Dr. Howard Fine, one of the leading cataract surgeons of our time, we have elected to include also a brief overview regarding the evolution and history of the cataract operation and the IOL. This not only serves to honor Sir Harold Ridley, who started it all, but also helps give credit to many other investigators and surgeons who have made today's accomplishments possible. Surgeons today, especially young residents in training, often take this procedure for granted, not realizing the ups and downs, dead ends, clinical disasters, and otherwise difficult times that surgeons, researchers, and, of course, patients have had during this evolutionary period. Our ability to insert foldable IOLs safely did not appear overnight. It was a long and arduous process. We all have short memories!

An understanding of the history, the many wrong turns, and the lessons they provided will be helpful in understanding how the cataract–IOL procedure evolved into what it is today. It has been a decade since the last detailed publication regarding the history of IOLs appeared.[1] That book was published just as the era of foldable lenses began to emerge. Readers are referred to this reference for additional details regarding the history of IOLs.

Implantation of foldable IOLs through a small incision after phacoemulsification implies a high-technology procedure performed in an industrialized world setting. Although this generally has been true until now, we confidently predict that implantation of foldable IOLs in the developing world will begin increasing in incidence in the near future.

Significant use of IOLs of any type or model in the developing world began at least a decade later (circa 1987) than occurred in the industrialized world (circa 1977), largely because of economic and logistical factors. This has turned around and a concerted effort is occurring to provide pseudophakia worldwide. The advantages of small-incision surgery and foldable IOLs are already being provided in large cities, private practices, and a few major centers in the developing world. With increased global communication and improved logistics and finances, this will undoubtedly expand over the next decade into more rural areas of the developing world.

In an attempt to help facilitate this expansion, we have recently completed a monograph focusing on cataract surgery in the developing world.[2] The main types of IOLs being implanted in the developing world are still one- and three-piece designs with rigid polymethyl methacrylate (PMMA) optics. These continue to provide excellent results. Because the PMMA designs are still used extensively in the developing world, the above mentioned monograph remains focused on rigid PMMA designs. There are introductory comments on foldable designs, but little detail is provided. However, as the transition from early types of precapsular surgery (often with can-open-

Figure P-2. Sir Harold Ridley (right) and the senior author (David J. Apple, MD; left), at home with Ridley in Stapleford (near Salisbury), United Kingdom. This photograph was taken in 1994 during preparation of Ridley's approved biography.[3]

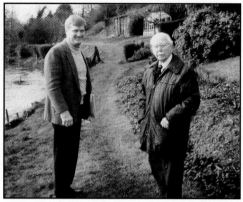

er anterior capsulotomy techniques), toward modern capsular surgery (with continuous curvilinear capsulorhexis or the envelope technique) continues at ever increasing rates, the use of foldable lenses will increase. It is timely and indeed inevitable that phacoemulsification and small-incision surgery with foldable lenses will be used more in the underprivileged world. We are therefore hopeful, as preparations for this transition occur, that this book on foldable lenses will be helpful to the developing world surgeon, especially in helping her or him navigate through the learning curve while choosing safe and efficacious IOL designs.

Widespread provision of high-quality pseudophakia throughout the developing world will be extremely pleasing to Sir Harold Ridley, to whom this book is dedicated in commemoration of the 50th anniversary of his invention of the implant and in celebration of his knighthood (see Dedication). We are delighted that he has lived to enjoy the fruits of his labor and has received several long-overdue honors. The senior author has had the honor and pleasure of writing his approved biography (Figure P-2).[3] Ridley has had a strong interest in developing world ophthalmology, first stimulated during the time of his work in tropical ophthalmology in Africa during World War II. Establishing widespread use of IOLs in the underprivileged world would be a joy to him and is in complete accord with a statement that he wishes to be placed on his epitaph—namely, that his greatest accomplishment was "the cure of aphakia."

REFERENCES

1. Apple DJ, Kincaid MC, Mamalis N, Olson RJ. *Intraocular Lenses: Evolution, Designs, Complications, and Pathology.* Baltimore, Md: Williams & Wilkins, 1989.

2. Apple DJ, Ram J, Foster A, Peng Q. Elimination of cataract blindness: a global perspective. *Surv Ophthalmol 2000* (supplement).

3. Apple DJ, Sims JC. Harold Ridley and the invention of the intraocular lens. *Surv Ophthalmol* 1995;40:279–292.

BIBLIOGRAPHY

Apple DJ, Ram J, Peng Q. The Fiftieth Anniversary of the Intraocular Lens and a Quiet Revolution. Editorial. *Ophthalmology.* 1999 [In Press].

Apple DJ. Harold Ridley. A Golden Anniversary Celebration and A Golden Age. Editorial. *Arch Ophthalmol.* 1999;117:827.

FOREWORD

The history of small incision cataract surgery and foldable IOL implantation is a spectacular clinical and intellectual adventure, combining the development of phacoemulsification and biomaterial technology with the rapid evolution in surgical technique and IOL design. These changes, taking place over a relatively short period of time, have resulted in dramatic improvements in surgical results and almost immediate visual rehabilitation for patients; goals which seemed impossible only 20 years ago. Many cataract surgeons practicing today don't know many of the details or the chronology of these changes.

The research of Dr. David Apple and his coworkers, first at the Center for Intraocular Lens Research in Salt Lake City, Utah, and more recently at the Center for Research on Ocular Therapeutics and Biodevices in Charleston, South Carolina, has contributed significantly to helping surgeons understand what constitutes good surgical technique and to helping the industry understand the anatomical and physiologic basis for proper lens design and biocompatability.

Some of the material in the following pages has been reported in the literature and discussed at scientific symposia. However, the text and illustrations derived from autopsy specimens, utilizing techniques developed at their laboratories, allow the authors to consolidate the material in a comprehensive and easily accessible form that will prove invaluable to the community of cataract and refractive surgeons.

I. Howard Fine, MD
Oregon Health Sciences University
Portland, Oregon
Oregon Eye Associates
Eugene, Oregon

Section
1

Background

Background

Introduction

Shortly after establishing the Center for Intraocular Lens Research in Salt Lake City, Utah in 1983, cofounders Randall Olson, MD, and the senior author, David J. Apple, MD, discussed how interesting it would be to be able to follow and perform long-term evaluations of the numerous intraocular lenses (IOLs) and IOL-related specimens that had been received for clinicopathologic analyses. Examination of pseudophakic eyes obtained postmortem, randomly accessioned from eye banks nationwide, would provide a unique opportunity to "autopsy" eyes containing IOLs. This would allow one to see which lenses, procedures, and other innovations had stood the test of time. That time has arrived. We present here a detailed pathology-based report on one of the most important innovations that has emerged during the last decade; namely, the field of small-incision cataract surgery with foldable lenses.

The judgment of time has confirmed many of the original findings derived from our database of IOL specimens. This includes confirmation of the efficacy of in-the-bag fixation, a topic that was highly controversial throughout much of the 1980s. Other surgical techniques[1] studied in the laboratory during this period, some of which now form the basis of modern small-incision surgery, include continuous curvilinear capsulorhexis (CCC) and hydrodissection. Many of these laboratory studies have helped confirm clinical discoveries and observations and have helped fine tune these techniques.

A series of pathologic analyses throughout the years has also helped identify a considerable number of IOLs that were substandard or even defective. Many of these are now memories. Simultaneously, while comparing the various IOL designs that have evolved throughout the last two decades, these laboratory investigations have also helped facilitate identification of the high-quality products that have survived. Among these are the foldable lenses and the surgical techniques that allow their successful implantation. Today's state of the art evolved during this period.

Clinicopathologic studies on IOLs have helped and continue to help researchers discern how we are doing with surgical techniques and outcomes. Much of the news today is very good. For example, with good surgical technique, significant IOL decentration has all but disappeared within the last few years. This success is based almost entirely on the ability of today's surgeons to achieve consistent and permanent capsular bag fixation. Only during the last 5 years has this become a consistent reality (see Figure 2-47).

Even more exciting, we can now report that appropriate surgical tools and high-quality IOLs have recently been developed, which when carefully applied helps to control posterior capsule opacification (PCO, secondary cataract). This complication used to occur at a rate of 30% to 50% during the 1980s and early 1990s; its incidence is now rapidly decreasing to 10% or less. This development has evolved almost without notice-a quiet revolution. It is of sufficient importance that we devote an entire chapter to it in this text (Chapter 7).

The development of foldable lenses, and perhaps even more important, the small-incision capsular surgical techniques that accompany them, has been instrumental in achieving the vast reduction of both of the above-mentioned complications. As we observe our specimen database, we take great pleasure in validating these improvements. The appearance of IOL specimens today, especially from eyes obtained postmortem containing IOLs, is vastly different from what was often seen even 5 to 10 years ago. Results are not yet perfect, but complications are far fewer. The evolutionary process leading to this is surveyed in Chapter 2.

The excellent optical and visual rehabilitory benefits of small incision phacoemulsification-foldable IOL surgery, including reduced astigmatism, quick recovery, and many other advantages, are well known. This modern procedure has achieved a state of not only vision restoration but also vision rehabilitation. Modern cataract surgery is now a genuine form of refractive surgery.

In addition to optical advantages, it is less well known and appreciated that this type of surgery has also done much to enhance the overall safety of the cataract operation-for instance, in decreasing morbidity to the eye. Good long-term tolerance of the eye to the IOL with far fewer complications is an actuality now, as compared with even one decade ago. One reason for this is that the modern small-incision technique, used with phacoemulsification, combined with insertion of a foldable IOL, has not only provided the above mentioned improvements in visual restoration but also has in essence guided the surgeon to perform what has become a much safer, more complication-free operation. The basic accomplishments we see now—most notably, consistent and secure in-the-bag fixation and thorough nuclear and cortical removal, which are helping to assure excellent centration and eliminate secondary cataract—have, almost without us realizing it, helped to almost eliminate these two long-standing, nagging complications that first appeared after Ridley's first operation.

This text provides us the opportunity to share the evidence we have accumulated that supports the quantum leap in safety and outcome-evidence that is clearly visible by examination of our series of pseudophakic eyes obtained postmortem. Our database of IOL-related specimens, including IOLs explanted for various clinical complications as well as eyes obtained postmortem containing IOLs, has grown steadily since we began the collection in 1982. As of the year 2000, this database has increased to about 16,000 specimens. Of these, over 7000 were eyes obtained postmortem with IOLs (Figure 1-1). Among the

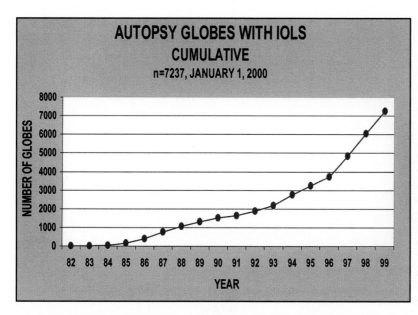

Figure 1-1. A total of 16,000 IOL specimens accessioned in the Center for Research on Ocular Therapeutics and Biodevices between 1982 and 2000. Of this total of 16,000, approximately 9000 were IOL explants obtained from complicated clinical cases, and the remaining 7000 were human eyes obtained postmortem containing IOLs. Accession of autopsy eyes containing IOLs has increased rapidly since 1996.

latter, over 800 were eyes containing foldable IOLs (Figure 1-2). Note in Figure 1-2 that the number of foldable IOLs arriving in our database is increasing exponentially. This allows us to present abundant and instructive illustrative material and also to offer clinical correlation and statistical analyses. For example, we are now able to compare rates of anterior and posterior capsule opacification among the various IOL styles, as will be discussed in detail in Chapter 7.

Examination of the foldable lens specimens over this period has shown a clear pattern of evolution. When the first foldable lenses were inserted in the late 1970s and early 1980s, the quality of lenses and surgical techniques were suboptimal. As foldable lenses continued to be implanted in the mid-1980s through the early 1990s, it appears that IOL development was sometimes ahead of the available surgical techniques. For various reasons, many surgeons rushed to insert foldable lenses before the proper techniques were in place. We have validated this tendency by observation on pathologic specimens from that period. There was a relatively high frequency of decentrations and PCO occurring at that time. The lenses today have improved, but most importantly, the surgical techniques have more than caught up and these complications are now rare.

The history of cataract surgery with IOLs is one of extensive trial and error, with many dead ends. By far the most important and basic element required for success with IOLs is fixation. Indeed, the generations of IOLs are named according to the type of fixation prominent during each era. Our conception of the "IOL Generation," first published in a review article from our laboratory in 1984[2] and later in more detail in 1989[3], is shown in Figure 2-1 and Tables 2-1 and 2-2. Six generations are identifiable. The continuous movement forward that created each new generation occurred as surgeons continuously attempted to improve IOL fixation. The move from Ridley's initial lens (Generation I) to the early anterior chamber lenses and iris fixated lenses (Generations II and III) were basically attempts to overcome decentration issues. In addition, the second move toward a sec-

Figure 1-2. Of the approximately 7000 autopsy globes with IOLs present in the Center's database, over 800 are foldable IOLs. Note the extremely rapid, almost exponential increase in specimens, beginning about 1993-1994. As the number of specimens increases, more precise evaluation of outcomes becomes increasingly possible.

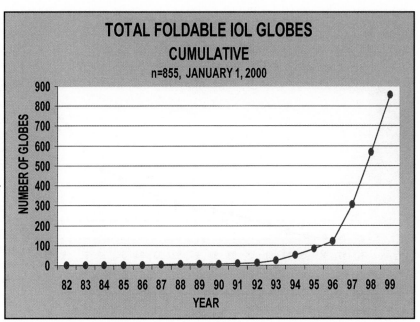

ond generation of anterior chamber lenses (Generation IV) was in part caused by a desire to avoid the secondary cataract (PCO) that often occurred after extracapsular cataract extraction (ECCE).

Today's small-incision operation is ready-made for implantation of foldable lenses (Generation VI) (Figure 2-2 and Table 2-2). Today's surgical techniques, based on information gained after numerous starts and stops that have occurred over the last 50 years, were not initially formulated with foldable IOLs in mind. However, by the early 1990s the techniques and foldable lenses ended up with a close-to-perfect partnership. It is useful to review some of the high and low points in this evolutionary process to help ophthalmologists, especially young surgeons in training (who have not had to struggle through this process), to understand where we are today. For this reason, we devote significant space in Chapter 2 to an overview of the history of cataract surgery and IOLs.

The posterior video/photographic technique pioneered by Dr. Kensaku Miyake of Nagoya, Japan in 1984 is our favored teaching tool. This technique was first used in the United States in our laboratory in Salt Lake City in 1987 and was modified and modernized by our group in 1992.[4] Use of what in 1998 Dr. Miyake himself designated and authorized as the Miyake-Apple posterior video/photographic technique-designed for examination of human eyes obtained postmortem containing PC IOLs-allows visualization from behind of structures not readily seen by clinical inspection. Examples are shown in a phakic eye (Figure 1-3), in an eye containing a generic rigid-optic all-polymethyl methacrylate (PMMA) PC IOL (Figure 1-4), and in an eye with a foldable hydrophobic acrylic design (Figure 1-5). This view is very helpful in exposing otherwise inaccessible and poorly visualized structures, thus allowing analysis of many features, including type of IOL fixation, centration/decentration, PCO, and many other factors. Although the view from behind in general provides the most information and is most educational, occasional study of the IOL and

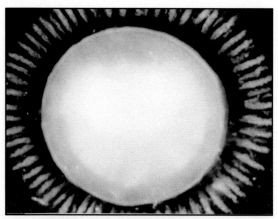

Figure 1-3. Gross photograph from behind of a human eye obtained postmortem (Miyake-Apple posterior photographic technique) showing a nonoperated eye containing an intact crystalline lens with cataractous change. This is the anatomic view that provides the basis of the technique we will see in operated eyes throughout this text.

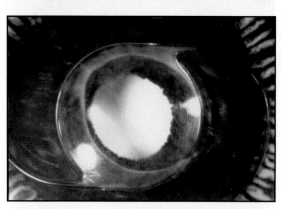

Figure 1-4. Gross photograph from behind of a human eye obtained postmortem (Miyake-Apple posterior photographic technique) showing the presence of a well-fixated generic one-piece all-PMMA posterior chamber IOL with excellent centration and clear media.

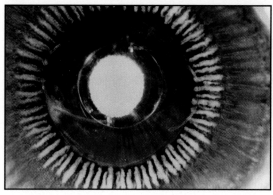

Figure 1-5. Gross photograph from behind of a human eye obtained postmortem (Miyake-Apple posterior photographic technique) showing an in-the-bag fixated, foldable, hydrophobic acrylic IOL (Alcon AcrySof) with excellent clarity of the media. This type of illustration will be used throughout this book to show both negative and positive outcomes of cataract surgery-IOL implantation.

Figure 1-6. Gross photograph of a human eye obtained postmortem. This view is from the front (anterior or surgeon's view), with cornea and iris removed. A good overview of the capsular bag is attainable with this view, but not nearly as much information can be derived with this technique compared with the Miyake-Apple posterior photographic technique illustrated in Figures 1-4 and 1-5.

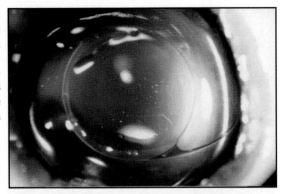

Figure 1-7. Gross photograph of a human eye obtained postmortem viewed with the "keyhole" technique of Assia and associates.[5] A one-piece all-PMMA IOL has been implanted in the capsular bag. The cornea and iris have been removed and a scleral window has been created, thus allowing an oblique view as seen here, as well as a sagittal or side view. This is an excellent teaching and research tool, supplementary to the Miyake-Apple posterior photographic technique (Figures 1-4 and 1-5) and the anterior or surgeon's view (Figure 1-6).

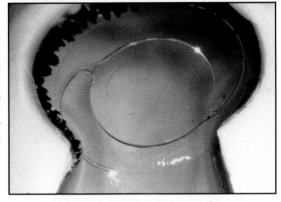

surrounding structures, such as the capsule-zonular complex from in front (anterior or surgeon's view) (Figure 1-6), can be accomplished by removing cornea and iris. In experimental surgery, we also use the technique for lens implantation through a closed-system technique designed by Dr. Gerd Auffarth and associates, as well as a side view (keyhole) technique developed in our laboratory by Dr. Ehud Assia and associates (Figure 1-7).[5]

In this book, we minimize the quantity of written text and allow the illustrations with their legends to speak for themselves. The goal is to help the reader understand the importance of establishing good surgical techniques and choosing the best available IOL design in order to achieve the fine results that we now almost take for granted.

Because the main focus of this text is to present information and illustrative material derived from our autopsy eye database, we necessarily must limit our detailed discussions of foldable lenses to those designs that have been or are actively implanted in the United States. Each foldable lens will be described in terms of general characteristics and specifications, normal features in uncomplicated cases, and general advantages and disadvantages characterizing each lens model. Our viewpoints are determined as much as possible from direct clinicopathologic correlation. Our interest is to avoid influence from manufacturers' marketing or other outside sources. The lenses available in our USA autopsy database are described in Section 2, Chapters 3 to 5. Foldable IOLs not in the USA autopsy database are briefly covered in Section 3, Chapter 6. Unfortunately, with the latter, we cannot provide pathology-derived details.

Virtually all of the foldable lenses described in this book that are still in clinical usage have been shown to be suitable for implantation and have provided good results. Some have been improved upon-for example, the small hole silicone plate IOL (Chapter 3), has been improved by substitution of large positioning holes. Surgeons and researchers are currently focusing on fine-tuning the technology of foldable IOLs, honing in on subtleties that may constitute either advantages or disadvantages to each given design. There is, of course, marked variation in a surgeon's preference among lenses, involving factors such as ease of insertion, possible minimum incision size, visual aberration issues such as glare, cost of the IOL, and relationship with the manufacturer or the local sale representative. These factors are very important. The information derived from the pathologic analyses in this text should provide an added tool for the surgeon in choosing an IOL.

After the general discussions of the foldable designs in Sections 2 and 3, Section 4 covers selected complications that may occur with any type of IOL, but most specifically for this discussion, those that are prone to occur with various foldable IOLs. As mentioned previously, the research activity on PCO has increased exponentially within the last few years, and marked success in its prevention can now be reported. This has become a hot topic, creating much interest and a huge literature. We have therefore elected to devote an entire chapter (Chapter 7) to a discussion of this complication. Chapter 8 covers selected miscellaneous complications of foldable IOLs that are also topics of current discussion and warrant special mention.

The tremendous advances that have occurred over the last few years allow us to omit discussions of many other complications that were commonplace as late as 1989, the time of our previous text on IOLs.[3] For example, with high-quality modern IOL surgery, complications such as pupillary capture; problems related to PC IOL malfixation, such as decentration; uveitis, glaucoma, hyphema (UGH) syndrome; cystoid macular edema (CME); toxic lens syndrome; various forms of postoperative inflammation; and various types of malpositions caused by disruption of the zonular-capsular apparatus are rare and need not be considered. A major cause of these vast improvements is that in the era of small-incision foldable lens surgery the incidence of in-the-bag fixation has jumped to over 90% (see Chapter 2, Figure 2-47). This is in sharp contrast to early success rates of only 30% in the 1980s and even only in the 60% range by the mid-1990s. It appears that the latter figure was about the maximum possible with classic large-incision extracapsular surgery. The good results now attainable with small-incision surgery allow us to dispense with discussion of fixation-related complications such as decentration.

As the reader moves forward, he or she is reminded that the goal of this book is to provide a relatively short written text for each chapter, and, most importantly, to let the tables and pictures with their legends speak for themselves in defining each foldable IOL style.

References

1. Apple DJ, Reidy JJ, Googe JM, et al. A comparison of ciliary sulcus and capsular bag fixation of posterior chamber intraocular lenses. *J Am Intraocul Implant Soc*. 1985;11:44-63.

2. Apple DJ, Mamalis N, Loftfield K, et al. Complications of intraocular lenses. A historical and histopathological review. *Surv Ophthalmol*. 1984;29:1-54.

3. Apple DJ, Kincaid MC, Mamalis N, Olson RJ. *Intraocular Lenses: Evolution, Designs, Complications, and Pathology.* Baltimore, MD: Williams & Wilkins; 1989.

4. Apple DJ, Lim ES, Morgan RC, et al. Preparation and study of human eyes obtained postmortem with the miyake posterior photographic technique. *Ophthalmology.* 1990;97:810- 816.

5. Assia EI, Castaneda VE, Legler UFC, et al. Studies on cataract surgery and intraocular lenses at the Center for Intraocular Lens Research. *Ophthalmol Clin N Amer.* 1991;4:251-266.

BIBLIOGRAPHY

Agarwal A, Fine I. *Phacoemulsification, Laser Cataract Surgery and Foldable IOLs.* Thorofare, NJ: SLACK Incorporated; 1998.

Apple DJ. Center for Intraocular Lens Research transfers to Medical University of South Carolina. *J Cataract Refract Surg.* 1988;14:481.

Apple DJ. Intraocular lens biocompatibility. *J Cat Refract Surg.* 1992;18(5):217-218.

Apple DJ. Utah Center for Intraocular Lens Research. *Proceedings of the Research to Prevent Blindness. Science Writer's Seminar.* Oct 1984: 35-36.

Apple DJ, Craythorn JM, Olson RJ, et al. Anterior segment complications and neovascular glaucoma following implantation of posterior chamber intraocular lens. *Ophthalmology.* 1984;91:403-419.

Apple DJ, Mamalis N, Brady SE, et al. Biocompatibility of implant materials: A review and scanning electron microscopic study. *J Am Intraocul Implant Soc.* 1984;10:53-66.

Apple DJ, Rabb MF. *Ocular Pathology, Clinical Applications, and Self-Assessment.* 5th ed. St. Louis, Mo: Mosby-Year Book, Inc.; 1998.

Apple DJ, Ram J, Peng Q. The fiftieth anniversary of the intraocular lens and a quiet revolution. *Ophthalmology.* 1999;10:1,2.

Apple DJ, Solomon KD, Tetz MR, et al. Posterior capsular opacification: A review. *Surv Ophthalmol.* 1992;37(2):73-116.

Auffarth G, Wesendahl T, Brown S, Apple D. Analysis of complications in explanted posterior chamber intraocular lenses. *Ger J Ophthalmol.* 1993;2(4/5):366.

Auffarth GU, Taso K, Wesendahl TA, Apple DJ. Pathology of autopsy eyes with implanted posterior chamber lenses. *Ger J Ophthalmol.* 1994;3(4/5):284.

Auffarth GU, Wesendahl TA, Brown SJ, Apple DJ. Grunde fhr die explantation von Hinterkammerlinsen. *Ophthalmologe.* 1994;91:507-511.

Auffarth GU, Wesendahl TA, Solomon KD, et al. Modified preparation technique for closed system ocular surgery of human eyes obtained postmortem: An improved research and teaching tool. *Ophthalmology.* 1996;103:977-982.

Borirak-Chanyavat S, Lindquist TD, Kaplan HJ. A cadaveric eye model for practicing anterior and posterior segment surgeries. *Ophthalmology.* 1995;102:1932-1935.

Brady DG, Giamporcaro JE, Steinert RF. Effect of folding instruments on silicone intraocular lenses. *J Cataract Refract Surg.* 1994;20:310-315.

Brint SF. Refractive cataract surgery. *Intl Ophthalmol Clin.* 1994;34:1-11.

Buratto L. *Phacoemulsification: Principles and Techniques.* Thorofare, NJ: SLACK Incorporated; 1998.

Chehade M, Elder MJ. Intraocular lens materials and styles: A review. *Aust N Z J Ophthalmol.* 1997;25:255-263.

Clayman HM. *Intraocular Lens Implantation.* Thorofare, NJ: SLACK Incorporated; 1985.

Corey RP, Olson RJ. Surgical outcomes of cataract extractions performed by residents using phacoemulsification. *J Cataract Refract Surg.* 1998;24:66-72.

Dick HB, Kohnen T, Jacobi FK, Jacobi KW. Long-term endothelial cell loss following phacoemulsification through a temporal clear corneal incision. *J Cataract Refract Surg.* 1996;22:63-71.

Duvall B, Lens A, Werner E. *Cataract and Glaucoma for Eyecare Professionals.* Thorofare, NJ: SLACK Incorporated; 1999.

Fine IH. *Phacoemulsification: New Technology and Clinical Application.* Thorofare, NJ: SLACK Incorporated; 1996.

Fine IH. *Clear Corneal Lens Surgery.* Thorofare, NJ: SLACK Incorporated;1998.

Fine IH, Agarwal A. *Laser Cataract Surgery and Foldable IOLs.* Thorofare, NJ: SLACK Incorporated; 1998.

Gayton JL. *Maximizing Results: Strategies in Refractive, Corneal, Cataract and Glaucoma Surgery.* Thorofare, NJ: SLACK Incorporated; 1996.

Gills JP. *Cataract Surgery: The State of the Art.* Thorofare, NJ: SLACK Incorporated; 1997.

Gills JP, Martin RG, Sanders DR. *Sutureless Cataract Surgery: An Evolution Toward Minimally Invasive Technique.* Thorofare, NJ: SLACK Incorporated;1991.

Gills JP, Sanders DR. Use of small incisions to control induced astigmatism and inflammation following cataract surgery. *J Cataract Refract Surg.* 1991;17(suppl):740-744.

Koch PS. *Simplifying Phacoemulsification: Safe and Efficient Methods for Cataract Surgery.* 5th ed. Thorofare, NJ: SLACK Incorporated; 1997.

Koch PS, Bradley H, Swenson N. Visual acuity recovery rates following cataract surgery and implantation of soft intraocular lenses. *J Cataract Refract Surg.* 1991;17:143-147.

Kohnen T, Dick B, Jacobi KW. Comparison of the induced astigmatism after temporal clear corneal tunnel incisions of different sizes. *J Cataract Refract Surg.* 1995;21:417-424.

Kohnen T, Lambert RJ, Koch DD. Incision sizes for foldable intraocular lenses. *Ophthalmology.* 1997;104:1277-1286.

Kohnen T. Complications and complication management with foldable intraocular lenses. *J Cataract Refract Surg.* 1998;24:1167-1168.

Kohnen T. The variety of foldable intraocular lens materials. *J Cataract Refract Surg.* 1996;22(suppl 2):1255-1258.

Martin RG, Gills JP, Sanders DR. *Foldable Intraocular Lenses.* Thorofare, NJ: SLACK Incorporated; 1993.

Mazzocco TR, Rajacich GM, Epstein E. *Soft Implant Lenses In Cataract Surgery.* Thorofare, NJ: SLACK Incorporated; 1986.

Obstbaum SA. Development of foldable IOL materials. *J Cataract Refract Surg.* 1995;21:233.

Obstbaum SA. Foldable intraocular lenses and vitreoretinal surgery. *J Cataract Refract Surg.* 1997;23:457.

Obstbaum SA. Intraocular lenses for small incision surgery. *J Cataract Refract Surg.* 1991;17:405.

Olson RJ, Crandall AS. Prospective randomized comparison of phacoemulsification cataract surgery with a 3.2-mm vs a 5.5-mm sutureless incision. *Am J Ophthalmol.* 1998;125:612-620.

Omar O, Mamalis N, Veiga J, Tamura M, Olson RJ. Scanning electron microscopic characteristics of small-incision intraocular lenses. *Ophthalmology.* 1996;103:1124-1129.

Oshika T, Tsuboi S, Yaguchi S, et al. Comparative study of intraocular lens implantation through 3.2-and 5.5-mm incisions. *Ophthalmology.* 1994;101:1183-1190.

Ram J, Apple DJ, Peng Q, et al. Update on fixation of rigid and foldable posterior chamber intraocular lenses (IOLs). Part I. Elimination of decentration to achieve precise optical correction and visual rehabilitation. *Ophthalmology.* 1999;106:883-890.

Ram J, Apple DJ, Peng Q, et al. Update on fixation of rigid and foldable posterior chamber intraocular lenses (IOLs). Part II. Choosing the correct IOL designs to help eradicate posterior capsule opacification. *Ophthalmology.* 1999;106:891-900.

Ram J, Auffarth GU, Wesendahl TA, Apple DJ. Miyake posterior view video technique: A means to reduce the learning curve in phacoemulsification. *Ophthalmic Prac.* 1994;12(5):206-210.

Ram J, Wesendahl TA, Auffarth GU, Apple DJ. Evaluation of phacoemulsification techniques: In situ fracture vs phaco chop. *J Cataract Refract Surg.* 1999;106:891-900.

Samuelson SW, Koch DD, Kuglen CC. Determination of maximal incision length for true small-incision surgery. *Ophthalmic Surg.* 1991;22:204-207.

Solomon KD, Apple DJ, Mamalis N, et al. Complications of intraocular lenses with special reference to an analysis of 2500 explanted intraocular lenses (IOLs). *Eur J Implant Refract Surg.* 1991;3:195-200.

Steinert RF, Brint SF, White SM, Fine IH. Astigmatism after small incision cataract surgery. A prospective, randomized, multicenter comparison of 4- and 6.5-mm incisions [published erratum appears in Ophthalmology 1997 Sep;104(9):1370]. *Ophthalmology.* 1991;98:417-423.

Steinert RF, Deacon J. Enlargement of incision width during phacoemulsification and folded intraocular lens implant surgery. *Ophthalmology.* 1996;103:220-225.

Yalon M. *Techniques of Phacoemulsification and Intraocular Lens Implantation.* Thorofare, NJ: SLACK Incorporated, 1992.

Evolution of Intraocular Lenses (Generations I to VI)

Apple and associates[1] have classified the development of IOLs into six generations (Table 2-1 and Figure 2-1). This categorization is based primarily on mode of IOL fixation (Figure 2-2). Each step forward, beginning with Ridley's 1949-1950 invention, represented an advance in both surgical technique and IOL design and quality. A brief overview of each generation, with a description of the numerous failures and successes occurring in each throughout this half century of development, is provided to help the reader understand how we have arrived at the excellent procedure that is available today.

Credit for the invention and first implantation of the IOL is given solely to Sir Harold Ridley of London (Figure 2-3). Details regarding Ridley and his invention are provided in a 1996 biography by Apple and Sims.[2] Peter Choyce of London (Figure 2-4), who was involved in many of the early procedures, was a colleague and supporter of Ridley, and played a significant role in guiding the implantation procedure through its evolutionary process. Ridley's first implant (Generation I, Figure 2-1) was implanted as a two-step procedure.[3] The ECCE was performed on November 29, 1949. Rather than permanently implanting the IOL, Ridley chose to wait and implant it secondarily a few months later, after the eye was quiet and suitable for implantation. The first permanent implantation was performed on February 8, 1950.

Ridley's first implant was manufactured by Rayner, Ltd., London, UK (Figure 2-5). The Ridley IOL was a biconvex disc that was designed in conjunction with Mr. John Pike, an optical scientist at Rayner. It was designed for implantation in the posterior chamber. Ridley filmed several of his early operations. Details extracted from footage of Case 8, a lens implanted at St. Thomas' Hospital in London on May 10, 1951, are shown in Figure 2-6.

From his very first cases, Ridley encountered the two major problems of lens implantation that have nagged ophthalmologists for half a century; namely, IOL malposition and PCO or secondary cataract. Regarding the malpositions, the main reasons for the decentrations were often attributed to excessive weight of the implant. However, two other important causes, which are directly applicable to the implantation procedure, were 1) the IOL had no appropriate fixation haptics, and 2) the anterior capsulotomy, in which he essentially opened and

Table 2-1.
Evolution of Intraocular Lenses

Generation	Dates and Types (approximate)
I	1949 - 1954 Original Ridley posterior chamber, PMMA* IOL manufactured by Rayner, LTD., U.K.
II	1952 - 1962 Early AC IOL
III	1953 - 1973 Iris-supported, including iridocapsular IOL implanted after ECCE
IV	1963 - 1992 Transition towards modern AC IOLs
V	1977 - 1992 Transition to and maturation of posterior chamber IOLS
VI	1992 - 2000 Modern IOLs

a) Capsular IOLs designed specifically for in-the-bag implantation.
i. Small, single-piece . modified C-loop designs.
ii. Foldable IOLs—designed for small incision surgery.

b) AC IOLs
- Kelman (flexibility)
- Choyce (footplates).
- Clemente (fine-tuning, no-hole, three-point fixation.

(c) Refractive IOLs
i. Phakic IOLs
  - Baikoff lens (anterior chamber)
  - Worst-Fechner iris claw (Artesen™ IOL) (iris)
  - Posterior chamber IOL (implantable contact lens
ii. Low power, + and - diopter IOLs designed for refractive correction, eg, after clear lens extraction.
iii. Multifocal IOLs.

*PMMA = polymethylmethacrylate

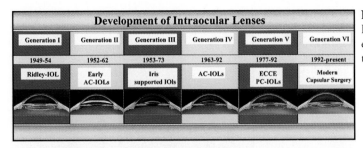

Figure 2-1. Six generations of IOLs, 1949 to present. Each generation is named according to the mode of IOL fixation.

Development of Intraocular Lenses					
Generation I	Generation II	Generation III	Generation IV	Generation V	Generation VI
1949-54	1952-62	1953-73	1963-92	1977-92	1992-present
Ridley-IOL	Early AC-IOLs	Iris supported IOls	AC-IOLs	ECCE PC-IOLs	Modern Capsular Surgery

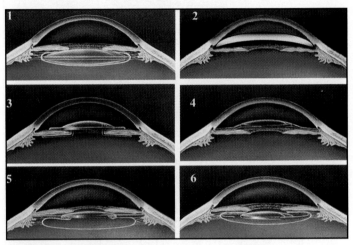

Figure 2-2. Schematic illustrations (sagittal views) of eyes with representative IOL types characteristic for each of the six generations (corresponding to the generation numbers in Table 2-1 and Figure 2-1).

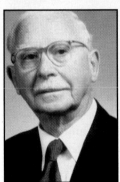

Figure 2-3. Sir Harold Ridley, circa 1990.

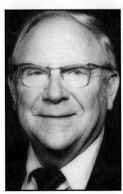

Figure 2-4. Peter Choyce, MD, a close colleague and supporter of Ridley since the beginning. He was an innovator in his own right, and an important advocate who did much to advance the cause of IOL implantation.

Figure 2-5. Ridley's original IOL was manufactured by Rayner, Ltd., UK. Note the early brochure describing the Ridley lens, a schematic illustration showing a sagittal section of the anterior segment of the eye with a Ridley IOL and a sketch of the Ridley IOL.

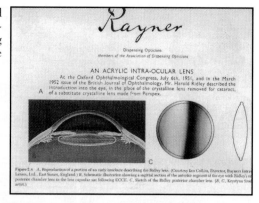

Figure 2-6. Selected frames from an original film made by Ridley of his eighth IOL implantation, St. Thomas' Hospital, London, May 10, 1951. The eye was entered via a von Graefe incision (frame at left center) and ECCE was performed. The lens, a biconvex disc made of PMMA, was inserted into the posterior chamber (two frames lower right).

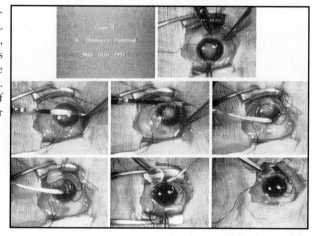

removed almost all of the anterior capsule in a very irregular fashion, was inefficient for good equatorial fixation of the edge of the lens. It did not permit stable and permanent fixation of the pseudophakos. These shortcomings have, of course, been overcome with modern surgery by the addition of appropriate haptics, and especially important, the invention and perfection of CCC. These, especially the CCC, came much later—not until the mid to late 1980s. The problem of lens decentration is largely solved now that high-quality surgical techniques are available.

After PCO developed in his first cases, Ridley quickly realized the need for copious irrigation and removal of lens substance. Not until the mid to late 1980s was the importance of this observation truly appreciated and applied, with the development of much better nucleus and cortical removal techniques. Especially important was the development of phacoemulsification and hydrodissection-enhanced removal of cortex (Generation VI) (see Table 2-1).

The movement toward Generation II, the early anterior chamber (AC) IOLs implanted after intracapsular cataract extraction (ICCE), was initiated to circumvent the two above mentioned complications of the Ridley lens-malposition and PCO.

This generation (Table 2-1; Figures 2-1, 2-7, and 2-8) represents the first attempt at implantation of various AC IOLs (Figure 2-7). The first AC IOL was implanted by Baron

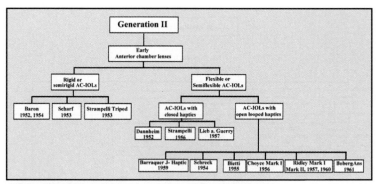

Figure 2-7. Generation II (most activity circa 1952 to 1962). Important pioneers of early rigid and flexible designs are noted here. For more details, see Reference No. 1.

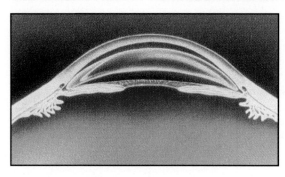

Figure 2-8. Generation II, the original AC IOL design of Baron (1952). This lens and other similar designs were immediately doomed to failure because of close proximity of the pseudophakos to the corneal endothelium, with inevitable subsequent corneal decompensation. It was during this generation that surgeons began to appreciate the fragility of corneal endothelium.

of France in 1952 (Figure 2-8). A quick glance at Figure 2-8 immediately explains why this lens failed; namely, because the excessive anterior vaulting of the entire pseudophakos caused inappropriate contact with the corneal endothelium. It was at this time that surgeons began to pay attention to the fragility of the corneal endothelium and the severe problem of corneal decompensation, a problem that has plagued all subsequent generations of IOL implantation. This was our predecessors' first lesson on avoidance of any type of intermittent or constant corneal touch with a pseudophakos. This is mandatory to prevent corneal decompensation (including pseudophakic bullous keratopathy [PBK]) and other secondary intraocular changes such as cystoid macular edema (CME). Corneal problems persisted well into Generations III and IV with many IOL designs and surgical techniques. Today's surgeon in training who is learning modern, high-quality PC IOL implantation of foldable lenses through a small incision is much better able to avoid cornea-related problems, but an awareness of the delicate nature of the corneal endothelium should always exist in one's mind, even today.

The move toward Generation III, iris-fixated IOLs (Figure 2-9), represented an attempt to fixate the IOL further posterior from the cornea to avoid the disastrous corneal problems of the previous decade. This step was an improvement. However, it was at this time that surgeons learned about the very delicate nature of the uveal tissues when brought into contact with elements of a pseudophakos. Physical contact of IOL haptics, especially metal haptics (Figure 2-10), with uveal tissue often caused inflammation and its sequelae, including corneal decompensation, CME, and membrane formation. Cornelius Binkhorst at this time made an important modification of his early four-loop iris clip lens, creating the two-loop iridocapsular lens. With the latter design he left the optical component in front of the

Figure 2-9. Generation III (most activity circa 1953 to 1973). In this generation, surgeons and researchers learned about the problems caused by contact of a foreign biomaterial with uveal tissue, including inflammation, PBK, and CME. Also, the development of Binkhorst's two-loop iridocapsular lens was a landmark in that this marked a return to ECCE and the beginnings of capsular (in-the-bag) fixation.

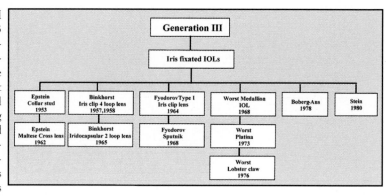

Figure 2-10. Iris-supported IOL (medallion style) with metal loops. Uveal contact of any haptic, especially haptics with metal loops such as these, caused sequelae derived from chafing or tearing of adjacent tissues and breakdown of the blood-aqueous barrier.

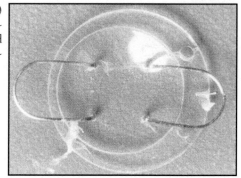

iris but the haptics were inserted into the capsular bag after ECCE (Figure 2-11). This step represented an important return to ECCE and capsular fixation; both had largely been abandoned since the time of Ridley's first implant.

Generation IV, a move again to the AC, was an attempt to avoid the complications of the iris fixated IOLs. This period, with most activity between 1963 and 1992, was a transitional period in which numerous designs were attempted, some successful but many ending in failure (Figures 2-12 to 2-16). Details regarding this process are documented in several references from our Center and need not be considered here.

This generation again called our attention to the problem of direct or indirect, constant or intermittent corneal contact. In addition, at this time problems of erosion of small-diameter round-loop fixation haptics into delicate uveal tissues were recognized (Figure 2-15). These were common with many of the closed-loop IOL designs of that era, and caused severe problems due to tissue contact and chafing. During this period, the concept of a protective membrane was recognized; ie, the usefulness of any sort of fibrous or hyaline-elastic membrane (callus) that could be situated between the fixation element of the IOL and delicate vascular tissues of the adjacent uveal tissues (see Figure 2-16A). With respect to AC IOLs, it was learned that Choyce-style footplates (Figures 2-16B and 2-17) provided markedly improved results. Stable fixation could be achieved whenever a fibrous scar or callus formed at the site of touch within the AC angle recess (Figure 2-16B). All successful modern AC

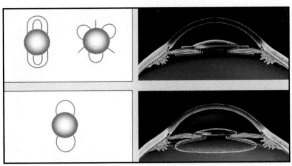

Figure 2-11. Schematic illustrations of two iris clip IOL designs (above) and Binkhorst's two-loop iridocapsular design (below), intended for placement of the posterior haptics into the capsular bag after ECCE.

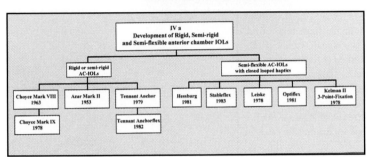

Figure 2-12. Several pioneers developed rigid designs, and others experimented with more flexible designs. In particular, the closed-loop (haptic) designs of the late 1970s to early 1980s were associated with very poor results. By 1987, most were withdrawn from the market.

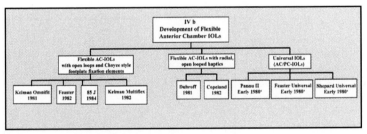

Figure 2-13. Development of improved flexible AC IOLs occurred during this era. Flexible AC IOLs with open loops and Choyce-style footplate fixation elements (on the left) formed the basis for the modern successful open loop AC IOLs used today (Generation IV, see Table 2-1).

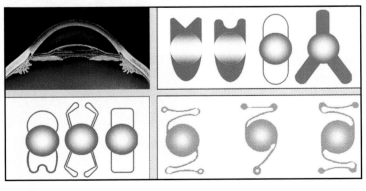

Figure 2-14. Myriad AC IOL designs were designed in Generation IV, with the transitional phase leading toward the open-loop flexible designs. The three- and four-point haptic (footplate) fixation element lenses noted in the lower right in this Figure were important advances. In the United States, the only no-hole AC IOLs had a four-point fixation; to date, a no-hole three-point fixation AC IOL is not yet available.

Figure 2-15A. In Generation IV, surgeons learned about problems related to fixation of small diameter, round, tubular fixation elements into the uveal tissues of the AC angle recess. These cause marked inflammation secondary to a "cheese cutter" effect. This figure shows a Leiske-style closed-loop AC IOL with round tubular haptics, circa 1978. Small diameter "cheese cutter"-like haptics were problematic when they eroded into the uveal tissue.

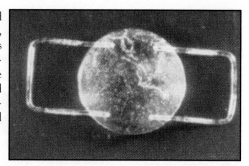

Figure 2-15B. In Generation IV, surgeons learned about problems related to fixation of small diameter, round, tubular fixation elements into the uveal tissues of the AC angle recess. These cause marked inflammation secondary to a "cheese cutter" effect. This figure shows a photomicrograph of the anterior segment of an eye containing a small diameter round closed-loop IOL (circular empty space) that eroded into the uveal stroma. Such a profile is associated with induced inflammation and an increased chance of PBK and CME. (Hematoxylin and eosin, original magnification x200.)

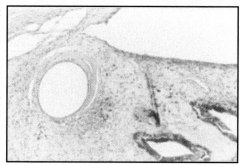

Figure 2-16A. Photomicrograph of the site of a Choyce-style footplate (empty space because the biomaterial dissolves out during processing). Note the formation of a fibrous membrane or callus, which formed shortly after the implantation. These effectively separate the pseudophakos biomaterial from direct contact with the adjacent uveal tissue of the AC recess. The barrier formed by this type of membrane is entirely analogous to that formed by the surrounding lens capsule in the case of in-the-bag fixation of PC IOLs (see Figure 2-19) (hematoxylin and eosin stain, original magnification x200).

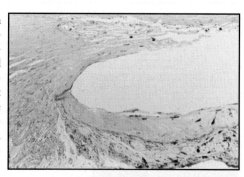

Figure 2-16B. Scanning electron micrograph showing the profile of fixation of a Choyce-style footplate. This is a well-polished, solid, tissue-friendly haptic or footplate (below, right; original magnification x75).

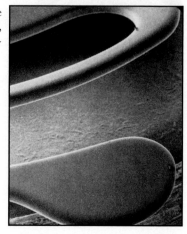

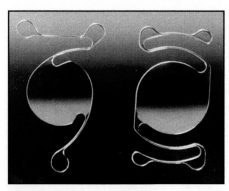

Figure 2-17. The one-piece open-loop AC IOL designs that were developed during Generation IV have evolved to the highly successful modern three- and four-point fixation AC IOLs that are now available, and indeed are classified with modern IOLs in Generation VI (see Table 2-1). The two IOL designs pictured here are characterized by excellent flexibility and the presence of no-hole Choyce-style fixation haptics. The latter provide very tissue-friendly contact with the angle recess when properly implanted.

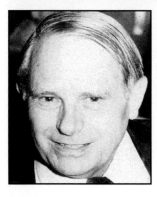

Figure 2-18. Cornelius Binkhorst, MD, of Holland, deserves credit for two important accomplishments that formed the basis for all modern PC IOL implantation, including foldable IOLs implanted via small incisions. These were 1) reintroduction and popularization of the ECCE technique in the 1960s and 2) research into and advocating capsular (in-the-bag) fixation.

IOLs now have solid Choyce-style haptics or footplates as fixation elements (see Figure 2-17). In contrast, the principle of a solid versus fenestrated haptic in the cases of modern silicone plate IOLs is based on another principle in which solid or small hole footplates are less satisfactory for establishing good fixation of the IOL in the capsular bag than are large hole footplates. This is discussed in Chapter 3.

The principle of the protective membrane has also become the basis for the success of modern PC IOL implantation, including foldable lenses. The lens capsular bag is a basement membrane that in effect provides a protective membrane between the pseudophakos and the adjacent delicate tissues of the iris and ciliary body. Therefore, the principles learned during early experiences with AC lenses, as well as later experiences with sulcus fixated lenses, were instrumental in helping surgeons evolve toward modern in-the-bag fixation, arguably one of the most important applications of bioengineering principles to IOL implantation. Experiences at that time helped renew awareness as to the advantages of the posterior chamber as the site of implantation. Generation V occurred as surgeons returned to ECCE and PC IOLs.

Cornelius Binkhorst of Holland (Figure 2-18) clearly deserves recognition as a visionary and thoughtful investigator who spearheaded the now permanent transition toward ECCE. Early on, he recognized the advantages of in-the-bag (capsular) fixation. This led to the important transition toward Generation V and subsequently the present Generation VI (Tables 2-1 and 2-2; Figures 2-1 and 2-19). Important features regarding PC IOL development during this era are charted in Figures 2-20 to 2-22. Further details regarding this were discussed by Apple and associates in 1989.[4] It is important to note that even in

Table 2-2.
Evolution Of Extracapsular Cataract Surgery

1977	1982	1987	1992	2000
V-a	**V-b**	**VI-a**	**VI-b**	
Beginning Phase	Transitional Period	Large Incision		Small Incision
Pre-Capsular Surgery		**Generations**	**Capsular Surgery**	
1) No viscoelastic 2) Can-opener anterior capsulotomy		1) Use viscoelastic 2) Continuous curvilinear Capsularhexis (CCC) or Envelope Technique (especially for large hard nucleus)		Same as Generation VI-a with increased use of ▶ phacoemulsi-fication and foldable IOLs inserted through a small incision
3) No hydrodissection 4) Manual ECCE 5) IOL Fixation with one or both haptics out of the bag	One or More elements of Generation V-a ▶ combined with one or more of the advances leading to Generation VI-a	3) Copious hydrodissection-enhanced cortical clean up 4) Manual or automated ECCE/ phaco 5) Consistent in-the-bag (capsular) haptic fixation		
6) Early 3-piece PC IOLs often poor designs and manufacture		6) High Quality PC IOLs Especially 1-piece all PMMA (capsular) designs.		
Complications were common, especially decentration and PCO			**Few Complications**	

*capsular-in-the-bag

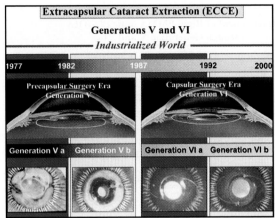

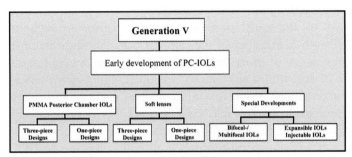

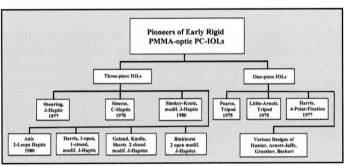

Figure 2-19. Generations V and VI (most activity circa 1977 to the present) form the basis for modern foldable IOL surgery following phacoemulsification via a small incision (see Table 2-1). Note that the generations are subdivided into two subgroups each, ranging from Generation V-a, the early years when ECCE-PC IOL implantation was first being attempted and researched (circa 1977 to 1982), to Generation V-b, the important transitional period when the modern capsular surgery techniques (see Table 2-1) were first being attempted (circa 1982 to 1987), culminating in the two subgroups of Generation VI (circa 1987 to 1992). Generation VI-a was the period when high-quality capsular surgery using mostly rigid lenses inserted via large incisions was common (circa 1987 to 1992). Generation VI-b (circa 1992 to present) is the era of small-incision phacoemulsification surgery with implantation of foldable IOL designs that we discuss here.

Figure 2-20. Generation V (marked activity circa 1977 to 1992) consisted not only of experimentation with PMMA PC IOLs, but also was a period of the first experimentation with soft lenses (which have evolved into today's modern foldable IOLs), as well as early experiments with special designs such as multifocal IOLs.

Figure 2-21. The return to the posterior chamber in Generation V, as Ridley originally began it (Generation I), was made possible by the efforts of many pioneers, some of whom are listed here (for further details see Reference 4).

Figure 2-22. This flow chart shows the evolution of rigid-optic PMMA IOLs from their early designs of the late 1970s and early 1980s to the modern capsular designs now available in Generation VI, including special designs such as those with surface modifications such as the Pharmacia-Upjohn heparin surface modified IOL design.

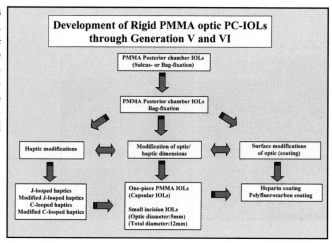

this early era, experimentation with soft lenses (see Tables 2-3 and 2-4) and other PC IOL types such as multifocal IOLs was commenced (see Figure 2-20).

Most fixation (Figure 2-23) of the early posterior chamber lenses throughout Generation V was uveal (one or both haptics out of the capsular bag). During this time surgeons learned the marked superiority of in-the-bag fixation, a fact that was not at all appreciated during the early 1970s and 1980s, and indeed, remained highly controversial even through the late 1980s. Successful transition toward in-the-bag fixation defines the transition from Generation V (precapsular surgery era) to Generation VI (capsular surgery era) (Table 2-1 and Figures 2-1 and 2-19).

During the 1980s, there was extensive experimentation with haptic fixation and PC IOL designs. After many false starts, the advantages of total in-the-bag fixation (Figure 2-23, no. 6) became apparent. This formed the basis of what is required for successful foldable implantation today. Indeed, one major false start with foldable lenses occurred in the mid to late 1980s. Some of the early foldable designs at that time were either intentionally or unintentionally implanted into the ciliary sulcus (usually one haptic in the bag and one haptic in the sulcus), creating an unnecessarily high incidence of complications. Apple and associates in their 1989 text[4] have described these in detail.

Figures 2-24 and 2-25 show examples of early Shearing-style J-loop IOL styles with implantation of the inferior haptic in the capsular bag and the superior haptic in the ciliary sulcus, an occurrence we found in more than 50% of cases analyzed during the early 1980s (see Figures 2-47). The histopathologic appearance of bag-sulcus fixation is illustrated in Figure 2-26A and B, respectively. Asymmetric fixation causes an almost automatic decentration of the IOL optic (Figures 2-24 and 2-27) and any contact with adjacent uveal tissues by either the IOL optic component or haptic component—very common in any form of "out-of-the-bag" fixation—has the potential to cause tissue changes due to chafing (Figure 2-28). This was very much exaggerated in the early 1980s when lens manufacture was poor, often with sharp edges to the IOL optic component (Figure 2-29A). Tissue chafing commonly caused transillumination defects with pigmentary dispersion. Subsequent breakdown of the blood-aqueous barrier could cause sequelae such as inflammation or even hemorrhage; e.g., the UGH syndrome. Improved polishing tech-

Table 2-3.

Foldable IOLs, Approved and Investigational, 2000
Available in the USA Autopsy Database

Design	Model (selected representative examples)	Company	Diameter (mm)	Optic Diameter (mm)	Water Content	Haptic Material
I. Silicone						
IA: Plate silicone lenses						
1 piece silicone plate lens (small holes)	Chiroflex C10UB	Bausch and Lomb Surgical, Inc.	10.5	Biconvex, 6.0	<1%	Silicone
1 piece silicone plate lens (large holes)	Chiroflex C11UB	Bausch and Lomb Surgical, Inc.	10.5	Biconvex, 6.0	<1%	Silicone
1 piece silicone plate lens (small holes)	AA-4203V	Staar Surgical Inc.	10.5	Biconvex, 6.0	<1%	Silicone
1 piece silicone plate lens (large holes)	AA-4203VF	Staar Surgical Inc.	10.5	Biconvex, 6.0	<1%	Silicone
1 piece silicone toric lens (large holes)	AA-4203TF	Staar Surgical Inc.	10.5	Biconvex, 6.0	<1%	Silicone
IB: Three-piece silicone lenses						
a) Staar — 3 piece silicone IOL	AQ1016/2010/2003	Staar Surgical Inc.	13.5/13.5/12.5	Biconvex, 6.3	<1%	Polyimide
b) Allergan Series — 3 piece silicone IOL	SI-30 NB	Allergan, Inc.	13.0	Biconvex, 6.0	<1%	Polypropylene
3 piece silicone IOL	SI-40 NB	Allergan, Inc.	13.0	Biconvex, 6.0	<1%	PMMA
3 piece silicone IOL	SI 55 NB	Allergan, Inc.	13.0	Biconvex, 5.5	<1%	PMMA
3 piece silicone IOL	SA 40 N	Allergan, Inc.	13.0	Biconvex, 6.0	<1%	PMMA
c) Bausch and Lomb — 3 piece silicone IOL	Soflex and LI Series	Bausch and Lomb Surgical, Inc.	13.0	Biconvex, 6.0	<1%	PMMA
II. Acrylics						
Hydrophobic (dry packed) 3 piece Acrylic IOL	AcrySof MA30BA/MA60BM	Alcon Laboratories, Inc.	12.5/30	Biconvex, 5.5/6.0	<2%	PMMA

Table 2-4.

Foldable IOLs, Approved and Investigational, 2000
Not Available in the USA Autopsy Database.

Design	Model (selected representative examples)	Company	Diameter (mm)	Optic Diameter	Water Content	Haptic Material
I. Silicone						
a. Pharmacia-Upjohn						
3-piece Silicone IOL	CeeOn (912)	Pharmacia & Upjohn, Inc.	12.0	Biconvex, 6.0	<1%	PVDF
3-piece Silicone IOL	CeeOn Edge	Pharmacia & Upjohn, Inc.	12.0	Biconvex, 5.50	<1%	
b. Bausch and Lomb						
3 piece Silicone IOL	Soflex, LI Series	Bausch and Lomb Surgical, Inc.	13.0	Biconvex, 6.0	<1%	PMMA
3 piece Silicone IOL (DomiLens Corp.)	Silens 6	Bausch and Lomb Surgical, Inc.	12.5	Biconvex, 6.0	<1%	PMMA
II. Acrylics						
a. Hydrophobic (dry packed)						
3 piece acrylic IOL	AR-40	Allergan, Inc.	13.0	Biconvex, 6.0	<1%	PMMA
b. Hydrophilic (wet packed) Bausch and Lomb						
3 piece Hydrogel IOL	Hydroview H55S/H60M	Bausch and Lomb Surgical, Inc.	12.0/12.5	Biconvex, 5.5/6.0	18%	PMMA
1-piece Acrygel IOL	EasAcryl1	Bausch and Lomb Surgical, Inc.	11.0	Biconvex, 6.0	26%	Acrygel
1-piece Acrygel IOL	HE26C	Bausch and Lomb Surgical, Inc.	12.0	Biconvex, 6.0	26%	Acrygel
Mentor						
3 piece Hydrogel IOL	Memory Lens U940A	Ciba Vision, Inc.	13.6	Biconvex, 6.0	20%	Polypropylene
Corneal						
1-piece Acrygel IOL	AC-55	Corneal, Inc.	10.5	Biconvex, 5.5-6.0	26%	Acrylgel
1-piece Acrygel IOL	HPFlex, HP 58	Corneal, Inc.	11.5–13.0	Biconvex, 5.8-6.0	26%	PMMA
1-piece Acrygel IOL	Quatro	Corneal, Inc.	11.25	Biconvex, 6.0	26%	Acrygel
1-piece Acrygel IOL	ACR6D Acrygel	Corneal, Inc.	12.0	Biconvex, 6.0	26%	Acrygel
1-piece Acrylgel IOL	M. 10 50	Corneal, Inc.	10.50	Biconvex, 5.75	26%	Acrygel
Rayner						
1-piece Acrygel IOL	Raysoft	Rayner, Ltd.	10.50	Biconvex, 5.75	26%	Acrygel

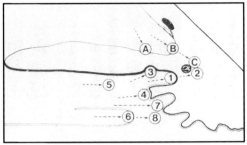

Figure 2-23. Developing an understanding of the importance and accomplishment of in-the-bag fixation (No. 6) was a significant landmark that opened the way to successful modern foldable IOL implantation. When a PC IOL is not within the capsular bag (No. 1-8 with the exception of 6), the surgeon cannot know where it is situated behind the iris. The way is therefore open for major complications such as decentration and PCO (see Chapter 7). In-the-bag fixation, which led to the transition to Generation VI (Table 2-1), is mandatory for small-incision surgery and foldable lens implantation. It has evolved so that it is now accomplished in over 90% of cases (see Figure 2-47). Note that letters A-C relate to AC IOLs, and connote A) AC IOL too short, B) proper sizing, and C) IOL too long.

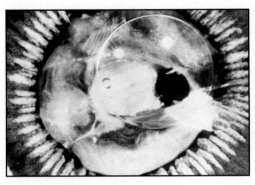

Figure 2-24. Gross photograph from behind, Miyake-Apple posterior photographic technique, showing an example of early Generation V-a implantation, with an asymmetrically implanted Shearing lens (right haptic in the pars plana, left haptic in the ciliary sulcus), with marked decentration so that the optic edge and positioning hole are within the visual axis. Also note the partial Soemmering's ring signifying incomplete cleanup. This surgery was done without the benefit of viscoelastics, capsulorhexis (CCC), hydrodissection, or the other modern techniques we enjoy today (see Table 2-2). This type of result was common in the early 1980s.

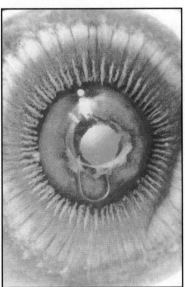

Figure 2-25A. The earliest flexible PC IOLs designed by Steve Shearing were designed to be implanted symmetrically within the ciliary sulcus. In reality, the vast majority were implanted with one loop in the capsular bag (usually inferior) and the opposite (superior) loop in the ciliary sulcus. This created an almost automatic decentration. This figure is a gross photograph from behind, Miyake-Apple posterior photographic technique, showing an asymmetrically implanted Shearing lens, early 1980s.

Figure 2-25B. Scanning electron microscope of an explanted Shearing lens in which the inferior loop was implanted in the capsular bag, remnants of which are seen in this photograph (lower left) wrapped around the haptic. The opposite haptic (upper right) had been enmeshed in uveal tissue of the ciliary sulcus (original magnification x8).This figure shows a photomicrograph illustrating in-the-bag (capsular and ciliary sulcus) PC IOL fixation.

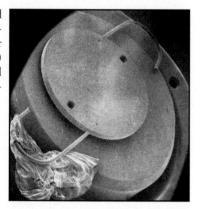

Figure 2-26A. Photomicrograph demonstrating basic PC IOL fixation, capsular fixation with the IOL haptic or loop (L) situated within the capsular bag. The IOL haptic biomaterial dissolves out during processing so the site of the haptic is always represented by an empty space. AC = anterior capsule; EC = equatorial capsule; PC = posterior capsule; I = iris; PE = posterior pigment epithelium of the iris; CS = ciliary sulcus; CB = main body of the ciliary body (hematoxylin and eosin stain, original magnification x100).

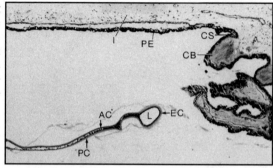

Figure 2-26B. Photomicrograph demonstrating basic PC IOL fixation. Ciliary sulcus fixation, with slight erosion of the haptic or loop empty space (L) into the stroma of the ciliary body (lower right). Because the biomaterial dissolves from the preparation, the loop is only seen as a clear circular space (hematoxylin and eosin stain, original magnification x125).

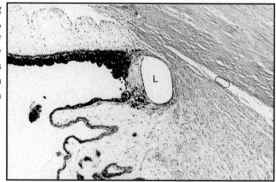

Figure 2-27. Gross photograph from behind, Miyake-Apple posterior photographic technique, showing an asymmetrically fixation modified J-loop (Sinskey-Kratz style) three-piece PC IOL with decentration as well as massive retained cortical material. These are characteristics of Generation V-a (Table 2-1 and Figure 2-23).

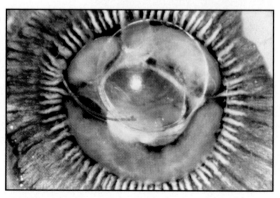

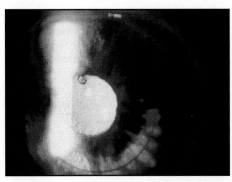

Figure 2-28. When uveal contact of any component of the pseudophakos (optic or haptic) occurred (as was often the case with sulcus-sulcus or asymmetric bag sulcus fixation), tissue chafing with significant clinical sequelae sometimes occurred. This clinical photograph shows a transillumination defect of the iris caused by chafing of the lens optic edge against the posterior iris pigment epithelium. This could create a pigmentary dispersion syndrome and even lead to pigmentary glaucoma. Such changes were particularly prone to occur with early, poorly polished IOLs (see Figure 2-29A).

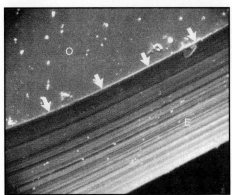

Figure 2-29A. Scanning electron micrograph of early and late PC IOL optic edges. Early PC IOLs (Generation V-a) were often poorly manufactured, and frequently had sharp edges due to poor polishing as shown in this scanning electron micrograph. The arrows show the razor-sharp junction between the optic (O) and the edge (E) of the optic. A sharp edge like this was a relatively common cause of clinical defects similar to those illustrated in Figure 2-32 (original magnification x50).

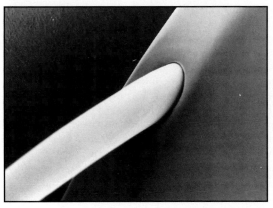

Figure 2-29B. Scanning electron micrograph of early and late PC IOL optic edges. By the late 1980s, much better polishing techniques were used, and high-quality lenses as noted here evolved. This high-power scanning electron micrograph shows the loop optic junction of a well-made three-piece PC IOL.

niques began to appear by the mid to late 1980s (Figure 2-29B). This, coupled with better in-the-bag fixation techniques, has largely solved this problem.

Intraocular decentration due to faulty asymmetric fixation, as seen in Figure 2-30A and B, should be distinguished from IOL malpositions due to surgical disruption of the zonular-capsular apparatus. The latter phenomenon was relatively frequent during the early years (Figure 2-31). Whereas the fixation-related malpositions were usually manifest as an upward decentration due to asymmetric fixation (the inferior haptic in the capsular bag) the superior haptic in the ciliary sulcus, (Sunrise syndrome, Figure 2-30A), the malpositions related to zonular-capsular disruption usually had inferior decentration (Sunset syndrome) (Figure 2-31).

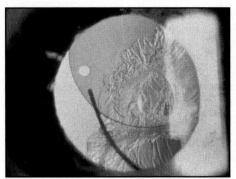

Figure 2-30A. Asymmetric implantation of PC IOLs. When the haptics of an asymmetrically implanted PC IOL were left in the vertical position, the decentration that often occurred was in an upward direction (Sunrise syndrome).

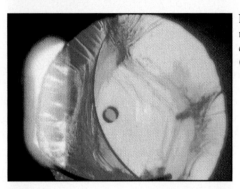

Figure 2-30B. When a PC IOL was implanted asymmetrically with the haptics in the horizontal meridian, the decentration that occurred was also in that meridian (East-West syndrome).

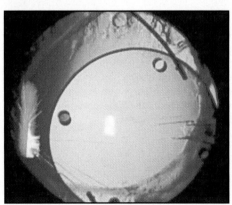

Figure 2-31. Decentrations caused by asymmetric implantation of haptics (Figure 2-30) should be sharply distinguished from decentrations caused by disturbance or rupture of the zonular capsular apparatus. Capsular and zonular ruptures were very common during the early years of ECCE PC IOL (Generation V-a, Figure 2-19). In most cases, zonular breakage led to inferior decentration of the pseudophakos. This is a severe case of the Sunset syndrome. The inferior decentrations have caused the edge of the IOL optics, the positioning holes, and the haptics to be situated within the visual axis. This was a common cause of visual aberrations and visual loss. With modern in-the-bag surgery and small-incision techniques available today (Generation VI-b), this complication has become very rare.

The severe problems illustrated in Figures 2-24 to 2-31 were examples of Generation V-a (Table 2-2 and Figure 2-19), the early period of precapsular surgery. As noted in Table 2-2, this era was characterized by a general lack of the modern techniques that we now take for granted with implantation of foldable lenses; namely, no viscoelastic, can opener anterior capsulotomy, no hydrodissection, manual ECCE, and malfixation of haptics of the early PC IOLs, which were often poorly designed and manufactured.

Figures 2-32 through 2-36 illustrate the advances that occurred during the transitional period (Generation V-b; Table 2-2, Figure 2-19) as surgeons moved from the early era (Generation V-a) toward modern capsular surgery (Generation VI). This era was an important transition period in which surgeons learned and began to apply one or more of the

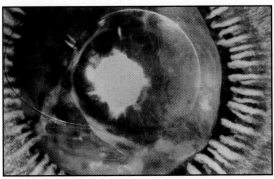

Figure 2-32. Generation V-b (Table 2-2, Figure 2-19) is a very important transitional period during which surgeons were gradually learning and applying the techniques of modern cataract surgery. Analysis of eyes from this generation showed significant improvement over Generation V-a. Some, but usually not all, of the essential tools were available, so a few improvements were achieved. This led to better results, but not those achievable in the mid Generation VI. This example is a gross photograph of a human eye obtained postmortem (Miyake-Apple posterior photographic technique). The cortical cleanup phase of the operation is somewhat improved over that typical of Generation V-a (eg, Figure 2-27). However, asymmetric haptic fixation is still evident, with one haptic in the sulcus (right) and one haptic in the capsular bag (left).

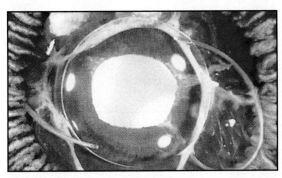

Figure 2-33. Gross photograph from behind of a human eye (Miyake-Apple posterior photograph technique) obtained postmortem showing a three-piece PC IOL implanted after relatively good cortical cleanup. However, in this case the right haptic is in the capsular bag, but the left one has escaped the capsular bag through two triangular radial tears of the anterior capsule (one to the left and one inferiorly) to become situated in the ciliary sulcus. This slippage of an IOL haptic out of the bag through a radial tear of the anterior capsule is termed "pea-podding." It was a common complication when the can opener anterior capsulotomy technique was used. Therefore, the technique in this particular case had not yet evolved toward capsulorhexis (CCC). Hence, it has not yet evolved toward Generation VI.

required elements needed to advance to Generation VI-a. This was a crucial era in which important new techniques began to be applied (Table 2-2). Most importantly, this transition to viscoelastics, CCC, hydrodissection-enhanced cortical cleanup, and modern Extracapsular cataract Extraction (ECCE) and phaco made possible the future implementation of foldable IOLs. In Generation VI-a (Table 2-2), the move toward consistent in-the-bag (capsular) fixation was underway. Each of the eyes shown in Figures 2-32 to 2-36 shows one or more of the criteria listed in Table 2-2 that define the transition toward Generation VI. During this transition, one or more of the essential factors was lacking, which by definition signifies a transition, but entrance into Generation VI (although not yet successful and complete) was underway.

    It is noteworthy that the first attempts at implantation of soft IOLs, the forerunners of today's modern foldable IOLs (see Tables 2-3 and 2-4), began during Generation V, from the later 1970s until the early 1980s (Figure 2-37). Examples from our database of a series of one-piece IOL designs (Figures 2-38 to 2-43), as well as multi-piece (three-

Figure 2-34. This illustration is a gross photograph from behind of a human eye (Miyake-Apple posterior photographic technique) obtained postmortem showing another move toward Generation VI; namely, the implantation of a one-piece all-PMMA IOL design. However, the same problems of Generation V-a are apparent, namely 1) poor cortical cleanup with a large Soemmering's ring formation and 2) asymmetric fixation with the right haptic in the capsular bag and the left haptic in the ciliary sulcus.

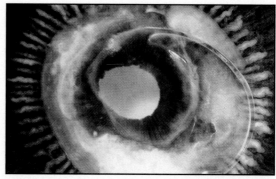

Figure 2-35. Gross photograph from behind of a human eye obtained postmortem (Miyake-Apple posterior photographic technique) showing success in transitioning toward Generation VI in two respects, namely 1) implantation of a well-manufactured one-piece all-PMMA IOL design and 2) good symmetric in-the-bag fixation with good centration. However, the hydrodissection-enhanced cortical cleanup phase of the operation still was lacking, as is evidenced by the large Soemmering's ring.

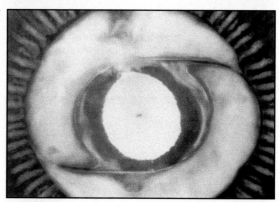

Figure 2-36. Gross photograph from behind of a human eye obtained postmortem (Miyake-Apple posterior photographic technique) showing a well-manufactured one-piece all-PMMA PC IOL. Note evidence of poor cortical cleanup and, most notably, PCO. A Nd:YAG laser secondary posterior capsulotomy had to be performed (central polygonal area).

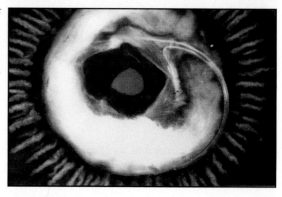

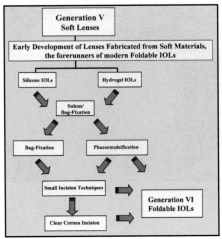

Figure 2-37. Early experimentation with soft IOL materials in Generation V, even dating back to the 1970s, provided important clinical and basic information that has made possible the development of today's modern foldable IOLs suitable for insertion via small-incision techniques. The soft lenses studied during this early period are the forerunners of today's modern foldable IOLs. Although there was much experimentation during this early period (Generation V), because of the rudimentary surgical techniques, including general lack of in-the-bag fixation, successful use of IOL implantation could only be accomplished much later, in Generation VI.

piece) foldable IOL designs, are illustrated in Figures 2-44 to 2-45. These are the designs that have culminated in modern foldable designs such as the plate styles (Figure 2-41), various modern three-piece silicone optic designs such as the Allergan SI-40 (Allergan Medical Optics, Irvine, CA) design (Figure 2-45A), and a modern hydrophobic acrylic design (Alcon AcrySof, Alcon Laboratories, Fort Worth, TX) (Figure 2-45B).

Cataract-IOL surgery as we know it began in the mid-1980s (Generation VI) (Tables 2-1 and 2-2, Figures 2-1, 2-19, and 2-46), and began in earnest about 1992. Application of the techniques listed in Table 2-2, leading to consistent in-the-bag fixation, has defined this era VI-a. It was then a small but significant step toward what we term Generation VI-b, which defines modern foldable lenses inserted through a small incision after phacoemulsification. Generation VI (defined as capsular surgery characterized by consistent, secure, and permanent in-the-bag fixation) has truly become a reality in the last few years with the advent of small-incision surgery. Note the chart from our database (Figure 2-47), which shows that a 90% plus success rate of in-the-bag fixation is now possible using small-incision techniques with foldable lenses. Two major hallmarks of Generation VI are, of course, CCC (Figures 2-48, A-C, and 2-49) and hydrodissection (Figure 2-50). Figure 2-49 summarizes what is now common knowledge; namely, that success in placing haptics within the capsular bag is inversely proportional to the number of radial tears of the anterior capsule. The issue of radial tears has been successfully resolved by the CCC technique (this being a very important factor in obtaining secure and permanent in-the-bag fixation). Hydrodissection (Figure 2-50) is not only useful and important in achieving safe surgery intraoperatively; it is very important in enhancing total lens epithelial cell removal. This is one of the most important factors in reducing the incidence of secondary cataract (PCO) (see Chapter 7).

The evolution toward Generation VI is characterized not only by the development of appropriate surgical techniques that enhance in-the-bag fixation (Table 2-2), but, equally important, by the development of lenses specifically designed for implantation within the capsular bag (Figure 2-51). Figure 2-51A shows an early and successful flexible circular IOL design by Dr. Aziz Anis of Omaha, Neb., and Figure 2-51B shows a rigid all-PMMA disc design by Dr. Albert Galand of Liege, Belgium. Both of these, designed to

Figure 2-38. Gross photograph from behind of a human eye obtained postmortem (Miyake-Apple posterior photographic technique) showing an early prototype hydrogel plate IOL design developed in the 1970s, a forerunner of modern foldable designs. One important lesson regarding fixation and PCO is illustrated here. We note in this text (Chapter 7) that prevention of secondary cataract (PCO) is strongly dependent on attainment of good in-the-bag fixation. In this illustration, the haptic on the left is situated in the capsular bag and no opacification is present. The haptic on the right was asymmetrically implanted in front of the capsular bag. Note here an ingrowth of retained cortex and lens epithelial cells has led to a secondary cataract on the right, subjacent to this area of out-of-the-bag fixation.

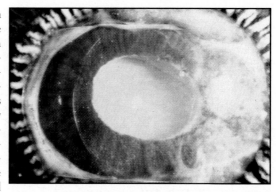

Figure 2-39. Early silicone plate IOL design (Mazaco Taco, 1980s). The quality of manufacture then was not comparable to what is available today. Note the sharp ragged edges of this IOL (scanning electron micrograph, original magnification x10).

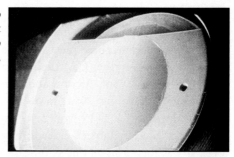

Figure 2-40A. In the late 1980s there was experimentation not only with various solid or small hole plate IOL designs, but also the design shown here. With this design, the outer haptics were too flimsy and stable fixation was difficult to achieve, so it was withdrawn. However, in some ways this design was the forerunner of modern large hole plate IOL designs that are currently being successfully implanted (see Figure 2-41, and 3-17 to 3-19). This is a gross photograph from behind of a human eye obtained postmortem (Miyake-Apple posterior photographic technique) showing experimental implantation of a closed-loop silicone design situated into the ciliary sulcus of a monkey eye (performed in our laboratory in Salt Lake City).

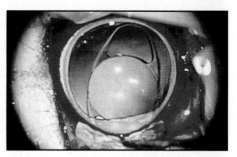

Figure 2-40B. In the late 1980s there was experimentation not only with various solid or small hole plate IOL designs, but also the design shown here. With this design, the outer haptics were too flimsy and stable fixation was difficult to achieve, so it was withdrawn. However, in some ways this design was the forerunner of modern large hole plate IOL designs that are currently being successfully implanted (see Figure 2-41, and 3-17 to 3-19). This is a gross photograph from behind of a monkey eye (Miyake-Apple posterior photographic technique) showing the same IOL as in Figure 2-40A, situated in the ciliary sulcus. This was not the correct fixation site.

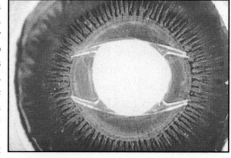

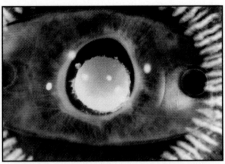

Figure 2-41. The plate silicone IOL designs illustrated in Figures 2-38 to 2-40 were the forerunners of the highly successful modern large hole silicone plate IOLs now manufactured by Staar Surgical and Bausch & Lomb Surgical (see Chapter 3). This is a gross photograph from behind of a human eye obtained postmortem (Miyake-Apple posterior photographic technique) showing successful implantation of a large hole plate lens in the capsular bag, with good centration and good clarity of the media.

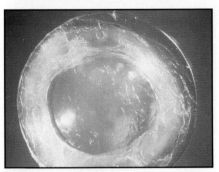

Figure 2-42. This is gross photograph of an explanted disc-style silicone IOL design, manufactured in Germany in the late 1980s. It was explanted within the surrounding capsular bag because of dislocation. This lens has been superseded by the modern plate and haptic style foldable IOL designs.

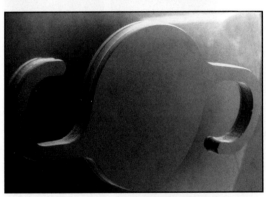

Figure 2-43. An early and very interesting attempt at manufacture of a one-piece, haptic style PC IOL fabricated from silicone (manufactured in China) is shown in this scanning electron micrograph. Note the rough edges and primitive lathe cut manufacturing technique of this early IOL (original magnification x10).

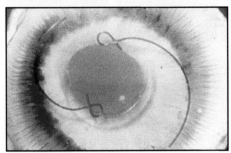

Figure 2-44A. Gross photographs from behind, Miyake-Apple posterior photographic techniques of two eyes with silicone IOLs. This is a rabbit eye experimentally implanted in our laboratory with an early prototype of a three-piece foldable IOL design, an early IOL of the SI series, manufactured by Allergan. It has a silicone optic and two polypropylene haptics. It evolved into later Allergan designs in the SI series, ranging from SI-13 to the SI-30. Note good fixation, good centration, and clarity of the media. This series of lens became the forerunner of the modern Allergan SI-40NB and SA-40 (Array) designs (see Figure 2-45; and Chapter 4 Figures 4-8 to 4-16).

Figure 2-44B. Gross photographs from behind, Miyake-Apple posterior photographic techniques of two eyes with silicone IOLs. This is a gross photograph from behind of a human eye obtained postmortem (Miyake-Apple posterior photographic technique) showing an early SI series Allergan silicone IOL implanted in the capsular bag. This illustration shows what we have observed in many cases; that the IOL itself sometimes appeared to be ahead of the surgical technique. The lens is securely implanted within the capsular bag, but retained cortex and fibrotic material have caused a contraction and crimping of the polypropylene loops and decentration of the IOL optic.

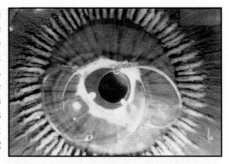

Figure 2-45A. Advances made throughout the early periods of soft IOLs have led to development of modern foldable IOLs, including silicone plate designs (Figure 2-41); modern three-piece IOL designs are seen here. This figure shows a clinical photograph showing the Allergan SI-30 design with polypropylene haptics (left) and the later SI-40NB design with PMMA haptics (right) (see Chapter 4).

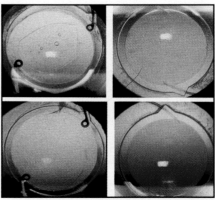

Figure 2-45B. Other foldable IOL materials were developed during this period, including the material that evolved into the modern Alcon AcrySof IOL design, which is being successfully implanted today. These four clinical photographs illustrate this lens. The two pictures on the left show an earlier AcrySof IOL design with the cruciate appearance of the haptic as it enters the optic. The later Acryset IOL design with a straight entrance into the optic by its PMMA haptics is shown on the right.

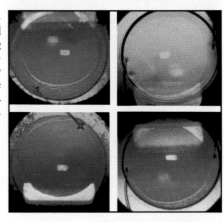

Figure 2-46. Generation VI (marked activity 1987 to present). Although IOL development—including soft IOLs, as noted previously—occurred rapidly, the entrance into Generation VI is characterized, indeed defined, by the ability to achieve secure and permanent in-the-bag fixation of the PC IOL (see Table 2-2 and Figure 2-19). This diagram shows the important subgroups of modern ECCE in PC IOL surgery. During this period, it was realized that IOL operation was not just removal of an opaque crystalline lens, but also a refractive procedure.

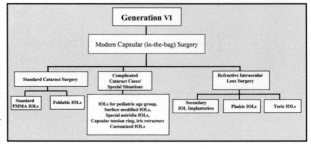

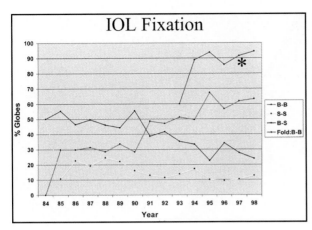

Figure 2-47. In-the-bag IOL fixation (red line, B-B fixation), the hallmark of Generation VI, improved slowly and gradually over the years, especially when used in association with standard ECCE and large incision-can opener anterior capsulotomy surgery. Note that the percentage of successful in-the-bag (B-B) fixation increased from about 30% in the early 1980s to a maximum of approximately 60% in the late 1990s. A quantum leap occurred in the late to mid-late 1990s with a transition to small-incision foldable IOL surgery-a surgical technique that demands meticulous in-the-bag fixation. Note that in-the-bag fixation is now being achieved in over 90% of cases in which foldable lenses are implanted via a small incision after phacoemulsification (blue line, asterisk).

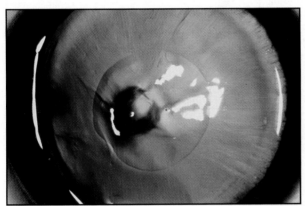

Figure 2-48A. The CCC technique is one of the most important hallmarks of Generation VI (Table 2-2 and Figure 2-19). CCC is viewed here on the lens of a human eye obtained postmortem (original magnification x50). This procedure more than any other accounts for secure and permanent fixation within the lens capsular bag. Avoidance of radial tears to the anterior capsule is the key advantage of this technique.

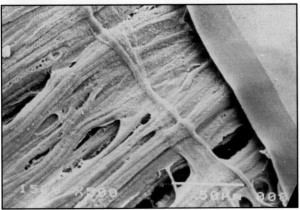

Figure 2-48B. These scanning electron micrographs of the capsulorhexis edge show the beautifully smooth edge that is attainable with the manual capsular tear technique (original magnification x100). In both figures, the edge of the torn anterior capsule was seen in the upper right.

Figure 2-48C. These scanning electron micrographs of the capsulorhexis edge show the beautifully smooth edge that is attainable with the manual capsular tear technique (original magnification x100). In these figures, the edge of the torn anterior capsule was seen in the upper right.

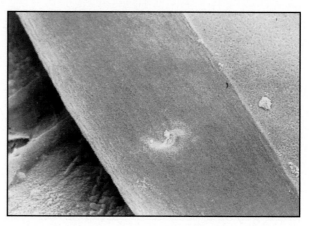

Figure 2-49. Diagram from Assia and associates showing the relationship of anterior radial tears and success of in-the-bag haptic placement. Successful in-the-bag fixation is best achieved by total avoidance of radial tears (and hence avoiding "pea podding") (see Figure 2-33). With multiple radial tears, as was common with the early can opener capsulectomy technique, stabilization of IOL haptics in the capsular bag was extremely difficult, indeed unlikely.

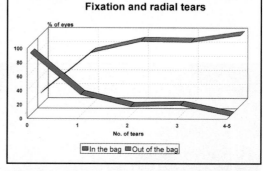

Figure 2-50. An unheralded surgical step that has played a major role in the transition to Generation VI has been the hydrodissection technique, shown here experimentally in a human eye obtained postmortem (Miyake-Apple posterior photographic technique). This technique is not only important in terms of achieving a safe, successful operation, with easy removal of lens nucleus, but equally important, it is instrumental in helping reduce the incidence of PCO. This technique is studied in further detail in Chapter 7.

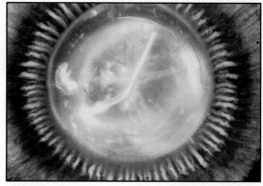

be implanted via the envelope technique, are successful examples of early lenses designed for the capsular bag.

During the 1980s, as most surgeons made the transition toward capsular fixation (Generation VI), the lens designs most commonly used were three-piece PMMA optic styles as illustrated in Figures 2-52 to 2-54. Also evolving concurrently throughout the 1980s were the one-piece all-PMMA designs (Figures 2-55 to 2-58). Studies in our laboratory have differentiated relatively rigid one-piece designs (Figure 2-55), in which the haptics come off from the optic in a relatively straight direction, from the much more flexible

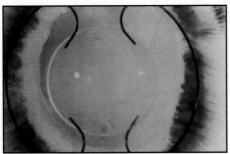

Figure 2-51A. As improved surgical techniques allowed for better in-the-bag fixation, IOL designers began designing IOLs especially for in-the-bag placement. The Anis IOL shown in this figure, designed by Aziz Anis of Lincoln, Neb in the early 1980s, is a flexible circular design, an excellent example of an early lens designed for in-the-bag placement. This photograph is of a rabbit eye after experimental implantation performed in our laboratory (Miyake-Apple posterior photographic technique).

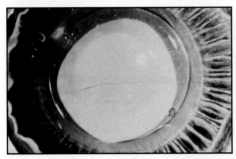

Figure 2-51B. As improved surgical techniques allowed for better in-the-bag fixation, IOL designers began designing IOLs especially for in-the-bag placement. This gross photograph from behind of an experimentally operated cat eye shows an experimental all-PMMA rigid disc IOL, designed by Albert Galand in Belgium, implanted in the capsular bag following the envelope technique. (Note two horizontal anterior capsular tears.) This IOL was implanted experimentally in our laboratory in the late 1980s. Lenses such as this and the Anis design were important for the development of in-the-bag techniques and other IOL designs for in-the-bag implantation, including foldables.

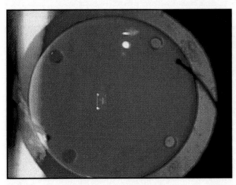

Figure 2-52. As the transition toward Generation VI (Table 2-1, Figure 2-19) occurred in the late 1980s, the majority of lenses implanted were three-piece PC IOL designs as shown in this illustration and in Figures 2-58, 2-60, and 2-61. This is a clinical photograph of an early three-piece design, with good centration following in-the-bag fixation. Note the four positioning holes, which were characteristic of many early PC IOL designs.

designs, where the C-shaped haptics come off the optic at an angle (Figures 2-56 to 2-58). This type of takeoff from the optic and the C configuration provide a highly flexible lens with a good fit within the capsular bag. This design remains the gold standard among rigid lenses today (Figure 2-58), and is the lens most commonly advocated in the developing world setting where small-incision techniques are not yet available.[5] By definition, these rigid, PMMA-optic lenses must go through a relatively large incision, and therefore comprise Generation VI-a.

The transition to Generation VI-b (Tables 2-1 and 2-2, and Figures 2-19 and 2-46) represents the definitive move toward the ability to insert specialized lenses such as foldable IOLs through a small incision after phacoemulsification. In addition to basic foldable lenses, to be described in subsequent chapters, this permitted development of several specialized types of IOLs, including refractive IOLs (Figures 2-59 to 2-63, Table 2-1) and lenses designed to restore accommodation (Figures 2-64 to 2-68).

Figure 2-53. Gross photograph of a human eye obtained postmortem (Miyake-Apple posterior photographic technique) showing an excellent result after implantation of a three-piece modified J-loop IOL into the capsular bag, with good cortical cleanup. This is a mid-1980s photograph.

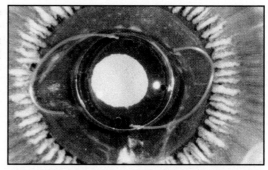

Figure 2-54. Gross photograph of a human eye obtained postmortem (Miyake-Apple posterior photographic technique) showing excellent implantation of a three-piece PC IOL into the capsular bag, with good results similar to those seen in Figure 2-58 (early 1990s photograph).

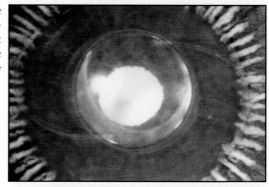

Figure 2-55. As Generation VI evolved, more and more implantations of one-piece all-PMMA designs occurred. Note excellent in-the-bag fixation and clarity of the media. This is a gross photograph of a human eye obtained postmortem (Miyake-Apple posterior photographic technique).

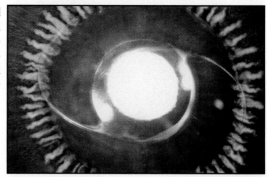

Figure 2-56. In experimental studies in our laboratory, we differentiated relatively rigid one-piece IOL designs, in which the haptic "take off" from the optic was relatively straight, from a design with a relatively flexible "take off" of the haptic. Note in this photograph, showing experimental implantation of an IOL in a human eye obtained postmortem (Miyake-Apple posterior photographic technique), that the haptic first comes to the left of the optic and then swings to the right in a C-shaped configuration. This configuration allows maximum flexibility and helps improve fitting of the lens into the capsular bag (see Figures 2-57 and 2-58).

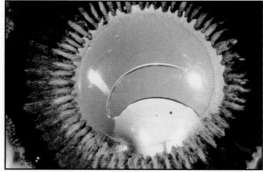

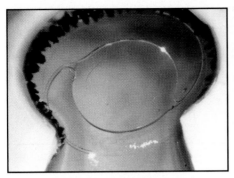

Figure 2-57. Oblique view showing an experimental implantation of the same type of lens as seen in Figure 2-26. This oblique or side view is made possible by the "keyhole" technique developed in our laboratory by Dr. Ehud Assia.[5] Note that the cornea and a scleral window have been removed to observe the lens within the lens capsular bag. The C-shaped configuration of this IOL, which is 12 mm in diameter, is ideal for most adult lens capsular bags.

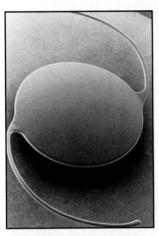

Figure 2-58. Scanning electron micrograph of the flexible modified C-loop PC IOL developed in our laboratory (same design as noted in Figures 2-56 and 2-57). This flexible design has become the gold standard of rigid all-PMMA designs and is still extremely important for implantations in areas where modern phacoemulsification and small-incision techniques are not available, especially the developing world (see reference 3). Note also that this design has been applied to a modern foldable IOL, the Pharmacia-Upjohn 911 CeeOn edge IOL (see Chapter 6, Figures 6-4 to 6-6).

To summarize, it is highly useful for the surgeon in training and the surgeon transitioning toward extracapsular surgery to be aware of the evolutionary process as outlined in Table 2-2 and Figure 2-1. Knowledge of these details allows a person to 1) to appreciate the mistakes of all of the early generations, especially the early phases of Generation V; 2) see the surgical and IOL improvements that were designed and implemented throughout the very important transition period of Generation V-b; and 3) apply the techniques and IOL designs of Generation VI-a initially and, finally, Generation VI-b. The pioneer surgeons and researchers who guided us through these last two decades were actually developing foldable IOL techniques prior to the development of the foldable IOLs themselves. They have been directly responsible for providing us and of course our patients, with the supreme results enjoyed today.

In the next sections (2 and 3, including Chapters 3 to 6), we provide a clinicopathologic discussion and illustrations of the major foldable IOL designs that have evolved through the 1990s and are accompanying us into the next century.

Table 2-3 lists foldable IOLs that are available in our United States autopsy eye database. In Section 3, Chapters 3 through 5, we provide a detailed clinicopathologic correlation on these IOLs and offer clinically relevant findings, tips and pearls that should be of use to the surgeon.

In Table 2-4 we listed a number of foldable lenses, some manufactured in the United States and some manufactured overseas, which for various reasons are not available to us

Figure 2-59. Although the use of IOLs for phakic implantation was attempted as early as the 1960s, increased activity in the field of refractive IOLs began in the 1980s. A wide variety of techniques devised specifically for refractive purposes emerged. Several general categories are listed in this diagram. Modern refractive IOLs also are classified as a component of Generation VI (see Table 2-1).

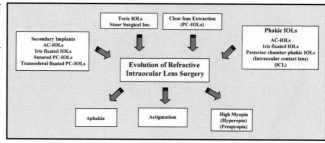

Figure 2-60A. The phakic IOLs designed for refractive purposes are classified into three categories based on fixation (see Table 2-2). These include AC lenses, iris fixation lenses, and phakic PC IOLs. The most commonly used AC lens to date is the four-point fixation designed by George Baikoff, MD, a modification of the Kelman multiflex design. This lens, of course, is a rigid PMMA design and is not foldable. The currently used iris fixation lens for refractive implantation is the Worst-Fechner Artesen IOL

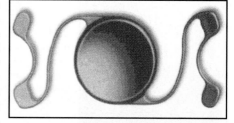

Figure 2-60B. The phakic IOLs designed for refractive purposes are classified into three categories based on fixation (see Table 2-2). These include AC lenses, iris fixation lenses, and phakic PC IOLs. The most commonly used AC lens to date is the four-point fixation designed by George Baikoff, MD, a modification of the Kelman multiflex design. This rigid PMMA IOL is under clinical investigation.

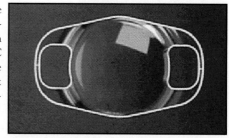

Figure 2-61. An important topic of research today concerns foldable phakic PC IOLs, which are undergoing worldwide investigation and scrutiny. We have had the opportunity to examine three explanted silicone phakic PC IOL designs manufactured by Adatomed in Germany. This IOL was well-polished, but in examining it, we learned various characteristics to avoid in design and manufacture of a lens of this style. These included too thick an anterior posterior dimension (1.15 mm with this IOL), fabrication from a poorly biocompatible silicone, and difficulty in obtaining the correct size and fixation site for this design.

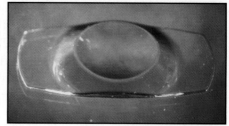

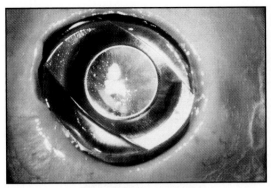

Figure 2-62. We implanted the Adatomed IOL (same IOL as in Figure 2-61) experimentally into human eyes obtained postmortem and verified the problems of this IOL; in particular, the excessive thickness in the anterior-posterior dimension as well as the excessive length of this IOL, which actually fixated into the zonular fibers. This lens has been withdrawn from the market.

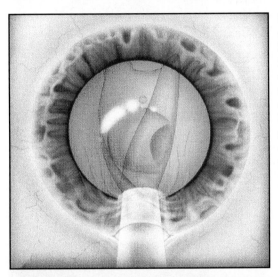

Figure 2-63A. The phakic PC IOL that has generated the most interest is the Staar Surgical hydrophilic plate IOL design termed the implantable contact lens. We have not had the opportunity to examine an explanted IOL or an autopsy globe containing this IOL, so we cannot comment on it directly. Clinical results seem to be very good in general, although complications such as complicated anterior subcapsular cataract and (secondary) glaucoma and pigmentary dispersion have been reported. Long-term investigations will be required to determine whether this lens is safe and effective for phakic refractive implantation. This figure shows a manufacturer's illustration of insertion and unfolding of the IOL.

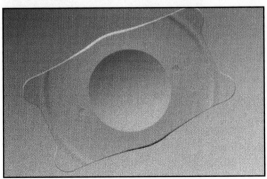

Figure 2-63B. The phakic PC IOL that has generated the most interest is the Staar Surgical hydrophilic plate IOL design termed the implantable contact lens. We have not had the opportunity to examine an explanted IOL or an autopsy globe containing this IOL, so we cannot comment on it directly. Clinical results seem to be very good in general, although complications such as complicated anterior subcapsular cataract and (secondary) glaucoma and pigmentary dispersion have been reported. Long-term investigations will be required to determine whether this lens is safe and effective for phakic refractive implantation. This figure is a manufacturer's illustration of the entire implantable contact lens.

Figure 2-64. As surgical techniques and modern foldable IOLs have vastly improved, there are now intense efforts toward developing IOLs suitable for restoration of accommodation. Several directions of research are listed on this chart.

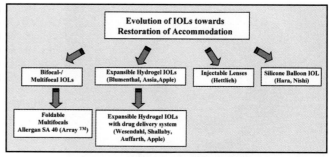

Figure 2-65. In association with Drs. Michael Blumenthal and Ehud Assia, we have experimented with development of an expansile hydrogel design. This is a disc-shaped IOL that in the dry state measures 2 x 7 x 7 mm and in the hydrated state measures 4 x 10 x 10 mm, thus filling the capsular bag. This malleable material therefore can modify its shape according to the action of the zonules and may be suitable as an accommodative IOL. Further research is necessary.

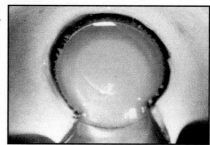

Figure 2-66. This early attempt at a bifocal IOL was a design of Dr. John Pearce of England. He designed a one-piece PMMA disc IOL with a bifocal add in the center of the lens. This was designed for implantation in the capsular bag. Overall, the optical quality was not satisfactory in terms of widespread clinical usage, and the lens has been abandoned.

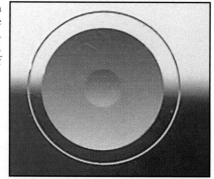

Figure 2-67. In the late 1980s, 3M Corporation developed a diffractive multifocal IOL technology, as shown here. Problems with this lens ensued—particularly problems related to fixation difficulties (common asymmetric fixation with decentration)—which were inherent with surgical techniques at that time (late 1980s). This is an example of an explanted 3M diffractive multifocal IOL that required removal and exchange because of decentration with subsequent decreased optical quality.

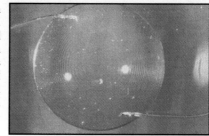

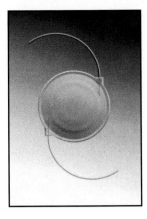

Figure 2-68. Manufacturer's illustration of the modern Allergan SA-40 (Array) design. The multifocal optical configuration is placed on their SI-40 design (see Chapter 4, Figures 4-14 to 4-19). To date, when appropriate patient selection is carefully accomplished, results with this lens have been excellent.

in our autopsy globe database. We have had the opportunity to study some in experimental animals and in experimental implantation with the Miyake-Apple posterior photographic technique. However, these lenses are too new to be available in large numbers on the American market. Therefore, in Section 3, Chapter 6, we can only list and catalog these lenses and offer general but not specific observations based on detailed pathologic analyses.

We do not provide the reader with our opinions of a preferred foldable IOL. However, with a careful perusal of the text, tables, photographs, and legends, this collection of material should provide additional data from a different perspective not generally available to the clinician that should help in choosing a suitable safe and effective design.

REFERENCES

1. Apple DJ, Rabb MF. *Ocular Pathology, Clinical Applications, and Self-Assessment.* 5th ed. St. Louis, Mo: Mosby Year-Book, Inc., 1998.

2. Apple DJ, Sims JC. Harold Ridley and the invention of the intraocular lens. *Surv Ophthalmol.* 1995;40:279-292.

3. Choyce P. Harold Ridley's first patient. *J Cataract Refract Surg.* 1999;25:731.

4. Apple DJ, Kincaid MC, Mamalis N, Olson RJ. *Intraocular Lenses: Evolution, Designs, Complications, and Pathology.* Baltimore, Md: Williams & Wilkins, 1989.

5. Apple DJ. Harold Ridley: A golden anniversary celebration and a golden age. *Arch Ophthalmol.* 1999;117(6):827.

6. Apple DJ, Ram J, Peng Q. The fiftieth anniversary of the intraocular lens and a quiet revolution. *Ophthalmology.* 1999;10:1,2.

BIBLIOGRAPHY

Allarakhia L, Knoll RL, Lindstrom RL. Soft intraocular lenses. *J Cataract Refract Surg.* 1987;13:607-620.

Anderson CJ, Sturm RJ, Shapiro MB, Ballew C. Visual disturbances associated with oval-optic poly (methyl methacrylate) and round-optic silicone intraocular lenses. *J Cataract Refract Surg.* 1994;20:295-298.

Anis AY. Hydrosonic intercapsular piecemeal phacoemulsification or the 'HIPP' technique. *Int Ophthalmol.* 1994;18:37-42.

Apple DJ. Center for Intraocular Lens Research transfers to Medical University of South Carolina. *J Cataract Refract Surg.* 1988;14:481.

Apple DJ. Intraocular lenses: Notes from an interested observer. *Arch Ophthalmol.* 1986;104:1150-1152.

Apple DJ. Lens Replacement. In: Yanoff M, Duker J. *Ophthalmology.* Philadelphia, Pa: Mosby-Year Book, Inc.; (In Press).

Apple DJ. Pathology of Intraocular Lenses: Polypropylene vs PMMA. In: Jeffe MS, ed. *Intraocular Lens Complications; Self-Study Program.* Module II. Proceedings of Symposium on IOL Complications. Stockholm, Sweden: Pharmacia; [monograph] 1985.

Apple DJ, Brems RN, Ellis GW, Spencer DA. A review of the histopathology of intraocular lens fixation. *Curr Can Ophthalmic Prac.* 1986;4:54-56,78-79.

Apple DJ, Cameron JD, Lindstrom RL. Loop fixation of posterior chamber intraocular lenses. *Cataract.* 1984;2(1):7-10.

Apple DJ, Craythorn JM, Olson RJ, et al. Anterior segment complications and neovascular glaucoma following implantation of posterior chamber intraocular lens. *Ophthalmology.* 1984;91:403-419.

Apple DJ, Gieser SC, Isenberg RA. *Evolution of Intraocular Lenses.* Salt Lake City, Ut: University of Utah Printing Services; 1985.

Apple DJ, Lichtenstein SB, Heerlein K, et al. Visual aberrations caused by optic components of posterior chamber intraocular lenses. *J Cataract Refract Surg.* 1987;13:431-435.

Apple DJ, Lim ES, Morgan RC, et al. Preparation and study of human eyes obtained post-mortem with the Miyake posterior photographic technique. *Ophthalmology.* 1990;97:810-816.

Apple DJ, Mamalis N, Brady SE. Biocompatibility of implant materials: A review and scanning electron microscopic study. *J Am Intraocul Implant Soc.* 1984;10:53-66.

Apple DJ, Mamalis N, Loftfield K, et al. Complications of intraocular lenses. A historical and histopathological review. *Surv Ophthalmol.* 1984;29:1-54.

Apple DJ, Morgan RC, Tsai JC. Histology of posterior chamber fixation. In: Percival SPB, ed. *A Colour Atlas of Lens Implantation.* London, England: Mosby Year Book; 1991.

Apple DJ, Osher RH, Lichtenstein SB, Koch DD. IOL *Materials and Complications.* Proceedings of Symposium on IOL Materials and Complications. Orlando, Fl, Coburn [monograph], 1986.

Apple DJ, Park SB, Merkley KH, et al. Posterior chamber intraocular lenses in a series of 75 autopsy eyes. Part I. Loop location. *J Cataract Refract Surg.* 1986;12:358-362.

Apple DJ, Ram J, Foster A, Peng Q. Elimination of cataract blindness: a global perspective. *Surv Ophthalmol.* 2000 (supplement).

Apple DJ, Reidy JJ, Googe JM, et al. A comparison of ciliary sulcus and capsular bag fixation of posterior chamber intraocular lenses. *J Am Intraocul Implant Soc.* 1995;11:44-63.

Apple DJ, Tetz MR, Hansen SO, et al. Intercapsular implantation of various posterior chamber IOLs: Animal test results. *Ophthalmic Prac.* 1987;5(3):100-104,132-134.

Apple DJ, Tetz MR, Hansen SO. Intercapsular (endocapsular) intraocular lens implantation: Results of animal studies. Proceedings of the Endocapsular Symposium, IOIS Meeting. Fukuoka, Japan: 1987, *Jpn IOL Soc J.* 1988;2(1):45-61.

Assia EI, Castaneda VE, Legler UFC, et al. Studies on cataract surgery and intraocular lenses at the center for intraocular lens research. In: Obstbaum SA, ed. *Cataract and Intraocular Lens Surgery; Ophthalmology Clinics of North America.* Vol 4, Num 2. Philadelphia, Pa: WB Saunders; 1991.

Auffarth G, Wesendahl T, Apple DJ. Surface characteristics of intraocular lens implants: An evaluation using scanning electron microscopy and quantitative three-dimensional non-contacting profilometry (TOPO). *J Long-term Effect Med Implants.* 1993;3(4): 321-331.

Auffarth GU, McCabe C, Tetz MR, Apple DJ. Die modifizierte Disk-Linse nach Anis: Befunde bei 15 menschlichen Autopsieaugen. In: Rochels R, Dunker G, Hartmann Ch, eds. *Transactions of the 9th Congress of the German Intraocular Lens Implant Society.* Kiel. Heidelberg, Berlin, New York: Springer Publ; 1995.

Auffarth GU, McCabe C, Tetz MR, Apple DJ. Clinicopathological findings in autopsy eyes with the Anis modified disc IOL. *J Cataract Refract Surg.* 1996;22(2):1471-1475.

Auffarth GU, Wesendahl TA, Solomon KD, Brown SJ, Apple DJ. Modified preparation technique for closed system ocular surgery of human eyes obtained post-mortem. An improved research and teaching tool. *Ophthalmology.* 1996;103:977-982.

Baldeschi L, Rizzo S, Nardi M. Damage of foldable intraocular lenses by incorrect folder forceps. *Am J Ophthalmol.* 1997;124:245-247.

Blaydes JE. Small incision intraocular lens: past, present and future. *Dev Ophthalmol.* 1989;18:107-110.

Borirak-Chanyavat S, Lindquist TD, Kaplan HJ. A cadaver eye model for practicing anterior and posterior segment surgeries. *Ophthalmology.* 1995;102:1932-1935.

Brems RN, Apple DJ, Pfeffer BR, et al. Posterior chamber intraocular lenses in a series of 75 autopsy eyes. Part III. Correlation of positioning holes and optic edges with the pupillary aperture and visual axis. *J Cataract Refract Surg.* 1986;12:367-371.

Cameron JD, Apple DJ, Sumsion MA, et al. Pathology of iris support intraocular lenses. *Eur J Imp Refract Surg.* 1987;5(1):15-24.

Chen TT. Clinical experience with soft intraocular lens implantation. *J Cataract Refract Surg.* 1987;13:50-53.

Choyce P. *Intraocular Lenses and Implants.* London, England: H.K. Lewis and Co., Ltd.; 1964.

Cornic JC, Pouliquen Y. First results with soft lens implants. *Dev Ophthalmol.* 1989;18:114-120.

Crandall AS, Richards SC, Apple DJ: Extracapsular cataract extraction. In-the-bag versus ciliary sulcus fixation. In: *Transactions of the Pacific Coast Oto-Ophthalmological Society* 1985;66:73-79.

Crawford JB, Faulkner GD. Pathology report on the foldable silicone posterior chamber lens. *J Cataract Refract Surg.* 1986;12:297-300.

Cusumano A, Busin M, Spitznas M. Bacterial growth is significantly enhanced on foldable intraocular lenses. *Arch Ophthalmol.* 1994;112:1015-1016.

Davison JA. A short haptic diameter modified J-loop intraocular lens for improved capsular bag performance. *J Cataract Refract Surg.* 1988;14:161-166.

Duncker GI, Westphalen S, Behrendt S. Complications of silicone disc intraocular lenses. *J Cataract Refract Surg.* 1995;21:562-566.

Fine IH, Robertson JE, Jr. Initial experience with the AMO PC-28LB (Phacofit) small-incision implant: a preliminary report. *J Cataract Refract Surg.* 1989;15:327-331.

Habal MB. The biologic basis for the clinical application of the silicones. a correlate to their biocompatibility. *Arch Surg.* 1984;119:843-848.

Hansen SO, Tetz MR, Solomon KD, et al. Decentration of flexible loop posterior chamber intraocular lenses in a series of 222 postmortem eyes. *Ophthalmology.* 1988;95:344-349.

Hettlich HJ, Kaufmann R, Harmeyer H, et al. In vitro and in vivo evaluation of a hydrophilized silicone intraocular lens. *J Cataract Refract Surg.* 1992;18:140-146.

Hoffman J. *A History of Modern IOLs.* Thorofare, NJ: SLACK Incorporated; (In Press).

Jacobi FK, Kammann J, Jacobi KW, Grosskopf U, Walden K. Bilateral implantation of asymmetrical diffractive multifocal intraocular lenses. *Arch Ophthalmol.* 1999;117:17-23.

Jacobi KW, Nowak MR. New materials for intraocular lenses. *Fortschritte der Ophthalmologie.* 1989;86:203-205.

Jaffe NS. New designs of intraocular lenses. *Transactions- New Orleans Academy of Ophthalmology.* 1988;36:269-277.

Kohnen T, Magdowski G, Koch DD. Scanning electron microscopic analysis of foldable acrylic and hydrogel intraocular lenses. *J Cataract Refract Surg.* 1996;22(suppl 2):1342-1350.

Kulnig W, Menapace R, Skorpik C, Juchem M. Optical resolution of silicone and polymethylmethacrylate intraocular lenses. *J Cataract Refract Surg.* 1987;13:635-639.

Levy JH, Pisacano AM, Anello RD. Displacement of bag-placed hydrogel lenses into the vitreous following neodymium: yag laser capsulotomy. *J Cataract Refract Surg.* 1990;16:563-566.

Levy JH, Pisacano AM. Clinical endothelial cell loss following phacoemulsification and silicone or poly-methylmethacrylate lens implantation. *J Cataract Refract Surg. 1988*;14:299-302.

Levy JH, Pisacano AM. Initial clinical studies with silicone intraocular implants. *J Cataract Refract Surg.* 1988;14:294-298.

Lindstrom RL, Allarakhia L, Knoll RL. Soft intraocular lenses. *Transactions-New Orleans Academy of Ophthalmology.* 1988;36:329-353.

Mackool RJ, Gupta A. New soft intraocular lens. *J Cataract Refract Surg.* 1988;14:691-692.

Mazzocco TR. Early clinical experience with elastic lens implants. *Transactions of the Ophthalmological Societies of the United Kingdom.* 1985;104:578-579.

Menapace R. Current state of implantation of flexible intraocular lenses. *Fortschritte der Ophthalmologie.* 1991;88:421-428.

Neumann AC, Cobb B. Advantages and limitations of current soft intraocular lenses. *J Cataract Refract Surg.* 1989;15:257-263.

Newland T, Auffarth G, Wesendahl T, et al. Pathology of Nd:YAG laser damage on explanted lenses with experimentally-produced lesions. *J Cataract Refract Surg.* 1994;20:527-533.

Nordlohne ME. The Intraocular Implant Lens Development and Results with Special References to the Binkhorst Lens. 2nd Ed. Baltimore, Md: Williams and Wilkins; 1975.

Obstbaum SA. Development of foldable IOL materials. *J Cataract Refract Surg.* 1995;21:233.

Packard RB, Garner A, Arnott EJ. Poly-hema as a material for intraocular lens implantation: A preliminary report. *Br J Ophthalmol.* 1981;65:585-587.

Park SB, Brems RN, Parsons MR, et al. Posterior chamber intraocular lenses in a series of 75 autopsy eyes. Part II. Post-implantation loop configuration. *J Cataract Refract Surg.* 1986;12:363-366.

Patel J, Apple DJ, Hansen SO, et al. Protective effect of the anterior lens capsule during extracapsular cataract extraction. Part II. Preliminary results of clinical study. *Ophthalmology.* 1989;96(5):598-602.

Popham JK, Apple DJ, Newman DA, et al. Advantages and Limitations of Soft Intraocular Lenses. A Scientific Perspective. In: Mazzocco TR, Rajacich GM, Epstein E, eds. *Soft Implant Lenses in Cataract Surgery.* Thorofare, NJ: SLACK Incorporated; 1986.

Ram J, Auffarth GU, Wesendahl TA, Apple DJ. Miyake posterior view video technique; a means to reduce the learning curve in phacoemulsification. Ophthalmic Prac. 1994;12 (5):206-210.

Refojo MF. Current status of biomaterials in ophthalmology. *Surv Ophthalmol.* 1982;26:257-265.

Skorpik C, Menapace R, Gnad HD, et al. Evaluation of 50 silicone posterior chamber lens implantations. *J Cataract Refract Surg.* 1987;13:640-643.

Skorpik C, Menapace R, Scholz U, et al. Experiences with disc lenses composed of silicone. *Klinische Monatsblatter fur Augenheilkunde.* 1993;202:8-13.

Solomon KD, Apple DJ, Mamalis N, et al. Complications of intraocular lenses with special reference to an analysis of 2500 explanted intraocular lenses (IOLs). *Eur J Implant Refract Surg.* 1991;3:195-200.

Solomon KD, Gwin TD, Hansen SO, et al. Preliminary report of ultrasound and laser energy applications to small incision cataract surgery: SEM and histopathologic study. *Ophthalmic Prac.* 1988;6(2):52-91.

Solomon KD, Gwin TD, O'Morchoe DJC, et al. Protective effect of the anterior lens capsule during extra-capsular cataract extraction. Part I: Experimental animal study. *Ophthalmology.* 1989;96(5):591-597.

Stenevi ULF, Gwin T, Anders H, Apple DJ. Demonstration of hyaluronic acid binding to corneal endothelial cells in human eye-bank eyes. *Eur J Implant Ref Surg.* 1993;5:228-232.

Wenzel MR, Imkamp EM, Apple DJ. Variations in manufacturing quality of diffractive multifocal lenses. *J Cataract Refract Surg.* 1992;18(2):153-156.

Zheng YR. Clinical report of transparent silicone intraocular lens implantation (author's transl). *Chung-Hua Yen Ko Tsa Chih.* 1981;17:17-20.

Section

2

Lens Evaluation, Clinicopathologic Correlation, and Intraocular Lenses in USA Autopsy Database

Chapter
3

Silicone Plate Intraocular Lenses

Staar Surgical and Bausch and Lomb Surgical

Foldable IOLs approved and investigational as of the year 2000 that are available in USA autopsy database are listed in Table 2-3. In this chapter, we consider silicone plate IOL designs (Table 3-1).

Development of one-piece soft or foldable IOL designs, including plate lenses (Figure 3-1), began in the 1970s and early 1980s (see Figures 2-37 to 2-41). These included both hydrogel designs (see Figure 2-38) and silicone designs. The early silicone plate IOL designs were difficult to manufacture (Figures 2-39, 3-2, and 3-3), and problems with molding, edge finishing (Figure 3-2), optic opalescence, and surface irregularities (Figure 3-3)[1] were not uncommon. The design of Dr. Thomas Mazzocco (Mazzocco Taco) appeared in the early 1980s and is the forerunner of the modern plate silicone IOL designs. In addition to problems related to manufacturing, these lenses were not specifically designed for in-the-bag implantation. They were purportedly designed for ciliary sulcus placement, but in actual fact the lenses were implanted asymmetrically, with one end in the capsular bag and the other in the ciliary sulcus. This caused a significant incidence of decentration and distortion of the pseudophakos.

By the late 1980s, the design and manufacture had markedly improved and modern foldable plate IOLs, first characterized by the presence of small positioning holes on either side of the optic, emerged (Tables 3-2 and 3-3, Figures 3-4 to 3-8). These became very popular, especially in the United States (Tables 3-2 and 3-3), because they were relatively easy to insert with an injector, could be placed within a very small incision, and were relatively inexpensive.

Figures 3-4 through 3-8 show examples of small hole silicone plate IOLs well implanted within the capsular bag of several eyes with excellent optical clarity. By necessity, a CCC of average diameter (5.0 to 6.5 mm are commonly encountered minimal and maximal extremes) overlies the anterior surface of the lens optic, so that the cut edge of the anterior capsular flap is in contact with the anterior silicone surface for 360° (Figure 3-5A through C). This creates a closed capsular bag where the pseudophakos is completely sequestered by the surrounding capsular membrane from the surrounding aqueous. Figures 3-4 to 3-5 are examples of the histopathologic appearance of silicone plate lenses implanted in cases in which complete cor-

Table 3-1.
Foldable IOLs, Approved and Investigational, 2000 Available in the USA Autopsy Database

Design	Model (selected representative examples)	Company	Diameter (mm)	Optic Diameter (mm)	Water Content	Haptic Material
I. Silicone						
IA: Plate silicone lenses						
1 piece silicone plate lens (small holes)	Chiroflex C10UB	Bausch and Lomb Surgical, Inc.	10.5	Biconvex, 6.0	<1%	Silicone
1 piece silicone plate lens (large holes)	Chiroflex C11UB	Bausch and Lomb Surgical, Inc.	10.5	Biconvex, 6.0	<1%	Silicone
1 piece silicone plate lens (small holes)	AA-4203V	Staar Surgical, Inc.	10.5	Biconvex, 6.0	<1%	Silicone
1 piece silicone plate lens (large holes)	AA-4203VF	Staar Surgical, Inc.	10.5	Biconvex, 6.0	<1%	Silicone
1 piece silicone toric lens (large holes)	AA-4203TF	Staar Surgical, Inc.	10.5	Biconvex, 6.0	<1%	Silicone
IB: Three-piece silicone lenses						
a) Staar						
3 piece silicone IOL	AQ1016/2010/2003	Staar Surgical, Inc.	13.5/13.5/12.5	Biconvex, 6.3	<1%	Polyimide
b) Allergan Series						
3 piece silicone IOL	SI-30 NB	Allergan, Inc.	13.0	Biconvex, 6.0	<1%	Polypropylene
3 piece silicone IOL	SI-40 NB	Allergan, Inc.	13.0	Biconvex, 6.0	<1%	PMMA
3 piece silicone IOL	SI 55 NB	Allergan, Inc.	13.0	Biconvex, 5.5	<1%	PMMA
3 piece silicone IOL	SA 40 N	Allergan, Inc.	13.0	Biconvex, 6.0	<1%	PMMA
c) Bausch and Lomb						
3 piece silicone IOL	Soflex and LI Series	Bausch and Lomb Surgical, Inc.	13.0	Biconvex, 6.0	<1%	PMMA
II. Acrylics						
Hydrophobic (dry packed)						
3 piece Acrylic IOL	AcrySof MA30BA/MA60BM	Alcon Laboratories, Inc.	12.5/30	Biconvex, 5.5/6.0	<2%	PMMA

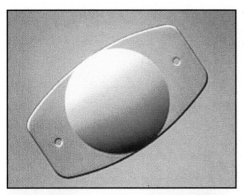

Figure 3-1. Small hole silicone plate IOL, manufacturer's illustration (see Tables 3-2 and 3-3 for specifications for this design).

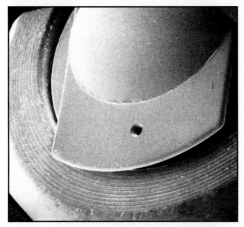

Figure 3-2A. The manufacturing quality of early silicone plate. This figure shows a scanning electron micrograph (original magnification x15).

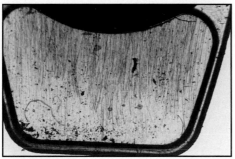

Figure 3-2B. High power gross photograph of an explanted silicone plate IOL from the late 1980s showing very poor surface finish.

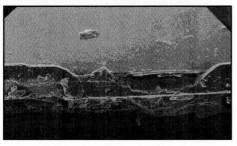

Figure 3-2C. Scanning electron micrograph high-power view of the edge of the IOL showing extensive molding flash and irregularities (original magnification x50).

Figure 3-3A. Some early silicone plate IOL designs showed opalescence of the IOL optic.

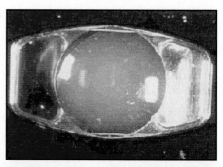

Figure 3-3B. The surface quality as measured by topographic analysis of some early plate silicone IOLs was sometimes less than optimal. Note IOL surface irregularity, as documented by distorted rings.

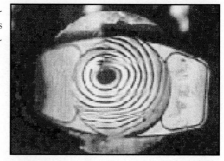

Figure 3-3C. Compare this control optic from a three-piece PMMA IOL showing excellent optical quality with concentric rings with distortions seen in Figure 3-3B.[2]

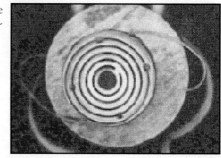

Table 3-2.
Chiroflex Small Hole Silicone Plate Lens
Bausch and Lomb Surgical, Inc.

Design	1-piece-silicone-IOL
Model	C10 UB (small holes 0.3mm)
Manufacturer	Bausch and Lomb Surgical, Inc. (Formerly Chiron Vision)
Overall diameter [mm]	10.5
Optic diameter [mm]	Biconvex 6.0
Optic material	Silicone polymer
Water content	<1%
Refractive index	1.413
Haptic material	Silicone
Haptic angulation	0°
A-constant	119
ACD [mm]	5.59
Diopter [range]	+4.0 to +31
Incision [mm]	3.2

Table 3-3.
Small Hole Silicone Plate Lens
Staar Surgical, Inc.

Design	1-piece-silicone-IOL
Model	AA-4203V (small holes 0.3mm)
Manufacturer	Staar Surgical, Inc.
Overall diameter [mm]	10.5
Optic diameter [mm]	Biconvex 6.0
Optic material	Silicone polymer
Water content	<1%
Refractive index	1.413
Haptic material	Silicone
Haptic angulation	0°
A-constant	118.5
ACD [mm]	5.26
Diopter [range]	+14.5 to +28.5
Incision [mm]	3.5

Figure 3-4A. Gross photograph from behind of human eye obtained postmortem (Miyake-Apple posterior photographic technique) showing well-centered silicone plate IOLs with good in-the-bag fixation and evidence of excellent cortical cleanup with no Soemmering's ring.

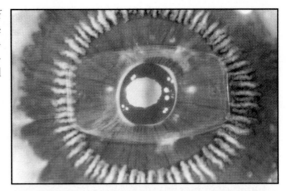

Figure 3-4B. Gross photograph from behind of human eye obtained postmortem (Miyake-Apple posterior photographic technique) showing well-centered silicone plate IOLs with good in-the-bag fixation and evidence of excellent cortical cleanup with no Soemmering's ring.

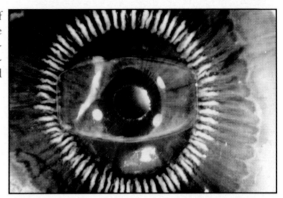

Figure 3-4C. Gross photograph from behind of human eye obtained postmortem (Miyake-Apple posterior photographic technique) showing well-centered silicone plate IOLs with good in-the-bag fixation and evidence of excellent cortical cleanup with no Soemmering's ring.

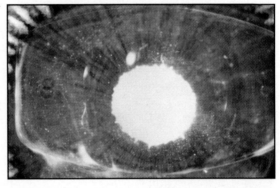

Figure 3-5A. Histopathologic appearance of fixation of plate IOLs. By definition, the anterior capsular CCC edge always rests on the anterior surface of the silicone IOL. This is a schematic illustration showing contact of the CCC edge on the optic (E = equatorial capsule).

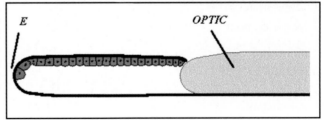

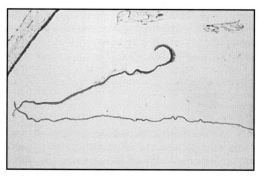

Figure 3-5B. Histopathologic appearance of fixation of plate IOLs. By definition, the anterior capsular CCC edge always rests on the anterior surface of the silicone IOL. This is a photomicrograph from two cases with small hole silicone plate IOLs. The silicone material dissolves from the section during processing. Note that the capsulorhexis edge rests on the site of anterior surface of the optic (hematoxylin and eosin stain, original magnification x25).

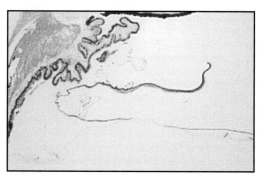

Figure 3-5C. Histopathologic appearance of fixation of plate IOLs. By definition, the anterior capsular CCC edge always rests on the anterior surface of the silicone IOL. This is a photomicrograph from two cases with small hole silicone plate IOLs. The silicone material dissolves from the section during processing. Note that the capsulorhexis edge rests on the site of anterior surface of the optic (hematoxylin and eosin stain, original magnification x25).

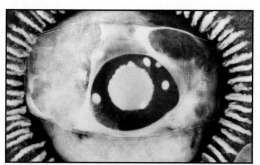

Figure 3-6A. Gross photograph from behind of a human eye obtained postmortem (Miyake-Apple posterior photographic technique) showing two examples of small hole silicone plate IOLs that are well centered in the capsular bag, but with evidence of retained lens epithelial cells. Note in both eyes that the optical region remains clear.

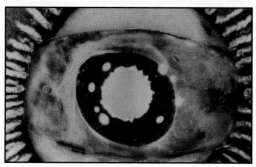

Figure 3-6B. Anterior capsular opacification with surrounding partial Soemmering's ring formation.

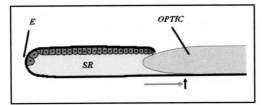

Figure 3-7A. Histopathologic appearance of a small hole plate IOL within the capsular bag, the scenario of incomplete cortical cleanup with residual Soemmering's ring formation. The CCC edge is on the anterior surface of the IOL and a Soemmering's ring (SR) composed of retained lens epithelial cells in cortex is present (E = equatorial lens capsule).

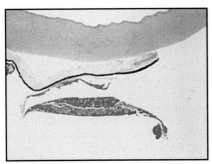

Figure 3-7B. Histopathologic appearance of a small hole plate IOL within the capsular bag, the scenario of incomplete cortical cleanup with residual Soemmering's ring formation. This is a photomicrograph of an eye with small hole plate IOLs (the silicone has dissolved out during sectioning) showing retained lens epithelial cells and cortex (Soemmering's ring), which stain red in the sections. The material is most apparent in the area behind the posterior aspect of the haptic. (Masson trichrome stain, original magnification x25.)

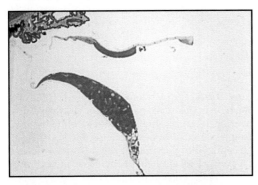

Figure 3-7C. Histopathologic appearance of a small hole plate IOL within the capsular bag, the scenario of incomplete cortical cleanup with residual Soemmering's ring formation. This is a photomicrograph of an eye with small hole plate IOLs (the silicone has dissolved out during sectioning) showing retained lens epithelial cells and cortex (Soemmering's ring), which stain red in the sections. The material is most apparent in the area behind the posterior aspect of the haptic. (Masson trichrome stain, original magnification x25.)

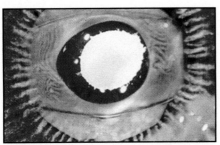

Figure 3-8A. Gross photograph from behind of a human eye obtained postmortem (Miyake-Apple posterior photographic technique) from a case of silicone small hole plate IOL with dense Soemmering's ring formation and extensive ACO.

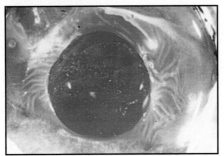

Figure 3-8B. Gross photograph from in front (surgeon's view, iris and cornea removed). Note the very thick anterior capsule around the capsulorhexis surface. Notice also the folds of the anterior capsule caused by contracture of the fibrous tissue.

tical cleanup was accomplished. In each case, the entire silicone IOL (both optic and haptic component) dissolved out during preparation is situated within a clean capsular bag and the entire edge of the capsulorhexis is in close contact to the anterior IOL surface.

The profile observed by gross examination when cortical cleanup is incomplete is illustrated in Figure 3-6. Again, the entire capsulorhexis edge rests on the anterior surface of the lens (Figure 3-7), but the space between equatorial anterior and posterior capsules is filled in by retained cortex—the Soemmering's ring (SR in Figure 3-37A). Figures 3-7 and 3-8 show histopathologic examples of two cases of small hole plate IOLs (again, note that the silicone biomaterial always dissolved out during tissue preparation) in which extensive Soemmering's ring material is present, especially on the posterior capsule. It is noteworthy that, although extensive Soemmering's ring is often seen in specimens with lenses of this type, in most cases the central optical zone remains clear (see Figures 3-6 and 3-8, and see also Figures 3-13A and 3-14A later in this chapter). This silicone material has a relatively low refractive index of about 1.4. Therefore, the anterior-posterior dimension of the lens optic is relatively thick. This puts the posterior optical surface in close contact with posterior capsule centrally, providing a substantial barrier effect. Indeed, the entire lens itself, which is relatively thick in the anterior-posterior dimension on all four sides, forms in and of itself a relatively large barrier effect against ingrowth of retained cortex (see also Chapter 7).

A noteworthy characteristic of silicone plate IOLs (both the small-hole design and the large-hole design to be described below), is a propensity for varying degrees of anterior epithelial cell proliferation and fibrosis (Figures 3-8 to 3-11).[3] A monolayer of cuboidal lens epithelial cells line the posterior surface of the anterior capsule (Figures 3-9). Most are retained following routine extracapsular surgery. Unlike the cells of the epithelial equatorial lens bow (Figure 3-9), which have a propensity to migrate posteriorly and form epithelial pearls, the anterior cells tend to undergo a pseudofibrous metaplasia and remain in place (in situ) when disturbed. This is the basis of the pathogenesis of anterior capsular fibrosis and opacification. This phenomenon, as seen in association with plate IOLs (especially common with plate designs in which a large surface area is in contact with the posterior capsule [Figure 3-12]), is demonstrated in Figures 3-8A and B, 3-10, 3-11B, 3-13, and 3-14. In addition to the outer Soemmering's ring in each case, there is a widening and thickening of the anterior capsule that is especially appreciated with the anterior view (Figure 3-8B).

Figure 3-10 is a low-powered photomicrograph of an eye with a small-hole plate IOL. The silicone lens material itself has dissolved from within the capsular bag, leaving an empty space. The posterior capsule is clear, but note the marked thickening of the anterior capsule. A thick band of subcapsular fibrosis extends from the capsulorhexis margin (right) in the direction of the equator towards the left. This is a frequent finding, both clinically and histopathologically. We recently completed a study to semi-quantitate this process, comparing various foldable IOLs. We have developed a scoring system ranging from 0, no thickening and opacification (Figure 3-11A) to 3, maximal opacification (Figure 3-11B). Figure 3-12, based on analysis of eyes obtained postmortem in our laboratory, tabulates scores of a group of eight PC IOLs—two rigid designs and six foldable designs. Most significantly, note that the silicone plate designs have the highest scores of anterior opacification. The Alcon AcrySof has the lowest score in this scale. This tabulation shows trends, but we will wait until the number of specimens is much larger to ascer-

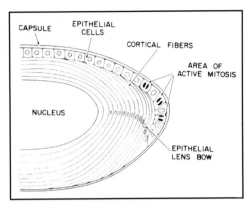

Figure 3-9. Schematic illustration showing the normal histology of the crystalline lens. The cuboidal epithelial cells underneath the anterior lens capsule (above in this image) are the cells that proliferate and undergo a pseudofibrous metaplasia forming the ACO. These are also termed A (anterior) cells, as noted in Chapter 7, Figure 7-6C.

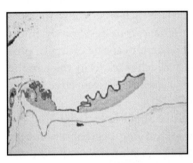

Figure 3-10. Photomicrograph through an eye with a small hole plate IOL (the silicone material is dissolved out in the preparation). Note the marked thickening of the anterior capsule in front of the IOL haptic. A fibrous contracture of the material has caused wrinkling of the anterior capsule (Periodic acid-Schiff stain x25).

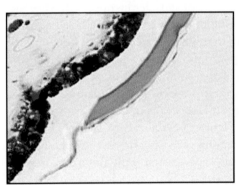

Figure 3-11A. Photograph showing the two extremes of ACO used in our scoring system, ranging from 0 to 3. A score of 0, in which there was virtually no lens epithelial proliferation underneath the anterior lens capsule. This is a high power photograph of the capsule at the capsulorhexis margin. The iris is above and to the left. (Periodic acid-Schiff stain x200.)

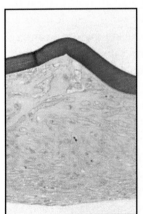

Figure 3-11B. Photograph showing the two extremes of ACO used in our scoring system, ranging from 0 to 3. This figure shows the anterior capsule from another case, showing a grade 3 fibrous thickening. Note the dense fibrous plaque below the lens capsule (see Figure 3-11A). (Periodic acid-Schiff stain x200.)

IOL Group	Sample Size	Mean
Anterior Capsule Opacification Scores **January 1988 thru August 1999** (From Apple and associates, 1999)		
3 PC Acrylic-PMMA (Acrysof)	96	.51
3 PC Silicone-Polyimide	40	.92
1 PC All-PMMA (Rigid)	50	.94
3 PC PMMA (Rigid)	51	1.07
3 PC Silicone-Prolene	92	1.09
3 PC Silicone-PMMA (Allergan SI 40)	24	1.21
1 PC Silicone Plate, Small Hole	67	1.28
1 PC Silicone Plate, Large Hole	40	1.77

Figure 3-12. Tabulation of scores of ACO noted in a comparative examination of eight IOL styles. This information is from a large database of human eyes obtained postmortem accessioned in our laboratory, compiled by Dr. Liliana Werner, Dr. Suresh Pandey, and Dr. Marcela Escobar-Gomez, Charleston, SC. Note that the silicone plate IOLs seem to have a slight tendency toward more anterior capsular opacification, whereas the lowest score was seen with the Alcon AcrySof IOL. The lower the ACO score, theoretically, the less likely the occurrence of deleterious sequelae of ACO, eg, decentration, CCC contraction, and problems with observation of the peripheral fundus during ophthalmoscopy.

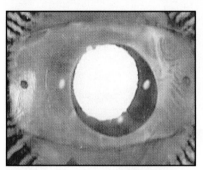

Figure 3-13A. Demonstration of a case with a small hole silicone plate IOL showing marked ACO. This is a gross photograph from behind of a human eye obtained postmortem (Miyake-Apple posterior photographic technique) showing dense opacification of the anterior capsule. This consists of the gray membrane surrounding the capsulorhexis orifice, which is completely clear. (Courtesy of Dr. Liliana Werner, Dr. Suresh Pandey, and Dr. Marcela Escobar-Gomez.)

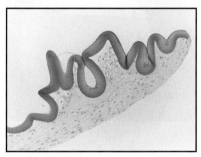

Figure 3-13B. Demonstration of a case with a small hole silicone plate IOL showing marked ACO. This is a photomicrograph from the same case as Figure 3-13A, showing the dense subcapsular fibrotic membrane, grade 2. Contraction of the membrane causes wrinkling of the anterior capsule (Figure 3-13A). (Periodic acid-Schiff stain, original magnification x200.) (Courtesy of Dr. Liliana Werner, Dr. Suresh Pandey, and Dr. Marcela Escobar-Gomez..)

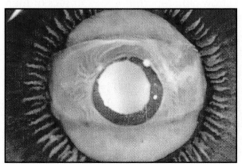

Figure 3-14A. Another case of ACO similar to that seen in Figure 3-13, also associated with extensive Soemmering's ring formation around the IOL. Gross photograph from behind of a human eye obtained postmortem (Miyake-Apple posterior photographic technique) showing the surrounding white Soemmering's ring and the dense gray membrane overlying the IOL itself. (Courtesy of Dr. Liliana Werner, Dr. Suresh Pandey, and Dr. Marcela Escobar-Gomez.)

Figure 3-14B. High-power photomicrograph through the anterior capsule of Figure 3-14A, showing the proliferation of fibrous tissue and loose interstitial matrix around the cells. (Periodic acid-Schiff stain, original magnification x200.) (Courtesy of Dr. Liliana Werner, Dr. Suresh Pandey, and Dr. Marcela Escobar-Gomez.)

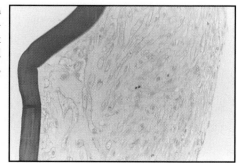

Figure 3-15A. Clinical photograph of upward decentration of a plate IOL sink movement grade 3 (decentration or dislocation) within the capsular bag is a not infrequent sequela of small hole silicone plate IOLs. This is caused by forces of contraction of the anterior capsule upon the IOL.

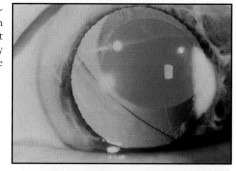

Figure 3-15B. Clinical photograph showing severe upward decentration so that the edge of the IOL haptic, as well as a positioning hole, are within the visual axis. Note the fibrous tissue subtending the anterior capsule visible in the lower area, just below the positioning hole.

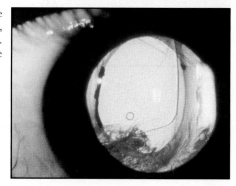

tain statistical significance. Figures 3-13 and 3-14 show clinicopathologic examples of high ACO scores associated with plate lenses. This probably correlates with the fact that the anterior surface plate lenses have more surface area of contact with the epithelial lining the anterior capsule than do three-piece designs. The score seen in Figure 3-13B is approximately 2, whereas the marked thickening seen in Figure 3-14B is a score of 3. Compare these with the control (score = 0) anterior capsule shown in Figure 3-11A.

Although the ACO described here is generally without major clinical significance, relatively dense opacification can impair an ophthalmologist's view into the retinal periphery. In addition, anterior capsular fibrosis may exert contractile forces on the IOL, leading to varying degrees of IOL decentration (Figure 3-15A and B), a not uncommon complication of plate IOLs. Anterior capsular fibrosis with contraction can also cause capsulorhexis orifice constriction (capsulorhexis contraction syndrome or capsular phimosis) (see Chapter

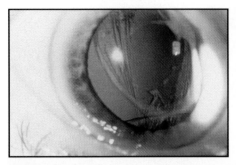

Figure 3-15C. Another complication that occasionally was seen with the small hole plate IOL design was dislocation (subluxation) occurring after Nd:YAG laser posterior capsulotomy. This clinical photograph shows this phenomenon, in which the superior tip of the IOL optic is barely visible at the inferior margin of the pupil. Note also the ruptured residual posterior capsule seen within the pupillary axis.

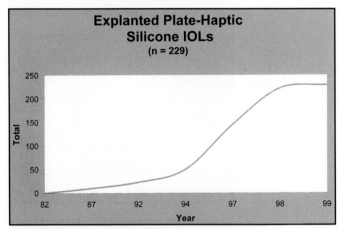

Figure 3-16A. By far the most common reasons for explantation of the small hole silicone plate IOLs were related to decentration or subluxation. As of 1999, 229 lenses had been accessioned in our laboratory. There was a marked increase in explantation rate between 1994 and 1998, the period of greatest usage of the small hole designs. This has now leveled off because of the overall change toward large hole plate designs.

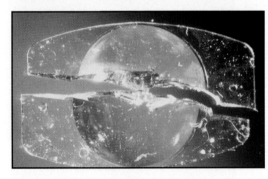

Figure 3-16B. By far the most common reasons for explantation of the small hole silicone plate IOLs were related to decentration or subluxation. This figure shows a gross photograph of a small hole silicone plate IOL explanted because of dislocation. The lens was bisected to facilitate removal.

7 and Figure 7-12). The small hole plate designs described here have been particularly susceptible to these complications, especially decentration (Figure 3-16A and B). This is the main reason that these have largely been replaced by the large hole plate IOL designs (Figures 2-40, 2-41 and 3-17 to 3-24). Apart from the main body of the lens itself, the small hole (no-hole) plate designs had no specific haptic elements designed for fixation. Not only were they therefore prone to decentration within the capsular bag (Figure 3-15), but also occasionally underwent significant dislocations when the surrounding capsular bag was disturbed, in particular following Nd:YAG laser posterior capsulotomy (Figure 3-15 C). In the mid 1990s, as implantations of the small hole plate lenses increased in number, the number of explants of this design accessioned in our laboratory following clinical malposition increased rapidly (Figure 3-16A). Figure 3-16B shows one of those lenses,

Figure 3-17. Although the widespread clinical use of large hole silicone plate IOLs is a very recent phenomenon, large hole designs had been experimented on in the 1980s (see also Figures 2-40A and B). This is a scanning electron micrograph of an experimental large hole silicone plate IOL from the 1980s that was never brought to market. (Original magnification x5.)

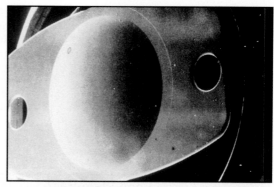

Figure 3-18A. Manufacturer's schematic illustration of a modern large hole silicone plate IOL. The diameter of the two holes in this IOL design has been increased from an original 0.3 mm to 1.15 mm. Tables 3-4 and 3-5 show the specifications of this model. The IOL has been modified for astigmatic correction.

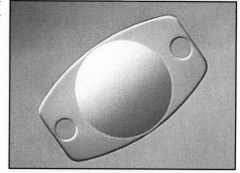

Figure 3-18B. Manufacturer's schematic illustration of a modern large hole silicone plate IOL (the Staar Surgical toric IOL, model AA-4203TF) (Table 3-6).

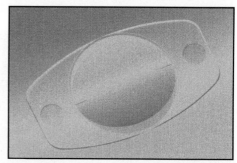

Figure 3-18C. Manufacturer's schematic illustration of a modern large hole silicone plate IOL (the Staar Surgical toric IOL, model AA-4203TF) (Table 3-6). This figure shows the critical dimensions of the toric IOL.

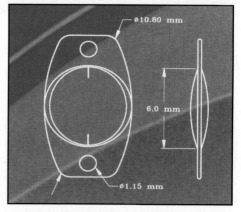

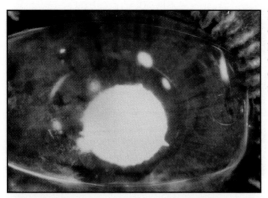

Figure 3-19A. Gross photograph from behind an eye obtained postmortem (Miyake-Apple posterior photographic technique) showing a well-implanted large hole silicone plate IOL with evidence of excellent cortical clean up, minimal Soemmering's ring formation, and minimal ACO.

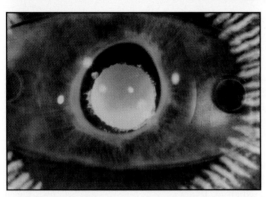

Figure 3-19B. Gross photograph from behind an eye obtained postmortem (Miyake-Apple posterior photographic technique) showing a well-implanted large hole silicone plate IOL with evidence of excellent cortical clean up, minimal Soemmering's ring formation, and minimal ACO.

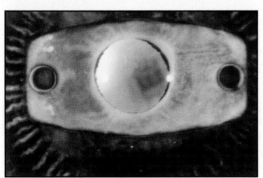

Figure 3-20A. Gross photograph from behind of a human eye obtained postmortem (Miyake-Apple posterior photographic technique) showing a well-implanted large hole silicone plate IOL with incomplete cortical clean up, Soemmering's ring formation, and moderate ACO.

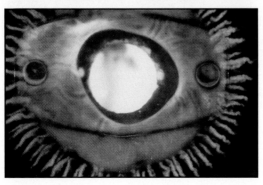

Figure 3-20B. Gross photograph from behind of a human eye obtained postmortem (Miyake-Apple posterior photographic technique) showing a well-implanted large hole silicone plate IOL with incomplete cortical clean up, Soemmering's ring formation, and moderate ACO.

Figure 3-21. Schematic illustration demonstrating the principle of growth through the large positioning hole of a plate haptic IOL. In effect, the peripheral rim of silicone forming the outer edge of the positioning hole (surrounded by a growth of tissue within the equatorial capsule fornix) functions as a fixation haptic (H). Two processes occur: 1) formation of a 360° synechiae by fibrous growth through the hole (as seen here); or 2) an actual direct fusion of the anterior and posterior capsules through the hole (not seen here). These processes enhance fixation. It generally requires 1 to 2 months for this to occur postoperatively, so the lens is still susceptible to rotation and movement prior to this time. This phenomenon does not occur in all cases, but does help enhance the long-term overall security of plate lenses.

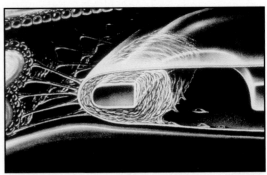

Figure 3-22A. Photomicrograph illustrating the principle of fusion of anterior and posterior capsule and growth of metaplastic lens epithelial cells and fibrous tissue through the large positioning holes, creating markedly enhanced fixation of the large hole silicone plate IOL. The silicone material washes out in sectioning, so that the silicone plate IOL is seen here as an empty space. The circular space surrounded by the equatorial capsule to the left in Figures 3-22A through E represents the outer silicone rim of the positioning hole, which in effect functions now as a small-diameter round haptic. In all photographs the anterior and posterior capsules are fused by growth of dense fibrous tissue through the hole. The CCC margin and site of the silicone optic component are located to the right in each photograph. (hematoxylin and eosin stain, original magnification x25.)

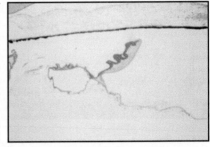

Figure 3-22B. Photomicrograph illustrating the principle of fusion of anterior and posterior capsule and growth of metaplastic lens epithelial cells and fibrous tissue through the large positioning holes, creating markedly enhanced fixation of the large hole silicone plate IOL. The silicone material washes out in sectioning, so that the silicone plate IOL is seen here as an empty space. The circular space surrounded by the equatorial capsule to the left in Figures 3-22A through E represents the outer silicone rim of the positioning hole, which in effect functions now as a small-diameter round haptic. In all photographs the anterior and posterior capsules are fused by growth of dense fibrous tissue through the hole. The CCC margin and site of the silicone optic component are located to the right in each photograph. (hematoxylin and eosin stain, original magnification x25.)

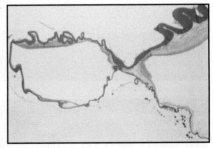

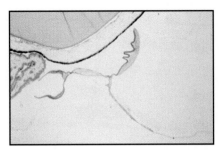

Figure 3-22C. Photomicrograph illustrating the principle of fusion of anterior and posterior capsule and growth of metaplastic lens epithelial cells and fibrous tissue through the large positioning holes, creating markedly enhanced fixation of the large hole silicone plate IOL. The silicone material washes out in sectioning, so that the silicone plate IOL is seen here as an empty space. The circular space surrounded by the equatorial capsule to the left in Figures 3-22A through E represents the outer silicone rim of the positioning hole, which in effect functions now as a small-diameter round haptic. In all photographs the anterior and posterior capsules are fused by growth of dense fibrous tissue through the hole. The CCC margin and site of the silicone optic component are located to the right in each photograph. (hematoxylin and eosin stain, original magnification x25.)

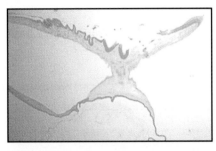

Figure 3-22D. Photomicrograph illustrating the principle of fusion of anterior and posterior capsule and growth of metaplastic lens epithelial cells and fibrous tissue through the large positioning holes, creating markedly enhanced fixation of the large hole silicone plate IOL. The silicone material washes out in sectioning, so that the silicone plate IOL is seen here as an empty space. The circular space surrounded by the equatorial capsule to the left in Figures 3-22A through E represents the outer silicone rim of the positioning hole, which in effect functions now as a small-diameter round haptic. In all photographs the anterior and posterior capsules are fused by growth of dense fibrous tissue through the hole. The CCC margin and site of the silicone optic component are located to the right in each photograph. (hematoxylin and eosin stain, original magnification x25.)

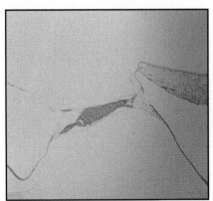

Figure 3-22E. Photomicrograph illustrating the principle of fusion of anterior and posterior capsule and growth of metaplastic lens epithelial cells and fibrous tissue through the large positioning holes, creating markedly enhanced fixation of the large hole silicone plate IOL. The silicone material washes out in sectioning, so that the silicone plate IOL is seen here as an empty space. The circular space surrounded by the equatorial capsule to the left in Figures 3-22A through E represents the outer silicone rim of the positioning hole, which in effect functions now as a small-diameter round haptic. In all photographs the anterior and posterior capsules are fused by growth of dense fibrous tissue through the hole. The CCC margin and site of the silicone optic component are located to the right in each photograph. (hematoxylin and eosin stain, original magnification x25.)

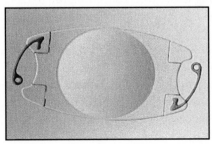

Figure 3-23A. An interesting variation of the silicone plate IOL is the prototype design seen here; namely, a silicone plate IOL with two mini-haptics (fabricated from yellow polyimide material) affixed to each end. Such an IOL provides the advantages of a classic plate IOL, namely, easy insertion through a small incision with an injector. In addition, the main advantage of the mini-haptic IOL would be to obtain better fixation by growth of intralenticular metaplastic fibrous cells and fibrous tissue around the mini-haptics. This figure shows a manufacturer's illustration of this IOL design.

Figure 3-23B. High-power gross photograph of the edge of this IOL experimentally implanted into the capsular bag of a rabbit, showing firm attachment of the mini-haptic to the equatorial lens capsule (right).

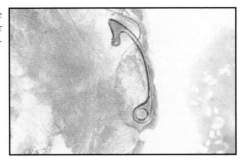

Figure 3-23C. Photomicrograph through the capsular bag of a rabbit implanted with the mini-haptic IOL design showing the yellow haptic in cross section. It is surrounded by retained equatorial lens epithelial cells and cortex, which firmly lock the lens in position. Rabbit cortex, of course, proliferates much more exuberantly than that of the human, but the concept applies in the human model.

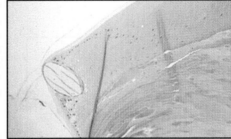

Figure 3-24. Explantation of the large hole silicone plate IOL designs is relatively unusual. Almost all cases of decentration have occurred in eyes in which the lens was in place for less than 6 weeks. This is the time required for completion of the fibrotic process that would help enhance fixation. In this case, the outer edge of the lens was cut to facilitate IOL removal.

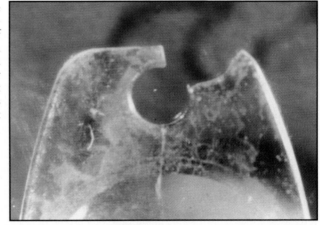

accessioned following post-Nd:YAG laser posterior capsulotomy dislocation into the vitreous. The lens was explanted by bisecting it in its long axis. Note also, in Figure 3-16A, that the rapid increase in explantation tapered off after 1998, at which time this IOL was largely replaced by the large hole plate lens design.

Finally, as noted above and in Chapter 7, the small hole plate lenses had an Nd:YAG laser posterior capsulotomy rate of approximately 20.7% as measured in our database of eyes obtained postmortem with PC IOLs. This ranked in the middle of those examined (see Figure 7-79 and 7-80), but the rate was higher than that noted with other modern foldable IOL designs. These included the large hole plate design (8.2%) and, most notably, the Alcon AcrySof design (Figure 7-78A, 7-79 and 7-80), which as of August of 1999 had a 1.7% Nd:YAG laser posterior capsulotomy rate.

Table 3-4.
Chiroflex Large Hole Silicone Plate Lens
Bausch and Lomb Surgical, Inc.

Design	1-piece-silicone-IOL
Model	C11 UB (large holes 1.15mm)
Manufacturer	Bausch and Lomb Surgical, Inc. (Formerly Chiron Vision)
Overall diameter [mm]	10.5
Optic diameter [mm]	Biconvex 6.0
Optic material	Silicone polymer
Water content	<1%
Refractive index	1.413
Haptic material	Silicone
Haptic angulation	0°
A-constant	119
ACD [mm]	5.59
Diopter [range]	+4.0 to +31
Incision [mm]	3.2

The significant incidence of the previously mentioned complications of small hole plate IOL designs-namely, decentration/dislocation, as well as the relatively significant PCO rate (20.7%), led to a search for specific improvements that addressed these complications. What followed was the introduction of a simple but highly significant alteration of the lens that offers much better results and has decreased the high incidence of explantation that occurred with the small hole plate design (Figure 3-16A). A simple increase in diameter of the two positioning holes from the previous 0.3 mm (Figure 3-1, Tables 3-2 and 3-3) to a diameter of 1.15 mm (Tables 3-4 to 3-6) has been shown to markedly improve the long-term results with this IOL design.

The idea of a large hole silicone plate IOL is not new. Figures 2-40A and B and 3-17 show an early prototype experimental design. The latter (Figure 3-17) is a large hole design, produced by CooperVision (Seattle, Washington) in the 1980s. Figure 3-18A is a manufacturer's illustration of the large hole design. Manufacturer's specifications of the large hole plate lenses manufactured by Bausch and Lomb Surgical Corporation and Staar Surgical Corporation, Monrovia, California, are listed in Tables 3-4 and 3-6.

An important modification of this design is illustrated in Figure 3-18B and C, namely, the toric IOL with correction cylinder added along the long axis of the IOL. This is marked on the surface of the lens optic (see manufacturer's illustration (Figure 3-18B). The dimensions of this lens are documented in a diagram from the manufacturers (Figure 3-18C) and specifications of the Staar Surgical AA-4203TF toric lens are shown in Table 3-6.

Table 3-5.
Large Hole Silicone Plate Lens
Staar Surgical, Inc.

Design	1-piece-silicone-IOL
Model	AA-4203VF (large holes 1.15mm)
Manufacturer	Staar Surgical, Inc.
Overall diameter [mm]	10.5
Optic diameter [mm]	Biconvex 6.0
Optic material	Silicone polymer
Water content	<1%
Refractive index	1.413
Haptic material	Silicone
Haptic angulation	0°
A-constant	118.5
ACD [mm]	5.26
Diopter [range]	+14.5 to +28.5
Incision [mm]	3.5

Table 3-6.
Toric Silicone Plate Lens
Staar Surgical, Inc.

Design	1-piece-silicone-IOL
Model	AA-4203TF (large hole 1.15mm)
Manufacturer	Staar Surgical, Inc.
Overall diameter [mm]	10.8
Optic diameter [mm]	Biconvex 6.0
Optic material	Silicone polymer
Water content	<1%
Refractive index	1.413
Haptic material Silicone	
Haptic angulation	0°
A-constant	
ACD [mm]	
Diopter [range]	
Incision [mm]	

Regarding the toric design, for it to be effective, the lens should not rotate within the eye after implantation. Rotation is relatively unusual but can occur during the first 4 to 6 weeks after implantation, prior to fibrosis around the lens and through the large positioning hole (see below). Such rotation is less likely after 4 to 6 weeks because the presence of the large hole adds to the security of the lens[4] and helps prevent long-term rotation as well as decentration and dislocation.

Figures 3-19A and B show examples of well-implanted large hole plate lenses in which centration is perfect and, because cortical cleanup was apparently very thorough, minimal retained cortex/lens epithelial cells are present.

Illustrations 3-20A and B demonstrate more typical cases in which retained cortex has led to formation of varying amounts of retained cortex/cells. Significant ACO is evident in both Figures 3-20A and B. The peripheral capsule is clear in Figure 3-20A, but a significant Soemmering's ring is present in Figure 3-20B. We noted previously that a high reactivity of the anterior capsule leading to ACO is a common occurrence with silicone plate IOLs, both large and small hole designs (see Figures 3-12 to 3-14). However, this only assumes clinical significance in instances where view of the peripheral retina may be diminished by the fibrosis, or in cases where excessive fibrosis and contraction occurs, creating decentration or capsulorhexis contraction syndrome (see Chapter 7). The design of this lens makes it almost automatic that the entire capsulorhexis edge and a large surface of the anterior capsule is in contact with the anterior lens epithelium. It follows that ACO is much more extensive with plate lens designs than with the three-piece silicone designs (see Figure 3-12), because of this broad area of contact.

The theoretical and actual rationale for the manufacture of two large positioning holes in the haptics of a plate IOL is illustrated in Figures 3-21 to 3-22. Figure 3-21 is a schematic illustration showing how retained lens epithelial cells in the region of the lens equator can proliferate and grow around and through the positioning hole, thus forming a partial or complete 360° synechia around the outer aspect of the hole. The silicone material in essence forms the outer rim of the hole, and in effect becomes a fixation haptic that enhances secure and permanent stabilization. This, as well as fusion of the anterior and posterior capsules through the large positioning hole, occur in a substantial percentage of cases. These tissue relations help stabilize the pseudophakos. This process does not occur in all cases and when it does, it cannot be expected until after 4 to 6 weeks postoperatively-the time when fibrotic process materializes.

These fibrotic phenomena help tightly wrap the anterior and posterior capsules onto the surface of the IOL and create a form of "shrink wrap" (see Chapter 7). One would expect this to efficacious in preventing PCO, and indeed analysis of the Nd:YAG laser posterior capsulotomy rate in our series of human eyes obtained postmortem for this lens design reveals a relatively low value of approximately 8.2%, considerably less than seen with the small hole designs (approximately 20.7%) (see Figures 7-79 and 7-80).

The relatively low PCO rate seen with the large hole plate lenses can probably be attributable to four factors: 1) the relatively thick anterior-posterior dimension of the lens optic (this silicone material has a relatively low index of refraction), which creates a tight contact of the posterior IOL optic against the posterior capsule, creating a substantial barrier effect (Figures 3-4, 3-6, 3-13A, 3-14A, and 3-20A and B; see also Chapter 7); 2) the large hole helps establish the above mentioned tight fit of the capsule around the lens (the shrink wrap), which also contributes to a "no-space-no cells" scenario (see Chapter 7); 3) by definition, the CCC edge is entirely anchored to the front of the silicone material for 360°, thus isolating the pseudophakos totally within the space of the closed compartment of the capsular bag, which sequesters it at least in part from some components of the surrounding aqueous. This helps protect it from potential inflammatory mediators; and 4) this lens design is relatively new, having been introduced after 1996—at a time when the quality of surgery, including cortical cleanup, was vastly improved over that present before the time when the small hole design had commonly been implanted.

An interesting variation of the large hole plate design that is in prototype stage only and has not reached the worldwide clinical market is the mini-haptic design shown in Figure 3-23. The mini-haptics are composed of yellow polyimide material. This modification of the lens allows for the same relatively easy insertion with an injector via a small incision that is possible with standard plate IOL, but has the advantage of the markedly enhanced fixation afforded by the two mini-haptics.[5] This tiny positioning hole or loop at the tip of the yellow haptic also enhances fixation. Figures 3-23B and C demonstrate in the rabbit model how the retained cortical material and cells wrap around the haptic. The rabbit model, of course, shows much more postoperative proliferation than does the human, but the principle applies to both.

SUMMARY

Because of their geometric profile (narrow and rectangular), plate IOLs are easy to fold and insert with an injector through a small incision. The early small hole plate lenses have largely been removed from the market because these occasionally decentered or dislocated after Nd:YAG laser posterior capsulotomy. They had a PCO rate of 20.7% as determined in our autopsy series (see Figure 7-79 and 7-80). Small hole designs have been superseded by the large hole plate designs, which in general fixate more securely in the capsular bag as the postoperative fibrotic process proceeds over 4 to 6 weeks. This has lowered the incidence of long-term IOL rotation (very important with the toric IOL), decentration, and dislocation. Explantation of a large hole plate IOL is very rare; virtually all cases of malposition that we have seen occurred prior to 4 to 6 weeks postoperatively (Figure 7-24). Although ACO is a common occurrence (Figure 3-12), the rate of central PCO as measured by the Nd:YAG laser posterior capsulotomy rate is relatively low (8.2%) see Figure 7-79 and 7-80). When implanted precisely in the bag after sufficient cortical cleanup, these IOLs provide salutary results.

REFERENCES

1. Newland TJ, Auffarth GU, Wesendahl TA, Apple DJ. Neodymium: YAG laser damage on silicone intraocular lenses. A comparison of lesions on explanted lenses and experimentally produced lesions. *J Cataract Refract Surg.* 1994;20:527-533.2.

2. Newman DA, McIntyre DJ, Apple DJ, et al. Pathologic findings of an explanted silicone intraocular lens. *J Cataract Refract Surg.* 1986;12:292-297.

3. Werner L, Pandey SK, Escobar-Gomez M, et al. Anterior capsule opacification: A histopathological study comparing different IOL styles. *Ophthalmology.* 2000;107:463-471.

4. Apple DJ. Enhancement of silicone plate IOL fixation by the use of positioning holes in the lens haptic. *J Cataract Refract Surg.* 1996;6[special issue; best paper of 1996 ASCRS Meeting]:21-25.RPB

5. Kent DG, Peng Q, Isaacs RT, et al. Mini-haptics to improve capsular fixation of plate-haptic silicone intraocular lenses. Part II. *Eur J Cataract Refract Surg.* 1998;24:666-671.

BIBLIOGRAPHY

Apple DJ, Blotnik C. Postoperative lens deposits. *J Cataract Refract Surg* 1993;19:441.

Apple DJ, Kent DG, Peng Q, et al. Verbesserung der befestigung von silikonschiffchenlinsen durch den gebrauch von positionierungslochern in der linsenhaptik, *Proceedings of the 10th Annual Deutche Gesellschaft fuer Intraokularlinsen Implantation Meeting.* Budapest, Hungary; 1996.

Auer C, Gonvers M. Silicone one-piece intraocular implant and anterior capsule fibrosis. *Klinische Monatsblatter fur Augenheilkunde.* 1995;206:293-295.

Auffarth GU, McCabe C, Wilcox M, et al. Centration and fixation of silicone intraocular lenses. An analysis of clinicopathological findings in human autopsy eyes. *J Cataract Refract Surg.* 1996;22(2):1281-1285.

Auffarth GU, Wesendahl TA, Brown SJ, Apple DJ. Häufigkeit und Art von Explantationsgrhnden von einstuckigen und dreistuckigen Hinterkammerlinsen. In: Wollensak J, et al, eds. *Transactions of the 8th Congress of the German Intraocular Lens Implant Society (DGII).* Berlin, Heidelberg, New York: Springer Verlag Pub; 1994;501-507.

Auffarth GU, Wilcox M, Sims JCR, et al. Analysis of 100 explanted one-piece and three-piece silicone intraocular lenses. *Ophthalmology.* 1995;102(8):1144-1150.

Auffarth GU, Wilcox M, Sims JCR, et al. Complications of silicone intraocular lenses. *J Cataract Refract Surg.* 1995;[special issue; best paper of 1995 ASCRS Meeting]:38-41.

Blotnick CA, Powers TP, Newland T, et al. Case report: Pathology of silicone intraocular lenses in human eyes obtained postmortem. *J Cataract Refract Surg.* 1995;21(4):447-452.

Brown DC, Grabow HB, Martin RG, et al. Staar Collamer intraocular lens: Clinical results from the phase I FDA core study. *J Cataract Refract Surg.* 1998;24:1032-1038.

Cook CS, Peiffer RL, Jr., Mazzocco TR. Clinical and pathologic evaluation of a flexible silicone posterior chamber lens design in a rabbit model. *J Cataract Refract Surg.* 1986;12:130-134.

Cumming JS. Postoperative complications and uncorrected acuities after implantation of plate haptic silicone and three-piece silicone intraocular lenses. *J Cataract Refract Surg.* 1993;19:263-274.

Cumming JS. Surgical complications and visual acuity results in 536 cases of plate haptic silicone lens implantation. *J Cataract Refract Surg.* 1993;19:275-277.

Dahlhauser KF, Wroblewski KJ, Mader TH. Anterior capsule contraction with foldable silicone intraocular lenses. *J Cataract Refract Surg.* 1998;24:1216-1219.

Faulkner GD. Early experience with STAAR silicone elastic lens implants. *J Cataract Refract Surg.* 1986;12:36-39.

Faulkner GD. Folding and inserting silicone intraocular lens implants. *J Cataract Refract Surg.* 1987;13:678-681.

Fogle JA, Blaydes JE, Fritz KJ, Blaydes SH, Mazzocco TR, Peiffer RL, Cook C, Wright E. Clinicopathologic observations of a silicone posterior chamber lens in a primate model. *J Cataract Refract Surg.* 1986;12:281-284.

Hwang IP, Clinch TE, Moshifar M, et al. Decentration of 3-piece versus plate-haptic silicone intraocular lenses. *J Cataract Refract Surg* 1998;24:1505-8

Kammann J, Cosmar E, Walden K. Vitreous-stabilizing, single-piece, mini-loop, plate-haptic silicone intraocular lens. *J Cataract Refract Surg.* 1998;24:98-106.

Kent DG, Peng Q, Isaacs RT, Whiteside SB, Barker DL, Apple DJ. Security of capsular fixation: Small- versus large-hole plate-haptic lenses. *J Cataract Refract Surg.* 1997;23(11):1371-1375.

Koch DD, Heit LE. Discoloration of silicone intraocular lenses. *Arch Ophthalmol.* 1992;110:319-320.

Kohnen T, Magdowski G, Koch DD. Surface quality of flexible silicone intraocular lenses. A scanning electron microscopy study. *Klinische Monatsblatter fur Augenheilkunde.* 1995;207:253-263.

Legler UF, Apple DJ. Comments on silicone intraocular lens discoloration. *Arch Ophthalmol.* 1991;109:1495-1496.

Mamalis N, Phillips B, Kopp CH, et al. Neodymium:YAG capsulotomy rates after phaco with silicone posterir chamber intraocular lenses. *J Cataract Refract Surg.* 1996;22(supp 2):1296-1302.

Mamalis N, Omar O, Veiga J, et al. Comparison of two plate-haptic intraocular lenses in a rabbit model. *J Cataract Refract Surg.* 1996;22 (supp 2):1291-1295.

Mazzocco TR. Early clinical experience with elastic lens implants. *Transactions of the Ophthalmological Societies of the United Kingdom.* 1985;104:578-579.

Milauskas AT. Capsular bag fixation of one-piece silicone lenses. *J Cataract Refract Surg.* 1990;16:583-586.

Miyake K, Ota I, Miyake S, Maekubo K. Correlation between intraocular lens hydrophilicity and anterior capsule opacification and aqueous flare. *J Cataract Refract Surg.* 1996;22(suppl 1):764-769.

Neumann AC, McCarty GR, Osher RH. Complications associated with STAAR silicone implants. *J Cataract Refract Surg.* 1987;13:653-656.

Omar O, Mamalis N, Veiga J, Tamura M, Olson RJ. Scanning electron microscopic characteristics of small-incision intraocular lenses. *Ophthalmology.* 1996;103:1124-1129.

Pisella PJ, Pietrini D, Limon S. Anterior cellular proliferation and silicone implant. Apropos of a case. *J Fr Ophthalmol.* 1996;19:615-618.

Popham JK, Apple DJ, Newman DA, Isenberg RA, Deacon J. Advantages and Limitations of Soft Intraocular Lenses: A Scientific Perspective. In: Mazzocco TR, Rajacich GM, Epstein E, eds. *Soft Implant Lenses in Cataract Surgery.* Thorofare, NJ, SLACK Incorporated; 1986:11-30.

Schipper I. Implantation of a Staar silicone intraocular lens with the anterior chamber maintainer. *J Cataract Refract Surg.* 1996;22:23-26.

Shepherd JR. Capsular opacification associated with silicone implants. *J Cataract Refract Surg.* 1989;15:448-450.

Shepherd JR. Continuous-tear capsulotomy and insertion of a silicone bag lens. *J Cataract Refract Surg.* 1989;15:335-339.

Shepherd JR. Small incisions and foldable intraocular lenses. *Int Ophthalmol.* 1994;34:103-112.

Tsai JC, Castaneda VE, Apple DJ, et al. Scanning electron microscopic study of modern silicone intraocular lenses. *J Cataract Refract Surg.* 18(5):232-235, 1992.

Tuft SJ, Talks SJ. Delayed dislocation of foldable plate-haptic silicone lenses after Nd:YAG laser anterior capsulotomy. *Am J Ophthalmol.* 1998;126:586-588.

Utrata PJ, Sanders DR, DeLuca M, Raanan MG, Ballew C. Small incision surgery with the Staar elastimide three-piece posterior chamber intraocular lens. *J Cataract Refract Surg.* 1994;20:426-431.

Watt RH. Discoloration of a silicone intraocular lens 6 weeks after surgery letter; comment. *Arch Ophthalmol.* 1991;109:1494-1495.

Watt RH. Pigment dispersion syndrome associated with silicone posterior chamber intraocular lenses. *J Cataract Refract Surg*. 1988;14:431-433.

Whiteside SB, Apple DJ, Peng Q, et al. Fixation elements on plate IOLs. Large positioning holes to improve security of capsular fixation. Part III. *Ophthalmology*. 1998;105:837-842.

Chapter 4

Three-Piece Silicone Intraocular Lenses

With Polyimide Haptics, Staar Surgical and Bausch and Lomb Surgical

The evolution of 3-piece foldable IOLs with haptics has been illustrated in Figures 2-43 and 2-44. The elastimide silicone three-piece IOL manufactured by Staar Surgical (Monrovia, Ca) and Bausch and Lomb Surgical (Irvine, Ca) is illustrated in Figures 4-1 and 4-2 (and the manufacturer's specifications of the Staar AQ 1016 series is shown in Table 4-2). The optic consists of a hydrophobic silicone polymer and the yellow haptic material is composed of polyimide. This haptic is slightly more rigid than prolene or PMMA haptic material. This substantial rigidity of this haptic material is probably an advantage in that it helps provide circumferential tension on and expansion of the capsular bag. This renders the posterior capsule more taught or drawn-like and thus helps provide a tight fit between the posterior aspect of the silicone optic and the anterior surface of the posterior capsule. This is a factor that is important in enhancing the barrier effect of the IOL optic against PCO (Table 4-1)(see Chapter 7, Table 7-3).

Figures 4-2A and B show examples of well-implanted lenses of this type, well-centered within the capsular bag, with apparent excellent cortical cleanup and little or no opacification of the media. Figures 4-2C and D show similarly well-centered elastimide lenses, but with varying degrees of retained cortex/cells forming substantial Soemmering's rings, as well as varying amounts of anterior capsular opacification or fibrosis (ACO). Regarding ACO, in Figure 3-12 we indicated that this, as well as most other three-piece silicone and acrylic IOL designs described in this text, generally undergo less ACO than do the plate IOLs described in Chapter 3. This is likely because the three-piece silicone IOL designs, having only the round silicone optic, have a lesser area of surface contact with the anterior capsule than does the silicone plate IOL.[1]

Figure 4-1. Clinical photograph of the elastimide design, a three-piece IOL with a silicone optic and a yellow polyimide haptic material that is manufactured by Staar Surgical and Bausch and Lomb Surgical (the latter is formally IOLab Corporation and Chiron Vision Corp.). The manufacturer's specifications of the Staar Surgical model, the AQ-1016 series, are listed in Table 4-2.

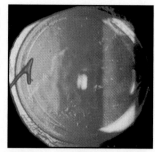

Figure 4-2A. Gross photographs from behind (Miyake-Apple posterior photographic technique) showing well-centered silicone optic/polyimide haptic IOLs in place within the capsular bag.

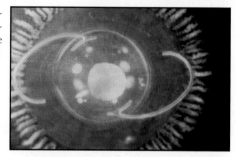

Figure 4-2B. This eye shows evidence of excellent cleanup of lens epithelial cells and cortex, with virtually no Soemmering's ring and minimal anterior capsular opacification (ACO).

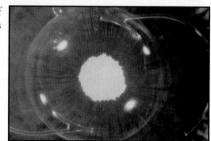

Figure 4-2C. Moderate ACO and mild Soemmering's ring formation.

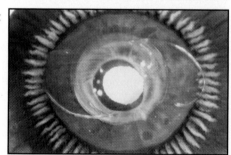

Figure 4-2D. Moderate ACO and extensive Soemmering's ring formation.

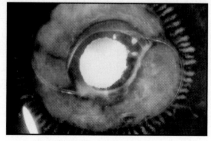

Table 4-1.
Foldable IOLs, Approved and Investigational, 2000
Available in the USA Autopsy Database

Design	Model (selected repre- sentative examples)	Company	Diameter (mm)	Optic Diameter (mm)	Water Content	Haptic Material
I. Silicone						
IA: Plate silicone lenses						
1 piece silicone plate lens (small holes)	Chiroflex C10UB	Bausch and Lomb Surgical, Inc.	10.5	Biconvex, 6.0	<1%	Silicone
1 piece silicone plate lens (large holes)	Chiroflex C11UB	Bausch and Lomb Surgical, Inc.	10.5	Biconvex, 6.0	<1%	Silicone
1 piece silicone plate lens (small holes)	AA-4203V	Staar Surgical Inc.	10.5	Biconvex, 6.0	<1%	Silicone
1 piece silicone plate lens (large holes)	AA-4203VF	Staar Surgical Inc.	10.5	Biconvex, 6.0	<1%	Silicone
1 piece silicone toric lens (large holes)	AA-4203TF	Staar Surgical Inc.	10.5	Biconvex, 6.0	<1%	Silicone
IB: Three-piece silicone lenses						
a) Staar						
3 piece silicone IOL	AQ1016/2010/2003	Staar Surgical Inc.	13.5/13.5/12.5	Biconvex, 6.3	<1%	Polyimide
b) Allergan Series						
3 piece silicone IOL	SI-30 NB	Allergan, Inc.	13.0	Biconvex, 6.0	<1%	Polypropylene
3 piece silicone IOL	SI-40 NB	Allergan, Inc.	13.0	Biconvex, 6.0	<1%	PMMA
3 piece silicone IOL	SI 55 NB	Allergan, Inc.	13.0	Biconvex, 5.5	<1%	PMMA
3 piece silicone IOL	SA 40 N	Allergan, Inc.	13.0	Biconvex, 6.0	<1%	PMMA
c) Bausch and Lomb						
3 piece silicone IOL	Soflex and LI Series	Bausch and Lomb Surgical, Inc.	13.0	Biconvex, 6.0	<1%	PMMA
II. Acrylics						
Hydrophobic (dry packed) 3 piece Acrylic IOL	AcrySof	Alcon Laboratories, Inc.	12.5/30	Biconvex,	<2%	PMMA

Table 4-2.
Elastimide IOL
Staar Surgical, Inc.

Design	3-piece-silicone-IOL
Model	AQ-1016/AQ-2010/AQ-2003
Manufacturer	Staar Surgical, Inc.
Overall diameter [mm]	13.5/13.5/12.5
Optic diameter [mm]	Biconvex 6.3
Optic material	Silicone polymer
Water content	<1%
Refractive index	N/A
Haptic material	Polyimide
Haptic angulation	10°
A-constant	119
ACD [mm]	5.55
Diopter [range]	+14.5 to +28.5
Incision [mm]	N/A

Figures 4-3A through C illustrate the histopathologic that correlates with the scenario of complete cortical cleanup (Figures 4-2A and B). In these cases, the capsulorhexis diameter is smaller than that of the optic so that in all three instances (A-C) the capsulorhexis edge rests on the surface of the optic. The silicone material of the optic has dissolved out in the processes, thus leaving an empty space.

Figures 4-4 and 4-5A through C illustrate the scenario where the capsulorhexis diameter is smaller than the lens optic and retained Soemmering's ring material exists (SR in Figure 4-4). In this scenario, cortical cleanup was incomplete, and the capsulorhexis edge rests on the IOL optic. Note also in Figure 4-4 that the optic of this IOL design is square or truncated, not unlike that of the Alcon AcrySof IOL (see Figures 5-8 and 5-9). This has been shown to be a positive factor in that it enhances the IOL optic's barrier effect against PCO (see Chapter 7). The square-edge effect is illustrated schematically in Figure 4-4 (arrow) and is seen in each histologic section in Figure 4-5 (A-C). The square or truncated edge of the optic (note that the silicone optic material has dissolved out in the tissue preparation) tends to abruptly block growth of cortical and cellular remnants within the Soemmering's ring toward the visual axis (right), leaving a clear posterior capsule (lower right in 4-5A through C). This IOL design has a relatively low explantation rate in our laboratory, (Figure 4-6) the most common reason being preoperative dioptric power miscalculation. The rate of decentration appears to be low following good surgery, as the relatively rigid haptic of this IOL fixates well in capsular bag and does not tend to crimp or move. The rate of PCO is relatively low (approximately 11.1% as shown in our database; see Figure 7-79 and 7-80). Again, this is partially explained by the presence of the relatively

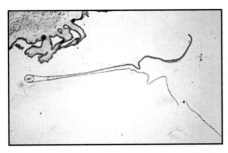

Figure 4-3A. Several possible fixation scenarios are possible with a three-piece IOL, including this model. When the capsulorhexis diameter is slightly larger than the IOL optic (see Figures 4-2A and B) and cortical cleanup is complete, the anterior and posterior capsules fuse together. In this scenario, we show a photomicrograph of a case with an elastimide-polyimide IOL in which cortical cleanup was complete, but the capsulorhexis diameter was smaller than the IOL optic. Therefore, the capsulorhexis edge in each case is adherent to the anterior surface of the IOL optic. The silicone optic of the IOL always washes out during preparation for histology; the haptic is seen as the small yellow circle.

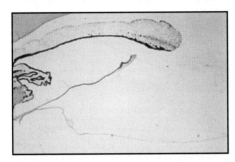

Figure 4-3B. Several possible fixation scenarios are possible with a three-piece IOL, including this model. When the capsulorhexis diameter is slightly larger than the IOL optic (see Figures 4-2A and B) and cortical cleanup is complete, the anterior and posterior capsules fuse together. In this scenario, we show a photomicrograph of a case with an elastimide-polyimide IOL in which cortical cleanup was complete, but the capsulorhexis diameter was smaller than the IOL optic. Therefore, the capsulorhexis edge in each case is adherent to the anterior surface of the IOL optic. The silicone optic of the IOL always washes out during preparation for histology; the haptic is seen as the small yellow circle.

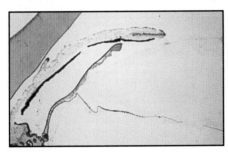

Figure 4-3C. Several possible fixation scenarios are possible with a three-piece IOL, including this model. When the capsulorhexis diameter is slightly larger than the IOL optic (see Figures 4-2A and B) and cortical cleanup is complete, the anterior and posterior capsules fuse together. In this scenario, we show a photomicrograph of a case with an elastimide-polyimide IOL in which cortical cleanup was complete, but the capsulorhexis diameter was smaller than the IOL optic. Therefore, the capsulorhexis edge in each case is adherent to the anterior surface of the IOL optic. The silicone optic of the IOL always washes out during preparation for histology; the haptic is seen as the small yellow circle.

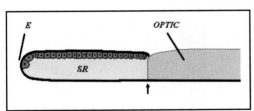

Figure 4-4. This figure represents the scenario when the capsulor-hexis diameter is slightly smaller than the IOL optic so that the capsulorhexis edge is on the optic, but the cortical cleanup is incomplete, leaving some lens and cortical material (Soemmering's ring [SR]). This schematic illustration shows that the optic edge of the elastimide IOL is square or truncated. It presents a good barrier against ingrowth of cells across the visual axis. The SR tends to remain in the periphery, being abruptly blocked by the square edge of the IOL optic (arrow).

Figure 4-5A. Photomicrograph of an eye with the silicone optic-polyimide haptic IOL showing how the square truncated edge of the silicone optic (dissolved out during processing) forms a barrier to growth of cells from the Soemmering's ring (large pink mass on the left) as they attempt to grow toward the visual access to the right. Note that the posterior capsule (lower right) is cell-free. The square truncated edge of the IOL optic appears to enhance the IOL's barrier effect (see also Chapter 7).

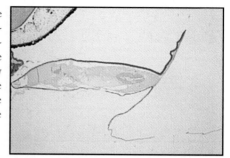

Figure 4-5B. Photomicrograph of an eye with the silicone optic-polyimide haptic IOL showing how the square truncated edge of the silicone optic (dissolved out during processing) forms a barrier to growth of cells from the Soemmering's ring (large pink mass on the left) as they attempt to grow toward the visual access to the right. Note that the posterior capsule (lower right) is cell-free. The square truncated edge of the IOL optic appears to enhance the IOL's barrier effect (see also Chapter 7).

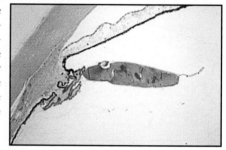

Figure 4-5C. Photomicrograph of an eye with the silicone optic-polyimide haptic IOL showing how the square truncated edge of the silicone optic (dissolved out during processing) forms a barrier to growth of cells from the Soemmering's ring (large pink mass on the left) as they attempt to grow toward the visual access to the right. Note that the posterior capsule (lower right) is cell-free. The square truncated edge of the IOL optic appears to enhance the IOL's barrier effect (see also Chapter 7).

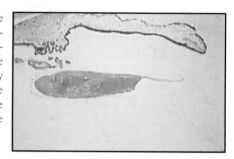

Figure 4-6. Relatively few elastimide-polyimide IOLs have been accessioned in our laboratory after explantation. Most explantations have been due to power miscalculations or difficulties in surgical techniques. This lens was removed because of a preoperative dioptric power miscalculation. Amputation of the IOL haptics and bisecting of the optic were necessary to facilitate explantation.

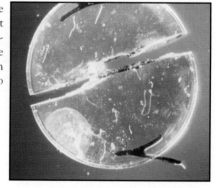

rigid polyimide haptics, which cause excellent expansion of the capsular bag, creating the tautness of the posterior capsule, which in turn enhances the IOL's barrier effect. In addition, the anterior-posterior diameter of this silicone IOL optic is relatively thick, also enhancing the barrier effect. Finally, this same barrier is also enhanced by the square, truncated edge of the IOL optic.

ALLERGAN SI SERIES (SI-9 TO SI-40 AND SA-40)

The Allergan, Inc. (Irvine, Calif) SI series, among the first three-piece foldable IOLs to be marketed successfully, was developed in the 1980s. All models have a silicone optic. Models up to the SI-30 (SI-9 to SI-30) had polypropylene haptics (Table 4-3). The most recent SI-40 has PMMA haptics (Table 4-4). The SI-30 model is shown in Figure 4-7 and the manufacturer's specifications of this lens are listed in Table 4-3. One of its predecessors, the SI-13, is shown in Figure 4-8, an early experimental implant in a rabbit eye done in our laboratory in Salt Lake City in the late 1980s. Figure 4-9 is a scanning electron micrograph of this series of three-piece designs showing the characteristic elevation of the optic around the base of the haptic at the site of take-off of the haptic from the optic. The development of the SI Series, especially the SI-30 design by the early 1990s, probably proceeded more rapidly than did the surgical techniques for implantation of these designs. Figure 4-10 shows a SI-30 IOL well fixated in the capsular bag. However, cortical cleanup was inadequate, leading to formation of a large Soemmering's ring from residual/retained/proliferative cortex and lens epithelial cells. This creates a high potential for PCO. Profiles of decentration and incomplete cleanup were commonly seen in the late 1980s and early 1990s with lenses of this type. At that time a complete transition toward the ultramodern capsular surgery now available (Generation VI, Figure 2-19, Tables 2-1 and 2-2) had not been universally applied.

More recent results are generally much different, as is readily demonstrated in Figure 4-11A through C. Incomplete cortical cleanup has lingered in a few instances (Figures 4-12A and B). This is not surprising as many of the SI series IOLs were implanted in the early to mid 1990s, prior to the era of complete transition toward optimal capsular surgery with complete cortical cleanup. Figures 4-13A through F demonstrate the histopathologic correlates of the scenario that occurs when complete and thorough cleanup is not accomplished and a Soemmering's ring forms. In each of these cases, the CCC orifice is smaller than the diameter of the IOL optic and the CCC rests totally on the anterior surface.

The histopathologic appearance of this IOL is partially related to reduced optic geometry. Note in the schematic illustration (Figure 4-13A) that the SI series of IOLs has a classic rounded optic edge, as opposed to the square, truncated optic edge noted with the elastimide-polyimide design (Figure 4-4) and Alcon AcrySof (see Chapters 5 and 7). Therefore, in some cases, but not all, growth of cells from the Soemmering's ring onto the outer periphery of the posterior capsule may occur with this design (Figures 4-13C through F). The rounded optic edge seems to provide less of a barrier effect than the square, truncated edge and permits growth of cells and tissue around the posterior lateral aspect of the IOL onto

Table 4-3.
SI 30 NB
Allergan, Inc.

Design	3-piece-silicone-IOL
Model	SI 30 NB
Manufacturer	Allergan, Inc.
Overall diameter [mm]	13.0
Optic diameter [mm]	Biconvex 6.0
Optic material	Silicone polymer
Water content	<1%
Refractive index	1.46
Haptic material	Polypropylene
Haptic angulation	10°
A-constant	117.4
ACD [mm]	4.4
Diopter [range]	+6.0 to +30.0
Incision [mm]	N/A

Table 4-4.
SI 40 NB
Allergan, Inc.

Design	3-piece-silicone-IOL
Model	SI 40 NB
Manufacturer	Allergan, Inc.
Overall diameter [mm]	13.0
Optic diameter [mm]	Biconvex 6.0
Optic material	Silicone polymer
Water content	<1%
Refractive index	1.46
Haptic material	PMMA
Haptic angulation	10°
A-constant	118
ACD [mm]	4.7
Diopter [range]	+6.0 to +30.0
Incision [mm]	N/A

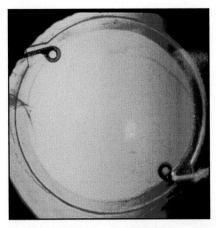

Figure 4-7. Allergan Corporation was the first successful manufacturer of foldable 3-piece silicone IOL designs, beginning with the prototype SI-9 and SI-13 designs in the early 1980s, continuing today with the successful SI- and SA-40 models. This is a clinical photograph of the SI-30 design, introduced in the early 1990s. The manufacturer's specifications of this design, which provided excellent results throughout the early mid 1990s and continues to do so today, are listed in Table 4-3.

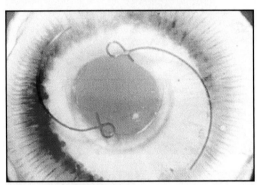

Figure 4-8. Early prototype Allergan SI design (SI-13) implanted experimentally in our research laboratory in a rabbit eye. Note the symmetric in-the-bag fixation with good centration. This design, introduced in the mid 1980s, was an important predecessor of today's SI-30 and SI (SA)-40 lenses. (Gross photograph from behind, Miyake-Apple posterior photographic technique.)

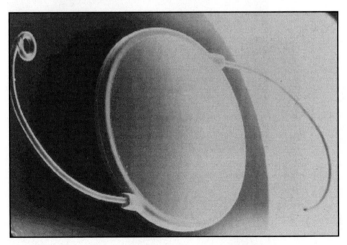

Figure 4-9. Scanning electron micrograph of an Allergan SI series three-piece IOL design (original magnification x10).

Figure 4-10. Gross photograph from behind (Miyake-Apple posterior photographic technique) showing an example of an Allergan SI series silicone optic IOL with polypropylene haptics that was inserted in the early 1990s. The complication seen here was not related to the IOL itself, but rather to variations in surgical technique. Note that the lens was implanted with good centration. However, the cortical cleanup was incomplete, and extensive residual/regenerate cortex and cells have formed an exuberant Soemmering's ring. The latter is a major precursor of PCO (see Chapter 7).

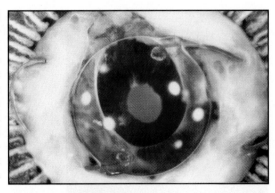

Figure 4-11A. Marked improvements in surgical techniques during the mid to late 1990s have vastly improved the success rate of the Allergan SI-30 design. This case of an eye obtained postmortem, viewed with the Miyake-Apple posterior photographic technique, shows a good example of well-fixated IOLs in the capsular bag associated with good cortical cleanup and excellent clarity of the media. The capsulorhexis margins are situated on the anterior surface of the IOL optic.

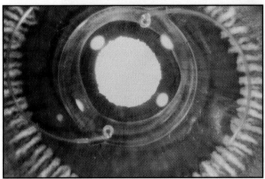

Figure 4-11B. Marked improvements in surgical techniques during the mid to late 1990s have vastly improved the success rate of the Allergan SI-30 design. This case of an eye obtained postmortem, viewed with the Miyake-Apple posterior photographic technique, shows a good example of well-fixated IOLs in the capsular bag associated with good cortical cleanup and excellent clarity of the media. The capsulorhexis margins are situated on the anterior surface of the IOL optic.

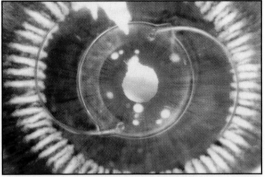

Figure 4-11C. Marked improvements in surgical techniques during the mid to late 1990s have vastly improved the success rate of the Allergan SI-30 design. This case of an eye obtained postmortem, viewed with the Miyake-Apple posterior photographic technique, shows a good example of well-fixated IOLs in the capsular bag associated with good cortical cleanup and excellent clarity of the media. The capsulorhexis margins are situated on the anterior surface of the IOL optic.

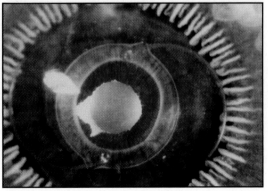

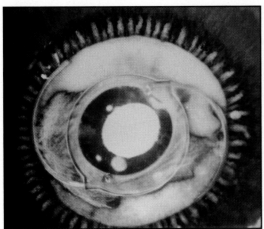

Figure 4-12A. Gross photograph from behind (Miyake-Apple posterior photographic technique) of a human eye obtained postmortem, showing an example of the SI-30 in which cortical cleanup was incomplete and extensive Soemmering's ring formation occurred. However, the central optic axis remained clear. In this case the capsulorhexis diameter was smaller than the lens optic, with the capsulorhexis edge on the anterior surface of the optic. In such cases with retained cortex, the barrier effect of the optic necessarily assumes a major role in preventing PCO (see Chapter 7).

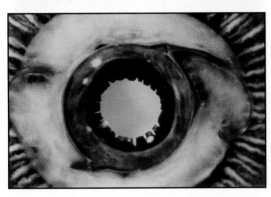

Figure 4-12B. Gross photograph from behind (Miyake-Apple posterior photographic technique) of a human eye obtained postmortem, showing an example of the SI-30 in which cortical cleanup was incomplete and extensive Soemmering's ring formation occurred. However, the central optic axis remained clear. In this case the capsulorhexis diameter was smaller than the lens optic, with the capsulorhexis edge on the anterior surface of the optic. In such cases with retained cortex, the barrier effect of the optic necessarily assumes a major role in preventing PCO (see Chapter 7).

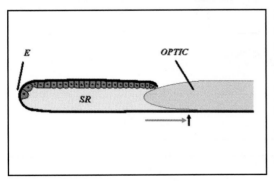

Figure 4-13A. Histopathologic appearance of the scenario illustrated in Figures 4-12 A and B. This is a schematic illustration showing the capsulorhexis diameter is smaller than the IOL optic so that the capsulorhexis edge rests on the anterior capsule. When the cortical cleanup is not complete, a large Soemmering's ring (SR) remains. The SI-30 has a round-edged optic, which typically may allow some growth behind the edge of the posterior peripheral aspect of the optic (arrow). This often creates a rim of opacification in the optic's periphery but the central axis usually remains clear.

Figure 4-13B. Histopathologic appearance of the scenario illustrated in Figures 4-12A and B. This figure is a photomicrograph showing the histopathologic appearance of an eye implanted with the SI-30 design. In this case, the capsulorhexis edge rests on the anterior side of the capsule. Retained cortex and cells forming a Soemmering's ring are present, represented by the pink mass on the left situated between the anterior and posterior capsule. There is extensive anterior capsular fibrosis but no growth of cells onto the posterior capsule.

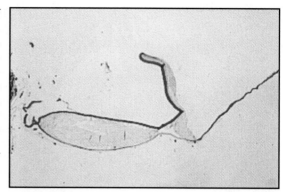

Figure 4-13C. Histopathologic appearance of the scenario illustrated in Figures 4-12A and B. In Figures 4-13C through F, the growth around the edge of each round optic onto the peripheral rim of the posterior capsule is seen in each case (corresponding to the region demarcated by the arrow in Figure 4-13A). Therefore, in contrast to an optic edge with a straight, square, truncated surface, a round edge sometimes allows some growth around the periphery. Hematoxylin and eosin stain. Original magnification x25.

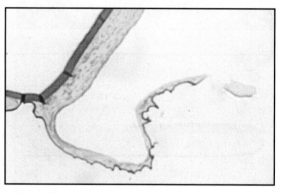

Figure 4-13D. Histopathologic appearance of the scenario illustrated in Figures 4-12A and B. In Figures 4-13C through F, the growth around the edge of each round optic onto the peripheral rim of the posterior capsule is seen in each case (corresponding to the region demarcated by the arrow in Figure 4-13A). Therefore, in contrast to an optic edge with a straight, square, truncated surface, a round edge sometimes allows some growth around the periphery. Hematoxylin and eosin stain. Original magnification x25.

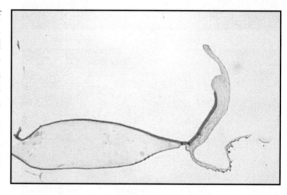

Figure 4-13E. Histopathologic appearance of the scenario illustrated in Figures 4-12A and B. In Figures 4-13C through F, the growth around the edge of each round optic onto the peripheral rim of the posterior capsule is seen in each case (corresponding to the region demarcated by the arrow in Figure 4-13A). Therefore, in contrast to an optic edge with a straight, square, truncated surface, a round edge sometimes allows some growth around the periphery. Hematoxylin and eosin stain. Original magnification x25.

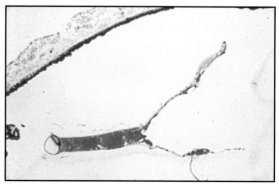

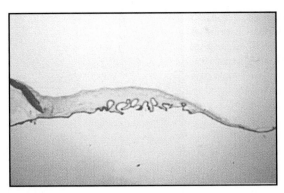

Figure 4-13F. Histopathologic appearance of the scenario illustrated in Figures 4-12A and B. In Figures 4-13C through F, the growth around the edge of each round optic onto the peripheral rim of the posterior capsule is seen in each case (corresponding to the region demarcated by the arrow in Figure 4-13A). Therefore, in contrast to an optic edge with a straight, square, truncated surface, a round edge sometimes allows some growth around the periphery. Hematoxylin and eosin stain. Original magnification x25.

the peripheral posterior capsule (Figure 4-13 [arrow]; see also Chapter 7). Histopathologic profiles, as seen in Figures 4-13C through F, provide evidence for the assertion that the square, truncated edge may serve to enhance the IOL barrier effect against PCO.

A major modification of the SI series of lenses occurred in the mid 1990s, when a PMMA haptic was substituted for the polypropylene haptic present on all previous designs in this series. This led to the development of the SI-40 series (Figure 4-14A and B). Selected specifications of this IOL are noted in Table 4-4 and specifications of the 5.5 mm optic SI-55 model are noted in Table 4-5.

Figure 4-15, a manufacturer's illustration, shows a very important modification of the SI-40 series; namely, the fabrication of a multifocal design, the SA-40. At the time of this writing, this was the only multifocal design available in the United States, and it has been undergoing successful implantation. The specifications of this design, termed the "Array," are listed in Table 4-6.

Figures 4-16A through C, are Miyake-Apple posterior views of several human eyes obtained postmortem containing the SI-40 IOL. Note the excellent appearance of all of these eyes, which has been the case in the vast majority of eyes with this IOL in our database. Recall that this is in contrast to the appearance of substantial numbers of the SI-30 design available in the earlier 1990s (e.g., Figures 4-10 and 4-12A and B), in which substantial Soemmering's rings were present and PCO occurred at a higher rate; namely, 19.1%. The reasons for the differences between the earlier SI-30 and the SI-40 are probably multifactoral. First,the surgery was not as consistently good during the early 1990s, the heyday of the SI-30; also, it is possible that the PMMA haptics of the later SI-40 design (as opposed to the prolene haptics of the early SI-30 design) provide a better haptic stability and stability to the lens capsular bag, which in turn enhances the IOL optic barrier effect and helps control the incidence of PCO. As is noted from our study of Nd:YAG rates of human eyes obtained postmortem in our database (Figures 7-79 and 7-80), the PCO rate of the earlier SI-30 design was 19.1%, whereas the PCO rate noted with the Allergan SI-40 design was 14.6%. It should be noted that these latter figures were based on an accession of relatively few specimens, so statistical significance cannot be claimed. However, there is no doubt that, subjectively speaking, the clinicopathologic profiles of the SI-40 globes (Figures 4-16A through C) are better than with the earlier SI-30 design. The SI-40 design clearly represents a major advance.

Figure 4-14A. The Allergan SI-40 series was introduced in the mid 1990s. The main feature was the substitution of PMMA haptics for the polypropylene haptics characteristic of the SI-30 and earlier series. Manufacturer's specifications of the modern Allergan silicone optic-PMMA designs, the SI-40 MB IOL, with a 6-mm optic size, and the SI-55 MB IOL, optic diameter 5.5-mm, are listed in Tables 4-4 and 4-5.

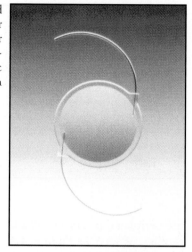

Figure 4-14B. Manufacturer's illustration of the SI-40. (B) Clinical photograph of a well-implanted, well-centered SI-40 IOL.

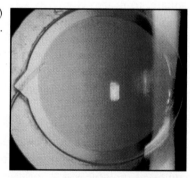

Table 4-5.
SI 55 NB
Allergan, Inc.

Design	3-piece-silicone-IOL
Model	SI 55 NB
Manufacturer	Allergan, Inc.
Overall diameter [mm]	13.0
Optic diameter [mm]	Biconvex 5.5
Optic material	Silicone polymer
Water content	<1%
Refractive index	1.46
Haptic material	PMMA
Haptic angulation	10°
A-constant	118
ACD [mm]	4.7
Diopter [range]	+6.0 to +30.0
Incision [mm]	2.6

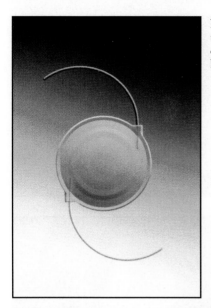

Figure 4-15. An important modification of the SI-40 series is the SA-40 multifocal design, which Allergan has marketed with considerable success during the late 1990s and continues to market. This is a manufacturer's illustration.

Table 4-6.
Array SA 40 N
Allergan, Inc.

Design	3-piece-silicone-IOL
Model	SA 40 N
Manufacturer	Allergan, Inc.
Overall diameter [mm]	13.0
Optic diameter [mm]	Biconvex 6.0
Optic material	Silicone polymer
Water content	<1%
Refractive index	1.46
Haptic material	PMMA
Haptic angulation	10°
A-constant	118
ACD [mm]	4.7
Diopter [range]	+16.0 to +24.0
Incision [mm]	3.0

Figure 4-16A. Examination of an eye in our database obtained postmortem containing the Allergan SI-40 foldable silicone IOL has shown excellent results. These three examples show perfect centration and good clarity of the media. (Miyake-Apple posterior photographic technique.)

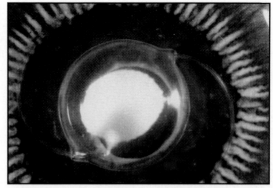

Figure 4-16B. Examination of an eye in our database obtained postmortem containing the Allergan SI-40 foldable silicone IOL has shown excellent results. These three examples show perfect centration and good clarity of the media. (Miyake-Apple posterior photographic technique.)

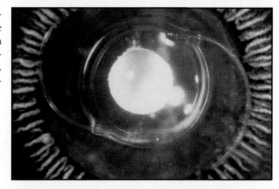

Figure 4-16C. Examination of an eye in our database obtained postmortem containing the Allergan SI-40 foldable silicone IOL has shown excellent results. These three examples show perfect centration and good clarity of the media. (Miyake-Apple posterior photographic technique.)

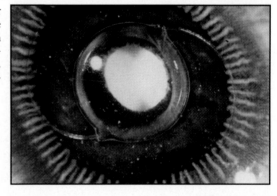

The different histopathologic scenarios that we have observed on examination of the SI-40 design are illustrated in Figures 4-17 to 4-19). In most cases, excellent cortical cleanup was evident (Figures 4-17 and 4-18). In the few cases where cortical cleanup was not complete, the barrier effect of the rounded optic was effective in blocking most migration, but some did occur onto the peripheral posterior capsule (see Figures 4-13C through F). With the SI-40 design, growth behind the round optic edge onto the posterior capsule has been much less than with the SI-30. This may be partly explained by the fact that the surgical cleanup with these eyes was measurably better than that noted with the earlier SI-30, and therefore there was less need for the second line of defense that the barrier effect of the optic comprises.

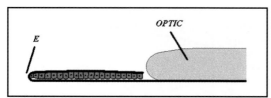

Figure 4-17A. Implantation of the SI-40 design with the capsulorhexis diameter larger than the IOL optic and good cortical cleanup. Note the fusion of anterior and posterior capsules. This figure is a schematic illustration (E = equatorial capsule).

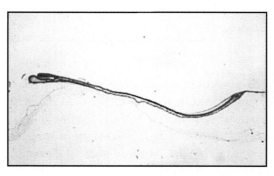

Figure 4-17B. Implantation of the SI-40 design with the capsulorhexis diameter larger than the IOL optic and good cortical cleanup. Note the fusion of anterior and posterior capsules. This figure is a photomicrograph showing that total cortical cleanup was achieved, so that the anterior and posterior capsules totally fused together, with no intervening Soemmering's ring (hematoxylin and eosin stain, original magnification x25).

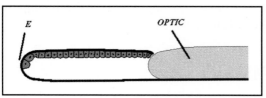

Figure 4-18A. This figure illustrates the scenario of implantation of the Allergan SI-40 design with 1) the capsulorhexis smaller than the optic diameter, leaving the capsulorhexis edge on the anterior surface of the optic, associated with 2) excellent cortical cleanup. This figure is a schematic illustration (E = equatorial cells).

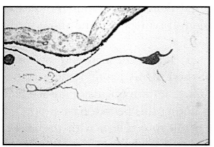

Figure 4-18B. This figure illustrates the scenario of implantation of the Allergan SI-40 design with 1) the capsulorhexis smaller than the optic diameter, leaving the capsulorhexis edge on the anterior surface of the optic, associated with 2) excellent cortical cleanup. This figure is a photomicrograph showing the anterior capsule resting on the anterior surface of the IOL optic (the silicone optic material dissolved out during preparation). (Hematoxylin and eosin stain; original magnification x25.)

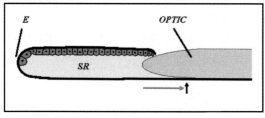

Figure 4-19A. Histopathologic appearance of the Allergan SI-40 in the presence of incomplete cortical cleanup. This figure shows a schematic illustration showing a potential space for cellular ingrowth behind the peripheral posterior aspect of the IOL optic (arrows).

Figure 4-19B. Histopathologic appearance of the Allergan SI-40 in the presence of incomplete cortical cleanup. This is a photomicrograph showing the presence of a Soemmering's ring because of an incomplete cortical cleanup. There is also growth of a narrow rim of cells onto the peripheral posterior capsule toward the visual axis (lower right). Such growth rarely extends to the center of the visual axis but usually remains in the periphery. (Hematoxylin and eosin stain; original magnification x25.)

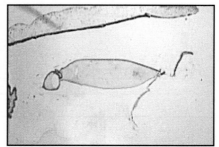

We have received very few explants of the SI-40 design, almost all of these being related to complications of surgical technique or power miscalculations rather than inherent problems with the lens. One problem that rarely affects silicone IOLs is silicone oil-silicone IOL adherence during retinal surgery, as described in Chapter 7. All cases we have seen have been associated with early cases; namely, the SI-30 design and earlier. Recognition of this condition during the last few years, about the time when the SI-40 was introduced, had made this an extreme rarity. It is important not to overweight the importance of this rare complication when choosing a IOL (Chapter 7).

SUMMARY

The elastimide-polyimide design of Staar Surgical and Bausch and Lomb Vision has provided excellent results with little need for explantation. It centers well and shows a relatively low rate of PCO to date.

The SI series of Allergan's silicone optic IOLs has shown constant improvement throughout the last decade, including introduction of the PMMA haptic leading to the model SI-40 and the SA ("Array") multifocal design. These improvements, in association with the improvement of surgical techniques evolving during this period, have produced results that have improved from very good with the SI-30 to excellent with the SI-40. From our limited database, the PCO rate is slightly higher than that noted with some of the models (see Figures 7-79 and 7-80), but the number of accessions is small, so further evaluation is necessary. The SI series of Allergan IOLs has had a tried-and-true history, with millions of lenses having been implanted over the years, and the SI-40 design, with its cousin the SA-40 "Array" multifocal, continues with this tradition.

REFERENCES

1. Auffarth GU, Wilcox M, Sims JCR, et al. Analysis of 100 Explanted One-Piece and Three-Piece Silicone Intraocular Lenses. *Ophthalmology.* 1995;102(8):1144-1150.(RPB)

2. Auffarth GU, Wilcox M, Sims JCR, et al. Complications of silicone intraocular lenses. *J Cataract Refract Surg.* 1995;(Special Issue) [Best Paper of 1995 ASCRS Meeting]:38-41.(RPB)

3. Werner L, Pandey SK, Escobar-Gomez M, et al. Anterior Capsule Opacification: A histopathological study comparing different IOL styles. *Ophthalmology.* 1999. [In Press]

BIBLIOGRAPHY

Apple DJ, Blotnik C. Postoperative lens deposits. *J Cataract Refract Surg*. 1993;19:441.

Apple DJ, Tsai JC, Castaneda VE, et al. Posterior chamber intraocular lens (PC-IOL): A clinical goal with bifocal and multifocal IOLs. In: Maxwell WA, Nordan LT, eds. *Current Concepts of Multifocal Intraocular Lenses.* Thorofare, NJ: SLACK Incorporated; 1991;219-231.

Auffarth GU, McCabe C, Wilcox M, et al. Centration and fixation of silicone intraocular lenses: An analysis of clinicopathological findings in human autopsy eyes. *J Cataract Refract Surg*. 1996;22(2):1281-1285.

Auffarth GU, Newland TJ, Wesendahl TA, Apple DJ. ND:Yag laser damage on silicone intraocular lenses confused with pigment deposits on clinical examination. *Am J Ophthalmo*l. 1994;118(4):526-528.

Auffarth GU, Newland TJ, Wesendahl TA, Apple DJ. Nd:YAG laser damage to silicone intraocular lenses confused with pigment deposits on clinical examination. *Am J Ophthalmol*. 118(4):526-530, 1994.

Auffarth GU, Wilcox CM, Sims JC, et al. Komplikationen von 100 explantierten Silikonhinterkammerlinsen. In: Rochels R, Dunker G, Hartmann Ch, eds. Transactions of the 9th Congress of the German Intraocular Lens Implant Society. Kiel, 1995. Heidelberg, Berlin, New York; Springer Publishing; 1995.

Blotnick CA, Powers TP, Newland T, et al. Pathology of silicone intraocular lenses in human eyes obtained postmortem. *J Cataract Refract Surg*. 1995;21(4):447-452.(RPB)

Brady DG, Giamporcaro JE, Steinert RF. Effect of folding instruments on silicone intraocular lenses. *J Cataract Refract Surg*. 1994;20:310-315.

Buchen SY, Richards SC, Solomon KD, et al. Evaluation of the biocompatibility and fixation of a new silicone intraocular lens in the feline model. *J Cataract Refract Surg*.1989;15:545-553.

Carlson D. Reduced vision secondary to pigmented cellular membranes on silicone intraocular lenses. *Am J Ophthalmol*. 1995;120:462-470.

Colin J, Mimouni F, Conrad H. Soft intraocular silicone lenses: Results after a one-year follow-up. *J Fr Ophthalmol*. 1988;11:257-260.

Davison JA. Modified insertion technique for the SI-18NB intraocular lens. *J Cataract Refract* Surg. 1991;17:849-853.

Deacon J, Buchen SY, Apple DJ. Evaluation of Silicone Intraocular Lenses in a Feline Model and Clinical Trials. In: *Proceedings of the Society for Biomaterials Symposium on Retrieval and Analysis of Surgical Implants and Biomaterials*. Snowbird, Ut; 1988.

Egan CA, Kottos PJ, Francis IC, et al. Prospective study of the SI-40NB foldable silicone intraocular lens. *J Cataract Refract Surg*. 1996;22:9(suppl 2):1272-1276.

Ernest PH, Lavery KT, Hazariwala K. Occurrence of pigment precipitates after small incision cataract surgery. *J Cataract Refract Surg*. 1998;24:91-97.

Fine IH, Robertson JE, Jr. Initial experience with the AMO PC-28LB (Phacofit) small-incision implant: a preliminary report. *J Cataract Refract Surg*. 1989;15:327-331.

Hayashi K, Hayashi H, Nakao F, Hayashi F. Corneal endothelial cell loss in phacoemulsification surgery with silicone intraocular lens implantation. *J Cataract Refract Surg*. 1996;22:743-747.

Hayashi K, Hayashi H, Nakao F, Hayashi F. Reduction in the area of the anterior capsule opacification after polymethylmethacrylate, silicone, and soft acrylic intraocular lens implantation. *Arch Ophthalmol*. 1998;123:441-447.

Hayashi K, Hayashi H, Nakao F, Hayashi F. Comparison of decentration and tilt between one piece and three-piece polymethyl methacrylate intraocular lenses. *Br J Ophthalmol*. 1998;82:419-422.

Hwang IP, Clinch TE, Moshifar M, et al. Decentration of 3-piece versus plate-haptic silicone intraocular lenses. *J Cataract Refract Surg*. 1998;24:1505-1508.

Keates RH, Sall KN, Kreter JK. Effect of the Nd:YAG laser on polymethylmethacrylate, hema copolymer, and silicone intraocular materials. *J Cataract Refract Surg.* 1987;13:401-409.

Kim MJ, Lee HY, Joo CK. Posterior capsule opacification in eyes with silicone or poly(methyl methacrylate) intraocular lens. *J Cataract Refract Surg.*1999;25:251-255.

Kimura W. Postoperative decentration of three-piece silicone intraocular lenses. *J Cataract Refract Surg.* 1996;22 (supp 2):1277-1280.

Koch DD, Heit LE. Discoloration of silicone intraocular lenses. *Arch Ophthalmol.* 1992;110:319-320.

Koch DD, Samuelson SW, Villarreal R, Haft EA, Kohnen T. Changes in pupil size induced by phacoemulsification and posterior chamber lens implantation: consequences for multifocal lenses. *J Cataract Refract Surg.* 1996;22:579-584.

Kohnen T, Ferrer A, Brauweiler P. Visual function in pseudophakic eyes with poly(methyl methacrylate), silicone, and acrylic intraocular lenses. *J Cataract Refract Surg.* 1996;22 (suppl 2):1303-1307.

Kohnen T, Koch DD. Experimental and clinical evaluation of incision size and shape following forceps and injector implantation of a three-piece high-refractive-index silicone intraocular lens. *Graefes Arch Clin Exp Ophthalmol.* 1998;236:922-928.

Kohnen T, Magdowski G, Koch DD. Surface quality of flexible silicone intraocular lenses. A scanning electron microscopy study. *Klin Monatsbl Augenheilkd.* 1995;207:253-263.

Kosmin AS, Wishart PK, Ridges PJ. Silicone versus poly(methyl methacrylate) lenses in combined phacoemulsification and trabeculectomy. *J Cataract Refract Surg.*1997;23:97-105.

Legler UF, Apple DJ. Comments on silicone intraocular lens discoloration. *Arch Ophthalmol.* 1991;109:1495-1496.

Lemagne JM. Results of the intraocular lens SI-30 implantation. *Bull Soc Belge Ophthalmol.* 1996;262:155-157.

Lemon LC, Shin DH, Song MS, et al. Comparative study of silicone versus acrylic foldable lens implantation in primary glaucoma triple procedure. *Ophthalmology.* 1997;104:1708-1713.

Liekfeld A, Pham DT, Wollensak J. Functional results in bilateral implantation of a foldable refractive multifocal posterior chamber lens. *Klin Monatsbl Augenheilkd.* 1995;207:283-286.

Linnola RJ, Holst A. Evaluation of a 3-piece silicone intraocular lens with poly(methyl methacrylate) haptics. *J Cataract Refract Surg.* 1998;24:1509-1514.

Mamalis N, Phillips B, Kopp CH, Crandall AS, Olson RJ. Neodymium:YAG capsulotomy rates after phacoemulsification with silicone posterior chamber intraocular lenses. *J Cataract Refract Surg.* 1996;22 (suppl 2):1296-1302.

Martin RG, Sanders DR, Van der Karr MA, DeLuca M. Effect of small incision intraocular lens surgery on postoperative inflammation and astigmatism. A study of the AMO SI-18NB small incision lens. *J Cataract Refract Surg.* 1992;18:51-57.

Menapace R. Evaluation of 35 consecutive SI-30 phacoflex lenses with high-refractive silicone optic implanted in the capsulorhexis bag. *J Cataract Refract Surg.* 1995;21:339-347.

Menapace R, Amon M, Papapanos P, Radax U. Evaluation of the first 100 consecutive phacoflex silicone lenses implanted in the bag through a self-sealing tunnel incision using the prodigy inserter. *J Cataract Refract Surg.* 1994;20:299-309.

Menapace R, Radax U, Vass C, Amon M, Papapanos P. In-the-bag implantation of the PhacoFlex SI-30 high-refractive silicone lens through self-sealing sclerocorneal and clear corneal incisions. *Eur J Implant Ref Surg.* 1994;6:143-152.

Milazzo S, Turut P, Artin B, Charlin JF. Long-term follow-up of three-piece, looped, silicone intraocular lenses. *J Cataract Refract Surg.* 1996;22(suppl 2):1259-1262.

Newland TJ, Auffarth GU, Wesendahl TA, Apple DJ. Neodymium:YAG laser damage on silicone intraocular lenses. A comparison of lesions on explanted lenses and experimentally produced lesions. *J Cataract Refract Surg.* 20:527-533, 1994.

Olson RJ. Crandall AS. Silicone versus poly(methyl methacrylate) intraocular lenses with regard to capsular opacification. *Ophthalmic Surg Lasers.* 1998;29:55-58.

Omar O, Mamalis N, Veiga J, Tamura M, Olson RJ. Scanning electron microscopic characteristics of small-incision intraocular lenses. *Ophthalmology.* 1996;103:1124-1129.

Oshika T, Tsuboi S, Yaguchi S, Yoshitomi F, Nagamoto T. Small incision cataract surgery-silicone intraocular lens vs poly(methyl methacrylate) intraocular lens. Nippon Ganka Gakkai Zasshi -*Acta Soc Ophthalmolo Jap.* 1994;98:362-368.

Popham JK, Apple DJ, Newman DA, Isenberg RA, Deacon J. Advantages and limitations of soft intraocular lenses: A scientific perspective. In: Mazzocco TR, Rajacich GM, Epstein E, eds. *Soft Implant Lenses in Cataract Surgery.* Thorofare, NJ: SLACK Incorporated: 1986:11-30.

Ravalico G, Parentin F, Pastori G, Baccara F. Spatial resolution threshold in pseudophakic patients with mono-focal and multifocal intraocular lenses. *J Cataract Refract Surg.* 1998;24:244-248.

Ravalico G, Parentin F, Sirotti P, Baccara F. Analysis of light energy distribution by multifocal intraocular lenses through an experimental optical model. *J Cataract Refract Surg.* 1998;24:647-652.

Rozsival P, Jiraskova N. Implantation of soft silicone intraocular lenses. *Cesk Slov Oftalmol* 1996;52:210-214.

Skorpik C, Menapace R, Gnad HD, Grasl M, Scheidel W. Evaluation of 50 silicone posterior chamber lens implantations. *J Cataract Refract Surg.* 1987;13:640-643.

Steinert RF, Bayliss B, Brint SF, et al. Long-term clinical results of AMO PhacoFlex model SI-18 intraocular lens implantation. *J Cataract Refract Surg.* 1995;21:331-338.

Steinert RF, Giamporcaro JE, Tasso VA. Clinical assessment of long-term safety and efficacy of a widely implanted silicone intraocular lens material. *Am J Ophthalmol.* 1997;123:17-23.

Steinert RF, Post CT, Jr., Brint SF, et al. A prospective, randomized, double-masked comparison of a zonal-progressive multifocal intraocular lens and a monofocal intraocular lens. *Ophthalmology.* 1992;99:853-860.

Strenn K, Menapace R, Vass C. Capsular bag shrinkage after implantation of an open-loop silicone lens and a poly(methyl methacrylate) capsule tension ring. *J Cataract Refract Surg.* 1997;23:1543-1547.

Tsai JC, Castaneda VE, Apple DJ, et al. Scanning electron microscopic study of modern silicone intraocular lenses. *J Cat Refract Surg.* 1992;18(5):232-235.

Watt RH. Discoloration of a silicone intraocular lens 6 weeks after surgery [letter; comment]. *Arch Ophthalmol.* 1991;109:1494-1495.

Watt RH. Pigment dispersion syndrome associated with silicone posterior chamber intraocular lenses. *J Cataract Refract Surg.* 1988;14:431-433.

Weghaupt H, Pieh S, Skorpik C. Visual properties of the foldable Array multifocal intraocular lens. *J Cataract Refract Surg.* 1996;22(suppl 2):1313-1317.

Wenzel M, Kammann J, Allmers R. Biocompatibility of silicone intraocular lenses. *Klin Monatsbl Augenheilkd.* 1993;203:408-412.

Werner L, Pandey SK, Escobar-Gomez M, et al. Anterior capsule opacification: A histopathological study comparing different IOL styles. *Ophthalmology.* 1999. [In Press]

Wesendahl TA, Hunold W, Auffarth GU, et al. Einfluss on Optikgeometrie und Haptikabwinklung auf die Lagebeziehungen on IOL und hinterem Kapselblatt. In: Gloor R, et al., eds. *Trans 7th Congress of the German Intraocular Lens Implant Society* (DGII). Zhurich; 1993:222-227.

Chapter 5

Hydrophobic Acrylic Intraocular Lenses

The Alcon AcrySof IOL (Figures 5-1A and B and Tables 5-1 and 5-2) was introduced in the early 1990s. Selected specifications of this IOL are listed in Table 5-2 and have been documented in detail by Koch.[1]

We have had the opportunity to accession 159 of these lenses as of August 1999. Most noteworthy, we have observed by both gross and microscopic examination that lens cellular reactivity within capsular bags implanted with this IOL is often very low. The capsule surrounding this IOL often remains very clear (Figures 5-2 to 5-5). This lens became available for implantation after 1992. By that time, significant improvements in surgical techniques had been attained, and almost without exception we have found that this lens centers well when carefully inserted in the capsular bag (Figure 5-2). Three histologic patterns are commonly observed with this IOL design. When the capsulorhexis diameter is larger than that of the IOL optic, and cortical cleanup is complete, the pattern is as noted in Figure 5-3. Note in this scenario the total fusion of anterior and posterior capsules peripheral to the IOL optic.

Another common profile, one we correlate with very good results, is illustrated in Figures 5-4 and 5-5. In this scenario, the capsulorhexis diameter is slightly smaller than the diameter of the IOL optic (eg, circa 5.25 to 5.5 mm when the optic diameter is 6.0 mm). When cortical cleanup is complete, as is seen in the sketch (Figure 5-5A) and micrographs shown in Figures 5-5B and C, the space between the anterior and posterior capsule remains open and contains the lens optic, without formation of a Soemmering's ring. Creation of this profile renders the capsular bag around the IOL optic a closed system and effectively sequesters it from the surrounding aqueous. In addition, this helps create a tight fit of the capsule around the optic—the "shrink wrap" phenomenon (see Chapter 7, Table 7-2 and 7-3) which we believe is helpful in reducing unwanted postoperative cellular proliferation and enhances the IOL optic's barrier effect against PCO (see Chapter 7).

When cortical cleanup is incomplete and unwanted retained/regenerate cortex and cells remain forming peripheral pearls and a Soemmering's ring (Figures 5-6 and 5-7), the barrier

Figure 5-1A. Clinical photograph of well-centered Alcon AcrySof foldable IOL. This lens has a foldable hydrophobic acrylic optic and PMMA haptics. Both of these lenses (Figures 5-1A and 5-1B) were implanted with a capsulorhexis that has a slightly smaller diameter than that of the IOL optic.

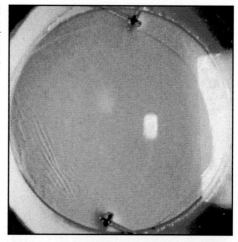

Figure 5-1B. Clinical photograph of well-centered Alcon AcrySof foldable IOL. This lens has a foldable hydrophobic acrylic optic and PMMA haptics. Both of these lenses (Figures 5-1A and 5-1B) were implanted with a capsulorhexis that has a slightly smaller diameter than that of the IOL optic.

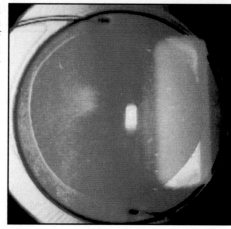

Table 5-1.

Foldable IOLs, Approved and Investigational, 2000
Available in the USA Autopsy Database

Design	Model (selected representative examples)	Company	Diameter (mm)	Optic Diameter (mm)	Water Content	Haptic Material
I. Silicone						
IA: Plate silicone lenses						
1 piece silicone plate lens (small holes)	Chiroflex C10UB	Bausch and Lomb Surgical, Inc.	10.5	Biconvex, 6.0	<1%	Silicone
1 piece silicone plate lens (large holes)	Chiroflex C11UB	Bausch and Lomb Surgical, Inc.	10.5	Biconvex, 6.0	<1%	Silicone
1 piece silicone plate lens (small holes)	AA-4203V	Staar Surgical Inc.	10.5	Biconvex, 6.0	<1%	Silicone
1 piece silicone plate lens (large holes)	AA-4203VF	Staar Surgical Inc.	10.5	Biconvex, 6.0	<1%	Silicone
1 piece silicone toric lens (large holes)	AA-4203TF	Staar Surgical Inc.	10.5	Biconvex, 6.0	<1%	Silicone
IB: Three-piece silicone lenses						
a) Staar						
3 piece silicone IOL	AQ1016/2010/2003	Staar Surgical Inc.	13.5/13.5/12.5	Biconvex, 6.3	<1%	Polyimide
b) Allergan Series						
3 piece silicone IOL	SI-30 NB	Allergan, Inc.	13.0	Biconvex, 6.0	<1%	Polypropylene
3 piece silicone IOL	SI-40 NB	Allergan, Inc.	13.0	Biconvex, 6.0	<1%	PMMA
3 piece silicone IOL	SI 55 NB	Allergan, Inc.	13.0	Biconvex, 5.5	<1%	PMMA
3 piece silicone IOL	SA 40 N	Allergan, Inc.	13.0	Biconvex, 6.0	<1%	PMMA
c) Bausch and Lomb						
3 piece silicone oil	Soflex and LI Series	Bausch and Lomb Surgical, Inc.	13.0	Biconvex, 6.0	<1%	PMMA
II. Acrylics						
Hydrophobic (dry packed) 3 piece Acrylic IOL	AcrySof MA30BA/MA60BM	Alcon Laboratories, Inc.	12.5/30	Biconvex, 5.5/6.0	<2%	PMMA

Table 5-2.	
AcrySof	
Alcon Laboratories, Inc.	
Design	3-piece-acrylic-IOL
Model	AcrySof MA30BA (5.5mm optic), MA60BM (6.0mm optic)
Manufacturer	Alcon Laboratories, Inc.
Overall diameter [mm]	12.5 and 13.0
Optic diameter [mm]	Biconvex 5.5 and 6.0
Optic material	Hydrophobic acrylic polymer
Water content	<0.5%
Refractive index	1.55
Haptic material	PMMA
Haptic angulation	5° and 10°
A-constant	118.9
ACD [mm]	5.49
Diopter [range]	+10 to +30 MA30BA +6 to +30 MA60BM
Incision [mm]	3.0 to 3.5 and 3.5 to 4.0

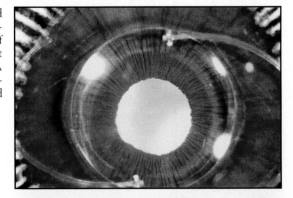

Figure 5-2A. Gross photograph from behind (Miyake-Apple posterior photographic technique) of a postmortem eye with an AcrySof IOL showing symmetric fixation and excellent centration. In all of these cases (Figures 5-2A through C), lens cortical removal was excellent and there is virtually no retained Soemmering's ring.

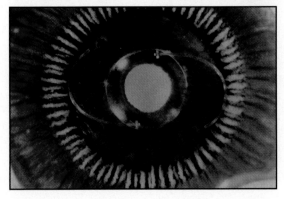

Figure 5-2A. Gross photograph from behind (Miyake-Apple posterior photographic technique) of a postmortem eye with an AcrySof IOL showing symmetric fixation and excellent centration. In all of these cases (Figures 5-2A through C), lens cortical removal was excellent and there is virtually no retained Soemmering's ring.

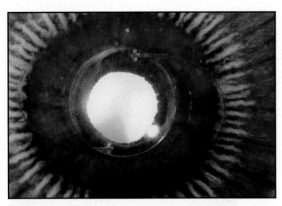

Figure 5-2C. Gross photograph from behind (Miyake-Apple posterior photographic technique) of a postmortem eye with an AcrySof IOL showing symmetric fixation and excellent centration. In all of these cases (FigureS 5-2A through C), lens cortical removal was excellent and there is virtually no retained Soemmering's ring.

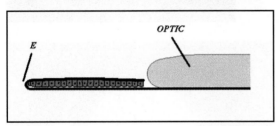

Figure 5-3A. Histopathologic scenario of implantation of an IOL with a capsulorhexis diameter larger than the IOL optic (as seen in Figures 5-2A through C). Note that cortical cleanup was excellent and the anterior and posterior capsules have fused, with no Soemmering's ring formation. This figure is a schematic illustration (E = equatorial capsule). Note that the Alcon AcrySof has a square edge, unlike the generic round edge shown here.

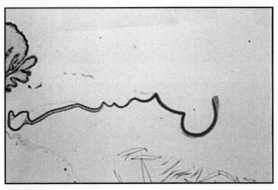

Figure 5-3B. Histopathologic scenario of implantation of the Alcon AcrySof IOL with a capsulorhexis diameter larger than the IOL optic (as seen in Figures 5-2 A-C). Note that cortical cleanup was excellent and the anterior and posterior capsules have fused, with no Soemmering's ring formation. This is a photomicrograph showing the histopathologic pattern demonstrated in Figure 5-3A, with total fusion of the anterior and posterior capsules following cortical removal (hematoxylin and eosin stain, original magnification x25).

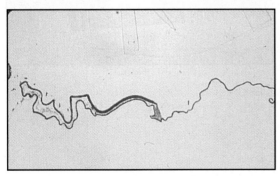

Figure 5-3C. Histopathologic scenario of implantation of the Alcon AcrySof IOL with a capsulorhexis diameter larger than the IOL optic (as seen in Figures 5-2A through C). Note that cortical cleanup was excellent and the anterior and posterior capsules have fused, with no Soemmering's ring formation. This is a photomicrograph showing the histopathologic pattern demonstrated in Figure 5-3A, with total fusion of the anterior and posterior capsules following cortical removal (hematoxylin and eosin stain, original magnification x25).

Figure 5-4A. Clinical photograph of an implantation of the Alcon AcrySof IOL, with a capsulorhexis diameter smaller than that of the IOL optic, allowing the cut edge of the capsulorhexis to rest on the anterior surface of the optic.

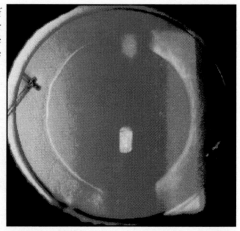

Figure 5-4B. Implantation of the Alcon AcrySof IOL, with a capsulorhexis diameter smaller than that of the IOL optic, allowing the cut edge of the capsulorhexis to rest on the anterior surface of the optic. This figure is a gross photograph of a human eye obtained postmortem, Miyake-Apple posterior photographic technique.

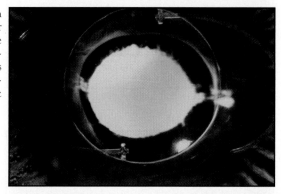

Figure 5-4C. Implantation of the Alcon AcrySof IOL, with a capsulorhexis diameter smaller than that of the IOL optic, allowing the cut edge of the capsulorhexis to rest on the anterior surface of the optic. This figure is a gross photograph of a human eye obtained postmortem, Miyake-Apple posterior photographic technique.

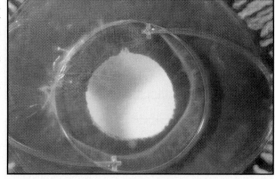

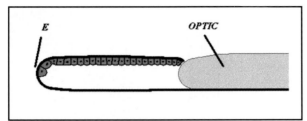

Figure 5-5A. Schematic illustration of implantation of an IOL with the capsulorhexis diameter slightly smaller than through C), associated with good cortical cleanup. Note the space between anterior and posterior capsules (E = equatorial capsule). This generic diagram shows a rounded edge as opposed to the square edge of the Alcon AcrySof.

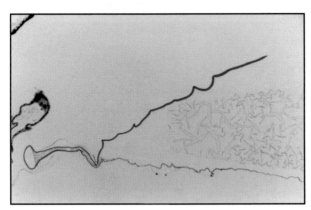

Figure 5-5B. Implantation of the Alcon AcrySof IOL with the capsulorhexis diameter slightly smaller than the IOL optic (as shown in Figures 5-4A through C), associated with good cortical cleanup. Photomicrograph showing the extension of the anterior capsulorhexis margin over the anterior surface of the IOL optic (note that the IOL optics have partially or totally dissolved out of the section, leaving the large space between the anterior capsular flap and the posterior capsule). Evidence of excellent cortical cleanup is provided by the fact that there is almost no Soemmering's ring material within the capsular bags. Note that the small round empty space in the bag at the left within the fornix of each capsule represents the site of each capsular-fixated haptic.

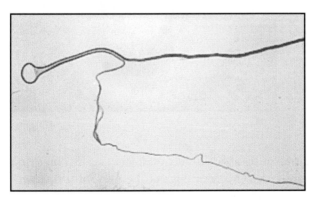

Figure 5-5C. Implantation of the Alcon AcrySof IOL with the capsulorhexis diameter slightly smaller than the IOL optic (as shown in Figures 5-4A through C), associated with good cortical cleanup. Photomicrograph showing the extension of the anterior capsulorhexis margin over the anterior surface of the IOL optic (note that the IOL optics have partially or totally dissolved out of the section, leaving the large space between the anterior capsular flap and the posterior capsule). Evidence of excellent cortical cleanup is provided by the fact that there is almost no Soemmering's ring material within the capsular bags. Note that the small round empty space in the bag at the left within the fornix of each capsule represents the site of each capsular-fixated haptic.

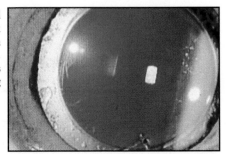

Figure 5-6. Even when cortical cleanup is incomplete and residual lens epithelial cells remain in the equatorial fornix of the capsular bag, the barrier effect of the optic forms a second line of defense to resist ingrowth of cells centrally. This is a clinical photograph showing the presence of pearls peripheral to the IOL optic. However, the zone subtending the entire optical component is almost cell-free.

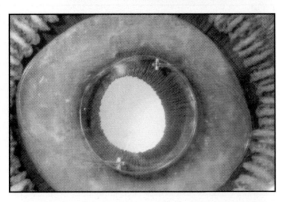

Figure 5-7A. Gross photograph from behind of a human eye obtained postmortem with an Alcon AcrySof IOL (Miyake-Apple posterior photographic technique) in which cortical cleanup was incomplete, resulting in formation of a Soemmering's ring. However, note the absence of growth across the posterior optic toward the visual axis, leaving a clear optical zone. The barrier effect formed by the square truncated edge of the optic helps protect against ingrowth. This barrier effect is demonstrated in Figures 5-8 throgh 5-10 and discussed in detail in Chapter 7.

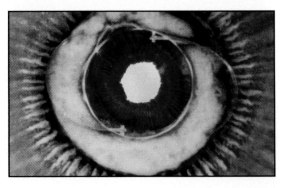

Figure 5-7B. Gross photograph from behind of a human eye obtained postmortem with an Alcon AcrySof IOL (Miyake-Apple posterior photographic technique) in which cortical cleanup was incomplete, resulting in formation of a Soemmering's ring. However, note the absence of growth across the posterior optic toward the visual axis, leaving a clear optical zone. The barrier effect formed by the square truncated edge of the optic helps protect against ingrowth. This barrier effect is demonstrated in Figures 5-8 throgh 5-10 and discussed in detail in Chapter 7.

effect of the IOL optic comes into play, forming a second line of defense against ingrowth over the posterior capsule into the optical axis. The optic edge of the AcrySof is square or truncated (Figure 5-8; see also Chapter 7), which we believe provides a maximal barrier effect against ingrowth of cells (Figures 5-8 to 5-10). This contributes to this IOL's extremely low PCO rate, as measured by a Nd:YAG laser posterior capsulotomy rate of 1.3% noted in a study in our laboratory as of August, 1999 (see Figures 7-79 and 7-80). Also attesting to the good biocompatibility of this IOL is the fact that anterior lens epithelial cell reaction appears to be low, leading to a low rate of ACO (Figure 3-12 and Figures 5-11 to 5-13). Data regarding various biocompatibility features of the Alcon AcrySof IOL are listed in Figure 5-13 (see also Chapter 7).

There is preliminary evidence that the Alcon AcrySof IOL biomaterial provides an enhanced adhesion of the capsule to the optic, as opposed to silicone and PMMA.[2-4] The

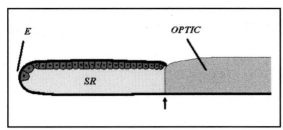

Figure 5-8. This schematic illustration demonstrates the concept of the barrier effect of the square edged or truncated optic (see also Figures 5-9 and 5-10, and Chapter 7). Note that even though a Soemmering's ring (SR) forms owing to incomplete cortical cellular removal, the square edge of the IOL optic, when firmly opposed to the posterior capsule (arrow), provides an effective barrier against ingrowth of cells from the Soemmering's ring onto the posterior surface of the capsule. (E = equatorial capsule.)

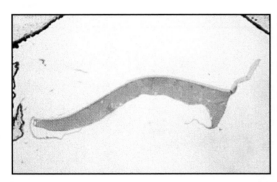

Figure 5-9A. Photomicrograph of the anterior segment of an eye containing an Alcon AcrySof IOL showing the effective barrier created by the square truncated edge. Note that the Soemmering's ring mass abuts against the square edge (right). Blockage of cells occurs directly at that point, leaving a cell-free posterior capsule (lower right). (Hematoxylin and eosin stain, original magnification x25.)

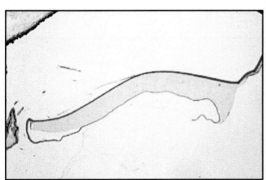

Figure 5-9B. Photomicrograph of the anterior segment of an eye containing an Alcon AcrySof IOL showing the effective barrier created by the square truncated edge. Note that the Soemmering's ring mass abuts against the square edge (right). Blockage of cells occurs directly at that point, leaving a cell-free posterior capsule (lower right). (Periodic acid-Schiff stain, original magnification x25.)

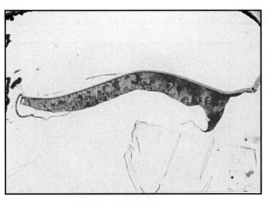

Figure 5-9C. Photomicrograph of the anterior segment of an eye containing an Alcon AcrySof IOL showing the effective barrier created by the square truncated edge. Note that the Soemmering's ring mass abuts against the square edge (right). Blockage of cells occurs directly at that point, leaving a cell-free posterior capsule (lower right). (Masson trichrome stain, original magnification x25.)

Figure 5-10A. A photomicrograph clearly demonstrating the barrier effect achieved with the square truncated edge of the Alcon AcrySof IOL optic. Note the interface between the relatively exuberant Soemmering's rings (pink-red material, left) and the IOL optic (clear space to the right). Note also the clear posterior capsule in lower right. (Hematoxylin and eosin stain, original magnification x40.)

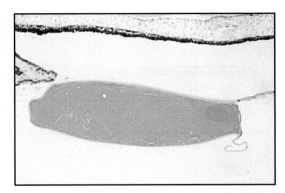

Figure 5-10B. A photomicrograph clearly demonstrating the barrier effect achieved with the square truncated edge of the Alcon AcrySof IOL optic. Note the interface between the relatively exuberant Soemmering's rings (pink-red material, left) and the IOL optic (clear space to the right). Note also the clear posterior capsule in lower right. (Masson's trichrome stain, original magnification x50.)

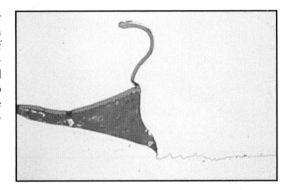

Figure 5-10C. A photomicrograph clearly demonstrating the barrier effect achieved with the square truncated edge of the Alcon AcrySof IOL optic. Note the interface between the relatively exuberant Soemmering's rings (pink-red material, left) and the IOL optic (clear space to the right). Note also the clear posterior capsule in lower right. (Hematoxylin and eosin stain, original magnification x50.)

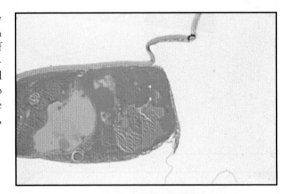

Figure 5-11A. Not only is the rate of PCO with the Alcon AcrySof IOL very low (see Chapter 7), the amount of ACO is also on average very low with this IOL (see Figures 3-12, 5-14). This figure is a AcrySof IOL gross photograph from in front (anterior or surgeon's view with cornea and iris removed), showing minimal opacification of the anterior capsule surrounding the capsulorhexis orifice.

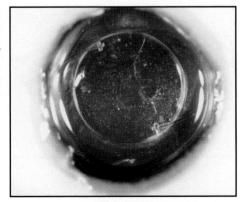

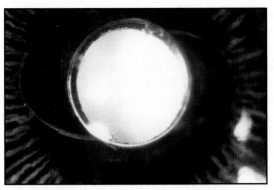

Figure 5-11B. Not only is the rate of PCO with the Alcon AcrySof IOL very low (see Chapter 7), the amount of ACO is also on average very low with this IOL (see Figures 3-12, 5-12). This figure is a gross photograph from behind (Miyake-Apple posterior photographic technique, same eye as Figure 5-11A) showing minimal reactivity of the anterior capsule (from Werner and associates).

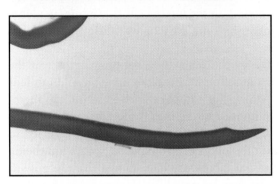

Figure 5-12. Photomicrograph of the Anterior capsule in an eye in which an Alcon AcrySof IOL had been implanted. This view of the capsulorhexis shows an ACO score of 0. Periodic acid-Schiff stain, original magnification x100 (from Werner and associates).

Summary of Alcon Acrysof™ Nd:Yag Rates and Biocompatibility Scores
(From Apple and assoc., 1999)

	Nd:Yag Laser Rates Range (0-100%)	Biocompatibility Score SRI X SRA Range (0-16)	Anterior Capsular Opacification (ACO) Scores Range (0-3)
Acrysof™ IOLs	1.7%	1.86	.51
Other Foldable IOLs	13.0%	4.03	1.23
Rigid IOLs	30.9%	6.92	1.00
All Other IOLs Since 1988	28.7%	4.70	1.16

Figure 5-13. According to our autopsy data, the Alcon AcrySof IOL not only has a low incidence of PCO (and hence requirement for Nd:YAG laser posterior capsulotomy), but also has low rates of Soemmering's ring formation and the lowest mean score of ACO among all lenses studied in our laboratory (Figure 5-12). Note that the value of 1.7% for the AcrySof IOL differs from our rate of 1.3% documented at a more recent date. (Courtesy of Dr. Liliana Werner and Dr. Nithi Visessook.)

concept of an IOL-capsule bio-adhesion was further supported by a study of RJ Linnola, who presented a bioactivity-based explanation for PCO, the "sandwich theory" (Linnola). Sandwich theory: bioactivity-based explanation for posterior capsule opacification.[5-7] According to the theory of Linnola and associates, if the IOL were of a bioactive material, it would allow a single lens epithelial cell to bond both to the IOL and the posterior capsule. This would produce a sandwich pattern including the IOL, the cell monolayer, and the posterior capsule. The sealed sandwich structure might prevent epithelial ingrowth behind the optic and thus inhibit PCO. Linnola, et al., have studied the proteins involved in the adhesion between the AcrySof lens and the capsule, 1) in vitro,[6,8] and more recently 2) in human globes obtained postmortem. Immunohistochemical staining of histological sections from pseudophakic human globes demonstrated that fribronectin and vitronectin were the major adhesion molecules present in the interface IOL-capsules in globes implanted with AcrySof lenses.[9,10] The protein-binding pattern was different in globes implanted with PMMA, silicone or hydrogel lenses.

Noting the low capsular reactivity induced by the Alcon AcrySof biomaterial and the low rates of PCO now being documented, the question immediately arises: would this lens be appropriate for pediatric implantation, where the complications of secondary membrane formation and PCO are major and common? During the last decade, application of adult surgical techniques to the treatment of congenital cataracts (Figure 5-14) has led to vast improvements in visual rehabilitation for this condition. Foldable lenses are now being successfully implanted in children. Studies in our laboratory have shown that the growth of the crystalline lens occurs very rapidly in the first 2 years of life (Figure 5-15). Based on this fact, and after analysis of experimental implantations of the AcrySof IOL in human eyes obtained postmortem in which a successful fit could be achieved (Figure 5-16), we believe at the time of this writing that this may be a potential lens of choice for pediatric implantation.

With its relatively flexible haptics, this lens is reasonably easy to insert. Some investigators believe that implantation of this lens may help avoid the necessity of a primary posterior capsulotomy, including a posterior continuous curvilinear capsulorhexis (PCCC), which heretofore has almost always been the case in pediatric cataracts. Figures 5-17A and B show examples of successful pediatric implantation of the AcrySof IOL performed by Dr. Abhay Vasavada of Ahamabad, India. Successful pediatric implantation in developing countries such as India is extremely important, as childhood cataracts are extremely common in many of these regions-much more common than in the industrialized world.

Explantation of the AcrySof IOL is extremely rare and in most cases documented in our laboratory has been related to surgical complications or dioptric miscalculations. In a few instances, the IOL has been explanted for various types of visual aberrations, including glare and halos. Reflections on the square truncated edge of the lens may play a role in creating these aberrations, but to date they have been reported rarely and the pathogenesis and nature require further study. Our current counsel is that the usefulness of this truncated edge in reducing the incidence of PCO would overpower the potential visual aberrations possibly induced by this IOL design, but final conclusions await further studies.

In rare instances, fine linear creases at the site of the fold on the acrylic optic as seen in Figures 5-18A and B have rarely caused visual sequelae that were sufficient to lead to IOL explantation and exchange. The lens illustrated in Figures 5-18A and B is a case where the

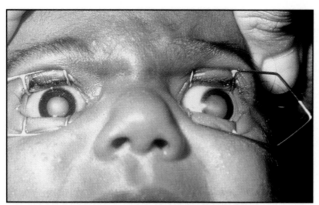

Figure 5-14. The finding of low capsular-epithelial reactivity of the AcrySof IOL suggests that this design may a useful IOL for treatment of congenital cataract as seen here. Secondary membrane and PCO formation are the most common complications of pediatric implantation and any design that would minimize these would be favorable. (Courtesy of Dr. Jagat Ram and Suresh K. Pandey.)

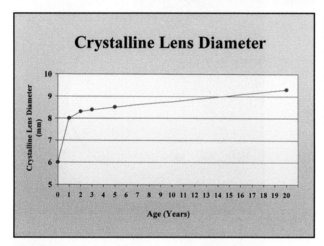

Figure 5-15A. Studies in our laboratory have shown that much (90%) of the growth of the human eye occurs during the first 2 months of life. This suggests that implantation of an adult-size IOL may be feasible in very young infants. (= crystalline lens diameter.) (Courtesy of Bluestein and associates.)

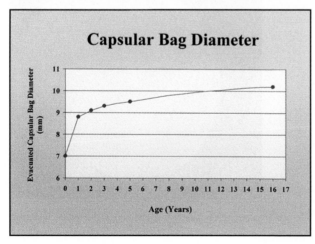

Figure 5-15B. Studies in our laboratory have shown that much (90%) of the growth of the human eye occurs during the first 2 months of life. This suggests that implantation of an adult-size IOL may be feasible in very young infants. (= capsular bag diameter.) (Courtesy of Bluestein and associates.)

Figure 5-16. Studies in our laboratory using the Miyake-Apple posterior photographic technique have shown that the Alcon AcrySof design fits satisfactorily in the eyes of very young children. This is a human eye obtained postmortem from a child who died at 21 days. There is a slight ovaling of the capsular bag, but generally a good fit (experimental surgery performed by Jagat Ram, MD).

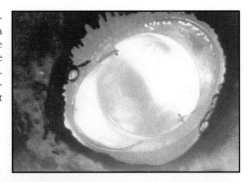

Figure 5-17A. An example of successful implantation of an Alcon AcrySof IOL into the eye of a young child. Note the posterior capsulorhexis in Figure 5-17B. (Courtesy of Abhay Vasavada, Ahmedabad, India.)

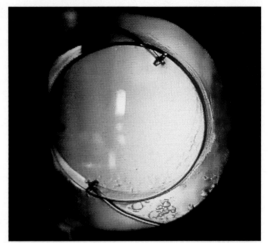

Figure 5-17B. An example of successful implantation of an Alcon AcrySof IOL into the eye of a young child. Note the posterior capsulorhexis. (Courtesy of Abhay Vasavada, Ahmedabad, India.)

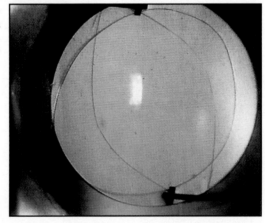

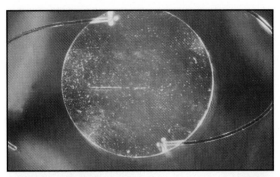

Figure 5-18A. Gross photograph of the entire lens. Complications requiring explantation of the Alcon AcrySof IOL are very rare. These figures illustrate the complication of a crease on the IOL caused by overzealous manipulation during insertion. This can be easily avoided with careful surgical technique and is rarely clinically significant. We have only seen two cases with symptoms that led to explantation and accession in our laboratory.

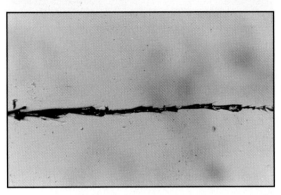

Figure 5-18B. High power gross photograph of the lens shown in Figure 5-18A showing details of the crease caused by the folding process. Complications requiring explantation of the Alcon AcrySof IOL are very rare. These figures illustrate the complication of a crease on the IOL caused by overzealous manipulation during insertion. This can be easily avoided with careful surgical technique and is rarely clinically significant. We have only seen two cases with symptoms that led to explantation and accession in our laboratory.

patient actually identified horizontal lines within the field of vision. This problem may be minimized by careful warming of the lens and very careful folding and insertion.

The issue of vacuoles ("glistenings") within the optical component of the AcrySof IOL has long been controversial (Figures 5-19 to 5-21). We first noticed this in an AcrySof IOL sent to our laboratory for analysis in 1994. A clinical photograph of this IOL is seen in Figure 5-19 (courtesy Dr. Louis Nichamin, Brookville, Pa). Our investigations have shown that the glistenings only occur under fluid, basically representing an influx of aqueous humor into the optic (Figure 5-21). The vacuoles can be induced in vitro by warming a lens to 37° and then cooling it to room temperature.

This may represent at least one factor in the pathogenesis of this condition. The Alcon AcrySof is often warmed before surgery. If allowed to cool in solution before insertion, the vacuoles may ensue. They have been reported in as many as 50% of cases in some series. The important fact regarding these is that, to our knowledge, very few cases have led to truly significant clinical consequences. To date, we have not seen any clinicopathologic correlation that would suggest that use of these lenses should be limited because of this problem. It should also be emphasized that formation of "glistenings" is not limited to the AcrySof IOL, but may be seen with PMMA IOLs (Figure 5-22) and silicone IOLs (Figure 5-23). As in the AcrySof, glistening in these latter biomaterials has not been shown to cause any adverse clinical sequelae.

Figure 5-19. The occurrence of vacuoles within the IOL optical component of the Alcon AcrySof IOL "glistenings" has been reported. These represent in-flow of aqueous fluid into the substance of the lens optic following implantation. In the overwhelming majority of cases these have been found not to be of clinical significance. This is a clinical photograph of glistenings in the optic of Alcon AcrySof IOL.

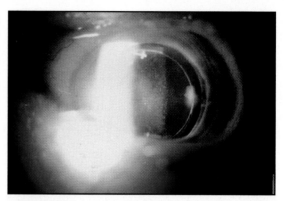

Figure 5-20A. Clinical photograph of another case showing the occurrence of vacuoles within an Alcon AcrySof IOL. The pathogenesis may be multifactorial, but we have found that preoperative warming and subsequent cooling of an immersed lens before implantation may initiate vacuole formation.

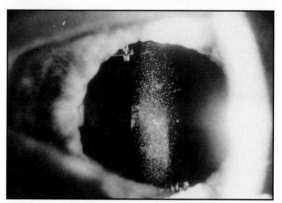

Figure 5-20B. High power gross photograph showing moderate numbers of the occurrence of vacuoles within an Alcon AcrySof IOL. The pathogenesis may be multifactorial, but we have found that preoperative warming and subsequent cooling of an immersed lens before implantation may initiate vacuole formation. These lesions can be found in a significant percentage of cases upon close inspection, but they rarely cause clinically significant visual problems.

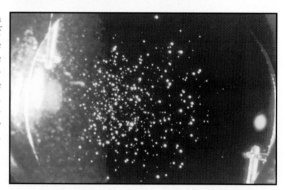

Figure 5-21. High power photomicrograph through the IOL optic of an Alcon AcrySof IOL showing the glistenings, which consist of tiny spaces within the substance of the polymer into which aqueous fluid has diffused (original magnification x400).

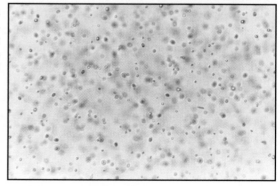

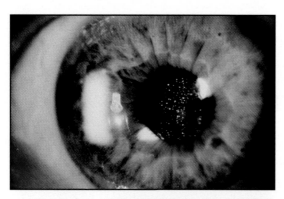

Figure 5-22. Vacuoles not only occur with the hydrophobic acrylic design, but have also been noted in other biomaterials such as PMMA, as noted in this clinical photograph. (Courtesy of Edmund Wilkins, MD, Kentucky.)

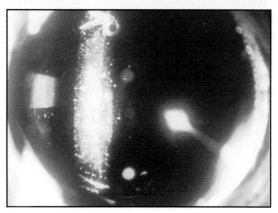

Figure 5-23. Vacuoles have also been demonstrated in eyes with silicone IOLs. Therefore, their occurrence is not entirely biomaterial-specific. It is important to emphasize that "glistenings" generally do not cause visual problems.

SUMMARY

The most notable characteristic of the AcrySof IOL is the apparent lack of lens epithelial cellular reactivity that occurs within the capsule and around the IOL. Cellular proliferation of both anterior and posterior capsule are the lowest that we have noted with any biomaterial (see Figure 5-13). Decreased reactivity of the anterior capsule is, of course, important in improving the view of the peripheral retina for the vitreoretinal surgeon, as well as preventing such sequelae as fibrosis-induced decentration and capsulorhexis contraction syndrome (capsular phimosis) (see Chapter 7). The lack of proliferation of cells across the posterior capsule is of paramount importance in helping reduce the incidence of PCO, which to date is the lowest among all lenses studied in or database. The apparently good biocompatibility of this IOL is probably related in part to its close adherence with both the anterior and posterior capsules. This material has an adhesive "sticky" characteristic. This helps explain the fact that, following apparent good removal of cells by hydrodissection-enhanced cortical cleanup, the vast majority of capsular bags associated with this design remains clear. The second line of defense against PCO, the square truncated optic edge probably represents an "icing on the cake" with this lens, helping to lower the observed incidence of PCO even further. The 1.3% Nd:YAG rate we have noted (Figures 7-79 and 7-80) represents the lowest Nd:YAG rate observed with any current or former

IOL. Complications (eg, visual disturbances) related to folding creases, "glistenings," and the square optic edge have been reported. However, these have been rare, and significant clinical sequelae are unusual.

REFERENCES

1. Anderson C, Koch DD, Green G, et al. Alcon Acrysof acrylic intraocular lens. In: Martin RG, Gills JP, eds. *Foldable Intraocular Lenses.* Thorofare, NJ: SLACK Incorporated; 1993.

2. Oshika T, Nagata T, Ishii Y. Adhesion of lens capsule to intraocular lenses of polymethyl-methacrylate, silicone, and acrylic foldable materials: An experimental study [see comments]. *British Journal of Ophthalmology.* 1998;82:549-553.

3. Nagata T, Minakata A, Watanabe I. Adhesiveness of AcrySof to a collagen film. *J Cataract Refract Surg.* 1998;24(3):367-370.

4. Ursell PG, Spalton DJ, Pande MV. Anterior capsule stability in eyes with intraocular lenses made of poly(methyl methacrylate), silicone, and AcrySof. *J Cataract Refract Surg.* 1997;23:1532-1538.

5. Linnola RJ. Sandwich theory: Bioactivity-based explanation for posterior capsule opacification. *J Cataract Refract Surg.* 1997;23:1539-1532.

6. Linnola RJ, Sund M, Ylonen R, Pihlajaniemi T. Adhesion of soluble fibronectin, laminin, and collagen type IV to intraocular lens materials. *J Cataract Refract Surg.* 1999 [In Press].

7. Linnola RJ, Salonen JI, Happonen RP. Intraocular lens bioactivity tested by rabbit corneal tissue cultures. *J Cataract Refract Surg.* 1999 [In Press].

8. Linola RJ. Acrylate intraocular lenses hinder posterior migration of epithelium; activity tested by corneal tissue cultures. XVth Congress of the ESCRS *Symposium on Cataract, IOL and Refractive Surgery.* Prauge, September 1997.

9. Linnola RJ, Werner L, Pandey SK, Escobar-Gomez M, Zuoyko S, Apple DJ. Adhesion of fibronectin, vitronectin, laminin, and collagen type IV to intraocular lens materials in human autospy eyes: Part I: histological sections. *J Cataract Refract Surg.* 1999 [In Press].

10. Linnola RJ, Werner L, Pandey SK, Escobar-Gomez M, Zuoyko S, Apple DJ. Adhesion of fibronectin, vitronectin, laminin, and collagen type IV to intraocular lens materials in human autopsy eyes: Part II: explanted IOLs. *J Cataract Refract Surg.* 1999 [In Press].

BIBLIOGRAPHY

Arshinoff S. Does a tight capsular bag cause glistenings? *J Cataract Refract Surg.* 1998;24:6.

Bluestein EC, Wilson ME, Wang XH, Apple DJ. Dimensions of the pediatric crystalline lens implications for intraocular lenses in children. *J Pediatric Ophthalmology Strabismus.* 1996;33:18-20.

Dhaliwal DK, Mamalis N, Olson RJ, et al. Visual significance of glistenings seen in the AcrySof intraocular lens. *J Cataract Refract Surg.* 1996;22:452-457.

Fry LL. Another possible cause of forceps-induced scratching of a foldable acrylic intraocular lens. *Arch Ophthalmol.* 1997;115:823.

Hayashi K, et al. Capsular capture of silicone intraocular lenses. *J Cataract Refract Surg.* 1996;22(supp 2):1267-1271.

Hayashi K, Hayashi H, Nakao F, Hayashi F. Reduction in the area of the anterior capsule opening after polymethylmethacrylate, silicone, and soft acrylic intraocular lens implantation. *Am J Ophthalmol.* 1997;123:441-447.

Hollick EJ, Spalton DJ, Ursell PG, Pande MV. Biocompatibility of poly(methyl methacrylate), silicone, and AcrySof intraocular lenses: randomized comparison of the cellular reaction on the anterior lens surface. *J Cataract Refract Surg.* 1998;24:361-366.

Kamiya H, Kozuka T. Comparison of postoperative inflammation in eyes with acrylic and heparin lens insertion in diabetics. *Jap J Cataract Refract Surg.* 1996;10:276-280.

Kohnen T, Magdowski G, Koch DD. Scanning electron microscopic analysis of foldable acrylic and hydrogel intraocular lenses. *J Cataract Refract Surg.* 1996;22(suppl 2):1342-1350.

Kohnen T. The variety of foldable intraocular lens materials. *J Cataract Refract Surg.* 1996;22(supp 2):1255-1258.

Kohnen S, Ferrer A, Brauweiler P. Visual function in pseudophakic eyes with poly(methyl metacrylate), silicone, and acrylic intraocular lenses. *J Cataract Refract Surg.* 1996;22(supp 2):1303-1307.

Lee GA. Cracked acrylic intraocular lens requiring explantation. *Aust NZ J Ophthalmol.* 1997;25:71-73.

Lemon LC, Shin DH, Song MS, et al. Comparative study of silicone versus acrylic foldable lens implantation in primary glaucoma triple procedure. *Ophthalmology.* 1997;104:1708-1713.

Mamalis N, Phillips B, Kopp CH, Crandall AS, Olson RJ. Neodymium:YAG capsulotomy rates after phacoemulsification with silicone posterior chamber intraocular lenses. *J Cataract Refract Surg.* 1996;22(supp 2):1296-1302.

Mengual E, Garcia J, Elvira JC, Ramon Hueso J. Clinical results of AcrySof intraocular lens implantation. *J Cataract Refract Surg.* 1998;24(1):114-117.

Milazzo S, Turut P, Blin H. Alterations to the AcrySof intraocular lens during folding. *J Cataract Refract Surg.* 1996;22(supp 2):1351-1354.

Mutlu FM, Bilge AH, Altinsoy HI, Yumusak E. The role of capsulotomy and intraocular lens type on tilt and decentration of polymethylmethacrylate and foldable acrylic lenses. *Ophthalmologica.* 1998;212:359-363.

Neuhann TH. Intraocular folding of an acrylic lens for explantation through a small incision cataract wound. *J Cataract Refract Surg.* 1996;22(suppl 2):1383-1386.

Oh KT. Optimal folding axis for acrylic intraocular lenses. *J Cataract Refract Surg.* 1996;22:667-670.

Omar O, Mamalis N, Veiga J, Maura M, Olson RJ. Scanning electron microscopic characteristics of small incision intraocular lenses. *Ophthalmology.* 1996;103(7):1124-1129.

Omar O, Pirayesh A, Mamalis N, Olson RJ. In vitro analysis of AcrySof intraocular lens glistenings in AcryPak and Wagon Wheel packaging. *J Cataract Refract Surg.* 1998;24:107-113.

Oshika T, Suzuki Y, Kizaki H, Yaguchi S. Two year clinical study of a soft acrylic intraocular lens. *J Cataract Refract Surg.* 1996;22(2):104-109.

Oshika T, Shiokawa Y. Effect of folding on the optical quality of soft acrylic intraocular lenses. *J Cataract Refract Surg.* 1996;22(supp 2):1360-1364.

Pfister DR. Stress fractures after folding an acrylic intraocular lens. *Am J Ophthalmol.* 1996;121:572-574.

Seward HC. Folding intraocular lenses: Materials and methods. *Br J Ophthalmol.* 1997;81:340-341.

Shugar J. Implantation of AcrySof acrylic intraocular lenses. *J Cataract Refract Surg.* 1996;22(supp 2):1355-1359.

Shugar J. Implantation of multiple foldable acrylic posterior chamber lenses in the capsular bag for high hyperopia. *J Cataract Refract Surg.* 1996;22(supp 2):1368-1372.

Ursell P, Spalton D, Pande MV, et al. Relationship between IOL biomaterials and posterior capsule opacification. *J Cataract Refract Surg.* 1998;24(3):352-360.

Vasavada A, Chauhan H. Intraocular lens implantation in infants with congenital cataracts, *J Cataract Refract Surg.* 1994;20:592-598.

Vrabec MP, Syverud JC, Burgess CJ. Forceps-induced scratching of a foldable acrylic intraocular lens. *Arch Ophthalmol.* 1996;114:777.

Werner L, Pandey SK, Escobar-Gomez M, Visessook N, Peng Q, Apple DJ. Anterior capsule opacification: A histopathological study comparing different IOL styles. *Ophthalmology.* 1999 [In Press].

Foldable Intraocular Lenses
Not in USA Autopsy Database

Section

3

Foldable Intraocular Lenses

Not in USA Autopsy Database

Chapter 6

Silicone, Acrylics, and Hydrogels

There are several foldable IOL designs manufactured in the United States and elsewhere that have not yet been implanted in a large series in the United States and are therefore not yet available in our USA autopsy globe database (Table 6-1). These include several silicone, hydrophobic and hydrophilic acrylic, and hydrogel designs that are still under investigation or have been very recently approved for use in the United States. Although we cannot directly comment on them, based on clinicopathologic correlation, we will catalog them in general and briefly illustrate them and list specifications. With the exception of a few cases currently available with clinicopathologic illustrations in our databases, most information here is derived from the manufacturers.

We recently developed a collaboration with Professor Ruediger Welt, Ludwigshafen, Germany, to form a sister center in Europe (Center for IOL Research, Europe), through which we hope to accession more specimens from that region. Such additional material in the database will help increase and broaden our knowledge of these lenses.

SILICONE

Figures 6-1A and B are examples of early silicone disc IOLs that were manufactured in Europe in the late 1980s. The explanted IOL in Figure 6-1A was removed in its entirety within the capsular bag following dislocation. The majority of these IOLs have proved satisfactory. However, they have largely been superseded by classic three-piece haptic designs, and especially in the United States, foldable silicone plate IOLs.

Table 6-1.

Foldable IOLs, Approved and Investigational, 2000
Not Available in the USA Autopsy Database

Design (selected representative examples)	Model	Company	Diameter (mm)	Optic Diameter (mm)	Water Content	Haptic Material
I. Silicone						
a. Pharmacia-Upjohn						
3 piece silicone IOL	CeeOn (912)	Pharmacia & Upjohn	12.0	Biconvex, 6.0	<1%	PVDF
3 piece silicone IOL	CeeOn Edge	Pharmacia & Upjohn	12.0	Biconvex, 5.5	<1%	
b. Baush and Lomb						
3 piece silicone IOL	Soflex, LI Series	Baush and Lomb Surgical, Inc.	13.0	Biconvex, 6.0	<1%	PMMA
3 piece silicone IOL	Silens 6 (DomiLens Corp.)	Baush and Lomb Surgical, Inc.	12.5	Biconvex, 6.0	<1%	PMMA
II. Acrylics						
a. Hydrophobic (dry packed)						
3 piece arylic IOL	AR-40	Allergan, Inc.	13.0	Biconvex, 6.0	<1%	PMMA
b. Hydrophilic (wet packed)						
Baush and Lomb						
3 piece Hydrogel IOL	Hydroview H55s/H60M	Baush and Lomb Surgical, Inc.	12.0/12.5	Biconvex, 5.5/6.0	<1%	PMMA
1-piece Acrygel IOL	EasAcryl1	Bausch and Lomb Surgical, Inc.	11.0	Biconvex, 6.0	26%	Acrygel
1-piece Acrygel IOL	HE26C	Bausch and Lomb Surgical, Inc.	12.0	Biconvex, 6.0	26%	Acrygel
Ciba Vision						
3 piece Hydrogel IOL	MemoryLensä U940A	Ciba Vision, Inc.	13.6	Biconvex, 6.0	20%	Polypropylene
Corneal						
1-piece Acrygel IOL	AC-55	Corneal, Inc.	10.5	Biconvex, 5.5-6.0	26%	Acrylgel
1-piece Acrygel IOL	HPFlex, HP 58	Corneal, Inc.	11.5 – 13.0	Biconvex, 5.8-6.0	26%	PMMA
1-piece Acrygel IOL	Quatro	Corneal, Inc.	11.25	Biconvex, 6.0	26%	Acrygel
1-piece Acrygel IOL	ACR6D Acrygel	Corneal, Inc.	12.0	Biconvex, 6.0	26%	Acrygel
1-piece Acrylgel IOL	M. 10 50	Corneal, Inc.	10.50	Biconvex, 5.75	26%	Acrygel
Rayner						
1-piece Acrygel IOL	Raysoft	Rayner, Ltd.	10.50	Biconvex, 5.75	26%	Acrygel

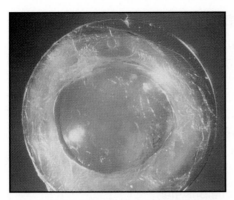

Figure 6-1. Several silicone disc IOL designs were fabricated and implemented in the late 1980s and early 1990s. This figure is a gross photograph of a silicone disc IOL that had subluxated. It was explanted with its surrounding capsule (Courtesy of Rueidger Welt, Ludwigshaften, Germany).

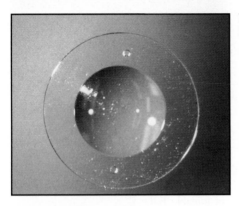

Figure 6-1B. Gross photograph of another silicone disk IOL explanted because of malposition.

PHARMACIA-UPJOHN 900 SERIES

In the mid 1990s, Pharmacia-Upjohn, Inc., Bridgewater, NJ, entered the foldable lens market with its 900 series of silicone three-piece designs. The CeeOn 912 design (Table 6-2 and Figures 6-2 and 6-3) is based on the general design of their flexible and very successful one-piece all-PMMA (Cap C) design, illustrated in Figures 2-56 and 2-58. Note in Figures 6-2 and 6-3 and Figures 2-56 to 2-58 how the haptic emerges directly off of the optic and then bends very shortly thereafter. The remaining haptic then is advantageously shaped so that it forms a smooth C-shaped configuration. This provides an excellent fit and configuration within the capsular bag. Selected manufacturer's specifications of the 912 IOL are listed in Table 6-2. We have little data on these lenses in our laboratory, but their clinical success has apparently been limited, partially owing to significantly high PCO rates.

PHARMACIA-UPJOHN CEEON EDGE 911

Use of the CeeOn 912 IOL is slowly being curtailed and they are being replaced by another new and very promising design from Pharmacia-Upjohn, the CeeOn Edge 911 IOL (Figures 6-4 to 6-6A). A manufacturer's illustration is provided in Figure 6-4 and selected specifications are listed in Table 6-3. In the United States, it is only available for

Table 6-2.
CeeOn (912)
Pharmacia-Upjohn, Inc.

Design	3-piece-silicone-IOL
Model	CeeOn 912
Manufacturer	Pharmacia-Upjohn, Inc.
Overall diameter [mm]	12.0
Optic diameter [mm]	Biconvex 5.5
Optic material	Silicone polymer
Water content	<1%
Refractive index	1.43
Haptic material	PMMA
Haptic angulation	6°
A-constant	117.8
ACD [mm]	4.6
Diopter [range]	+10.0 to +30.0
Incision [mm]	N/A

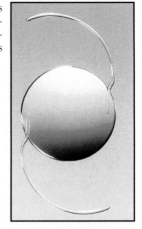

Figure 6-2. Pharmacia-Upjohn has manufactured a series of foldable IOLs with silicone optics, the CeeOn 900 series. Note in this manufacturer's illustration that this IOL has a design and unique haptic configuration that is similar to their popular capsular rigid PMMA design (Cap C design) (See Figures 2-56 to 2-58). (Courtesy of Pharmacia & Upjohn, Bridgewater, NJ.)

Figure 6-3. Gross photograph of an explanted CeeOn 912 IOL, removed because of surgery-related complications.

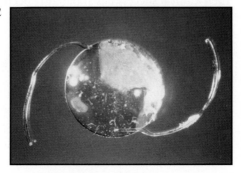

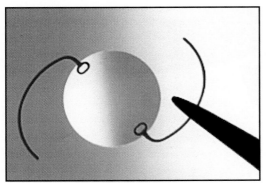

Figure 6-4. A more recent foldable IOL in the Pharmacia-Upjohn CeeOn 900 series is the CeeOn 911 Edge design lens, not yet available for general implantation in the United States. It has a silicone optic and a polyvinylidene haptic (see Table 6-3). This is a manufacturer's illustration, showing the characteristic capsular C-shaped haptic configuration (see Figures 6-2 and 2-56 to 2-58).

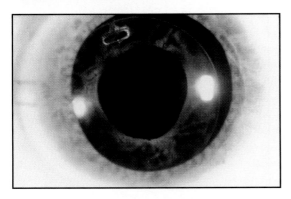

Figure 6-5A. Widespread implantation of the Pharmacia-Upjohn CeeOn Edge 911 design has not yet occurred in the USA, so specimens are not available for autopsy analysis. However, some lenses have been implanted for experimental and investigational studies. Note that they were implanted with a relatively small capsulorhexis so that the diameter of the capsulorhexis was smaller than that of the IOL optic. The lens is recognizable owing to the oval-rectangular looping configuration of the tips of the haptics at the site where they enter the peripheral optic. This is a clinical photograph. (Courtesy of Kerry D. Solomon, MD, Charleston, SC.)

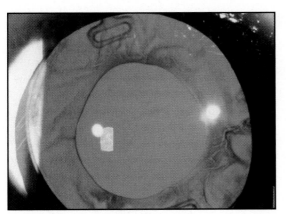

Figure 6-5B. Widespread implantation of the Pharmacia-Upjohn CeeOn Edge 911 design has not yet occurred in the USA, so specimens are not available for autopsy analysis. However, some lenses have been implanted for experimental and investigational studies. Note that they were implanted with a relatively small capsulorhexis so that the diameter of the capsulorhexis was smaller than that of the IOL optic. The lens is recognizable owing to the oval-rectangular looping configuration of the tips of the haptics at the site where they enter the peripheral optic. This is a clinical photograph with transillumination. (Courtesy of Kerry D. Solomon, MD, Charleston, SC.)

Figure 6-6A. The CeeOn Edge 911 IOL has a square truncated edge. This scanning electron micrograph shows a side (sagittal) view of the optic. The square edge and a small portion of the haptic are seen on the left (original magnification x50).

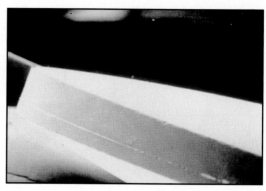

Figure 6-6B. The CeeOn Edge 911 IOL has a square truncated edge. This is a photomicrograph of a portion of a capsular bag of a rabbit following an experimental implantation of the Pharmacia-Upjohn CeeOn 911 Edge IOL. The large mass of red material is a massive Soemmering's ring and the capsule fornix is to the left in this illustration. Cortex extends towards the visual axis (right) but has been abruptly and totally blocked by the edge of the optic. The optic biomaterial has dissolved out during tissue preparation. The posterior capsule (lower right) is cell free. Experimental surgery prepared by Qun Peng, MD, Charleston, South Carolina. (Hematoxylin and eosin stain, x150.)

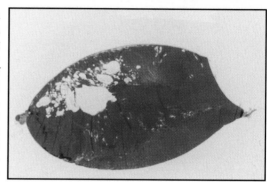

Table 6-3.
CeeOn Edge
Pharmacia-Upjohn, Inc.

Design	3-piece-silicone-IOL
Model	CeeOn Edge
Manufacturer	Pharmacia-Upjohn, Inc.
Overall diameter [mm]	12.0
Optic diameter [mm]	Biconvex 6.0
Optic material	Silicone polymer
Water content	<1%
Refractive index	1.46
Haptic material	PVDF (polyvinylidene flouride)
Haptic angulation	6°
A-constant	118.3
ACD [mm]	4.9
Diopter [range]	+12.0 to +28.0
Incision [mm]	N/A

limited investigational implantation and has therefore not surfaced in an autopsy database. Figures 6-5A and B show the CeeOn Edge 911 IOL in a patient implanted in an investigational study by Dr. Kerry Solomon of Charleston, SC. Note the circular capsulorhexis situated centrally on the lens optic. The lens is easily identifiable by noting the rectangular looping configuration of the haptic where it inserts into the substance of the optic.

Our only laboratory experience with this lens is in experimental rabbit implantation studies. The edge of the optic is square or truncated (Figure 6-6A), similar to that previously described with the three-piece elastimide-polyimide IOL (Chapter 4, Figure 4-1, 4-2A and B), as well as the Alcon AcrySof IOL (Chapter 5, Figures 5-2A through C). As will be discussed in Chapter 7, this geometric shape is efficacious in enhancing the optic's barrier effect, helping to reduce the incidence of PCO. The histopathologic profile noted by the square-edged optic of the CeeOn Edge 911 lens, as seen in our experimental rabbit study (Figure 6-6B), is identical to that seen with the elastimide-polyimide IOL (Figures 4-1 and 4-2A and B) and the Alcon AcrySof IOL (Figures 5-2A through C and 5-8 to 5-10).

In summary, based on its design, the use of a tried and true, well-established silicone material for the optic, the use of a unique polyvinylidine fluoride haptic material, with favorable "memory" features, the well-designed Cap C haptic configuration design of this lens, the favorable optic edge geometry of this lens, and results obtained in European clinical studies, this is a markedly improved lens over the early CeeOn 912.

BAUSCH AND LOMB SURGICAL

Solflex, LI Series (Formerly IOLab Corporation) and Silens Series (Formerly DomiLens Corporation)

Modern silicone lenses manufactured by Bausch and Lomb Surgical are illustrated in Figures 6-7 to 6-9. These represent lens designs previously manufactured by IOLab Corporation (Figures 6-7 and 6-8 are Tables 6-4 and 6-5) and DomiLens Corporation (Figure 6-9 and Table 6-6). Only a handful are available in our autopsy series. Examples are shown in Figure 6-8.

Figure 6-7. Bausch and Lomb Surgical manufactures a silicone optic IOL in their Solflex series. This is a manufacturer's diagram with dimensions (see Tables 6-4 and 6-5).

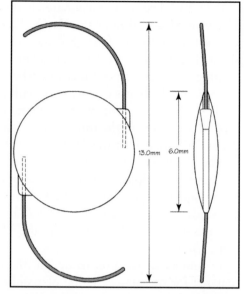

Figure 6-8A. The Solflex Series of Bausch and Lomb silicone IOLs (previously IOLab Corporation) have only rarely been accessioned in our laboratory. This figure shows an example of these eyes, in a human eye obtained postmortem. (Miyake-Apple posterior photographic technique.) This figure shows mild retention of cortex and formation of Soemmering's ring.

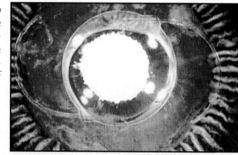

Figure 6-8B. The Solflex Series of Bausch and Lomb silicone IOLs (previously IOLab Corporation) have only rarely been accessioned in our laboratory. This figure shows an example of these eyes, in a human eye obtained postmortem. (Miyake-Apple posterior photographic technique.) This figure shows more advanced Soemmering's ring formation around the IOL.

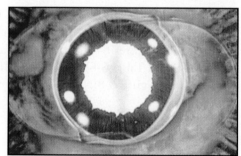

Figure 6-8C. The Solflex Series of Bausch and Lomb silicone IOLs (previously IOLab Corporation) have only rarely been accessioned in our laboratory. This figure shows an example of these eyes, in a human eye obtained postmortem. (Miyake-Apple posterior photographic technique.) This figure shows extensive Soemmering's ring formation around the implant.

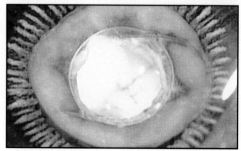

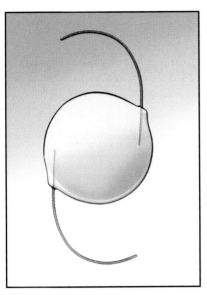

Figure 6-9. Bausch and Lomb also manufacturers a silicone lens designated as the Silens series (previously DomiLens Corporation). This is a manufacturer's illustration. (See also Table 6-6).

Table 6-4.	
Soflex	
Bausch and Lomb Surgical, Inc.	
Design	3-piece-silicone-IOL
Model	Soflex LI 61U
Manufacturer	Bausch & Lomb Surgical, Inc.
Overall diameter [mm]	13.0
Optic diameter [mm]	Biconvex 6.0
Optic material	Silicone polymer
Water content	<1%
Refractive index	1.43
Haptic material	PMMA
Haptic angulation	5°
A-constant	118
ACD [mm]	5.0
Diopter [range]	+5.0 to +30.0
Incision [mm]	N/A

Table 6-5.
Soflex 2
Bausch and Lomb Surgical, Inc.

Design	3-piece-silicone-IOL
Model	Soflex 2
Manufacturer	Bausch & Lomb Surgical, Inc.
Overall diameter [mm]	12.5
Optic diameter [mm]	Biconvex 6.0
Optic material	Silicone polymer
Water content	<1%
Refractive index	
Haptic material	PMMA
Haptic angulation	0°
A-constant	118.1
ACD [mm]	4.75
Diopter [range]	+0.0 to +30.0
Incision [mm]	3.2 to 3.5

Table 6-6.
Silens 6
Bausch and Lomb Surgical, Inc.

Design	3-piece-silicone-IOL
Model	Silens 6
Manufacturer	Bausch & Lomb Surgical, Inc.
Overall diameter [mm]	12.5
Optic diameter [mm]	Biconvex 6.0
Optic material	Silicone polymer
Water content	<1%
Refractive index	
Haptic material	PMMA
Haptic angulation	0°
A-constant	118.1
ACD [mm]	4.75
Diopter [range]	+10.0 to +30.0
Incision [mm]	N/A

ACRYLICS AND HYDROGELS

The term acrylic is a generic term with little specific meaning. For example, Ridley termed his original PMMA lens designs as "acrylic." With the modern acrylic IOLs it is important to subdivide these into the hydrophobic and hydrophilic groups. The hydrophobic (dry packed) group includes the Alcon AcrySof IOL (see Chapter 5) and a more recently introduced design from Allergan Corporation-the AR—40 IOL. The latter has not yet been implanted in large numbers in the United States. In contrast to the hydrophobic acrylics, there is a large category of lenses that are fabricated from biomaterials that are hydrophilic. These necessarily are packed in fluid (wet packed). These are designated as hydrophilic acrylics or hydrogels. Two early examples of wet-packed hydrophilic lenses, illustrated later in this chapter include an early prototype hydrogel lens (see Figure 6-19 later in this chapter) and the Alcon IOGel IOL from the late 1980s (see Figure 6-20 later in this chapter). We had the opportunity to study the latter lens in experimental Miyake-Apple insertion studies. We determined that some of the early models were oversized, with a poor fit in the capsular bag. This IOL was highly biocompatible, but problems with dislocation from the capsular bag after Nd:YAG laser posterior capsulotomy necessitated removal from the market.[1]

The terms "hydrophilic acrylic" and "hydrogel" are often used interchangeably. There are significant basic differences but we describe these as a group in this section.

HYDROPHOBIC (DRY-PACKED)

Allergan AR-40

This is the only IOL (Figures 6-10 to 6-11) in this section that is hydrophobic. Manufacturer's specifications are listed in Table 6-7. We have done preclinical experimental rabbit studies with this lens and found good biocompatibility, with good design and manufacturing quality. Autopsy eyes with this lens in our database are not available.

HYDROPHILIC (WET-PACKED)

Bausch and Lomb Surgical Hydroview Hydrogel Intraocular Lens

This IOL (Figures 6-12 to 6-14) has many unique features. It is the only lens on the market with a foldable hydrophilic optic and PMMA haptic. It is manufactured in such a way that it basically looks like and functions as a one-piece design (Figure 6-12). Manufacturer's specifications are listed in Table 6-8. The only two autopsy specimens we have received have been from Italy (courtesy of Dr. G. Ravilico, Trieste, Italy; Figures 6-13A and B). These two examples show good results. We have received eight explants (Figure 6-14), and have noted calcuim deposits on the surface of five of these lenses, a phenomenon somewhat analogous to that which occurs on hydrogel contact lenses. Further

Figure 6-10A. The only other hydrophobic acrylic IOL, in addition to the Alcon AcrySof IOL (Chapter 5), is the Allergan AR-40 design, composed of an acrylic polymer optic with PMMA haptics. This IOL is not yet available in our USA autopsy database. This is a manufacturer's diagram with dimensions (Figure 6-10B) (see also Table 6-7).

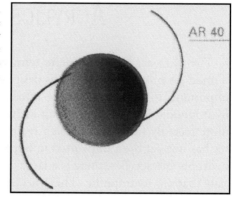

Figure 6-10B. The only other hydrophobic acrylic IOL, in addition to the Alcon AcrySof IOL (Chapter 5), is the Allergan AR-40 design, composed of an acrylic polymer optic with PMMA haptics. This IOL is not yet available in our USA autopsy database. This is a manufacturer's diagram (Figure 6-10A) with dimensions (see also Table 6-7).

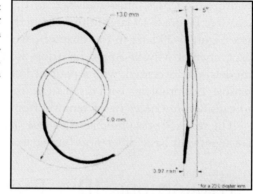

Figure 6-11. Clinical photograph of the AR-40 well-centered in an eye. We do not have clinicopathologic data regarding this IOL.

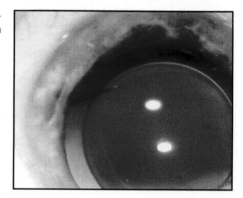

Table 6-7. AR-40 Allergan, Inc.	
Design	3-piece-acrylic-IOL
Model	AR-40
Manufacturer	Allergan, Inc.
Overall diameter [mm]	13.0
Optic diameter [mm]	Biconvex 6.0
Optic material	Hydrophobic acrylic polymer
Water content	N/A
Refractive index	1.47
Haptic material	PMMA
Haptic angulation	5°
A-constant	118.4
ACD [mm]	5.2
Diopter [range]	+10 to +30
Incision [mm]	3.2

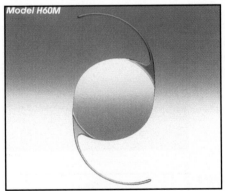

Figure 6-12A. Bausch and Lomb Surgical, Inc. manufactures a hydrophilic hydrogel design, the Hydroview H-55S and H60M series. This was approved by the Food and Drug Administration (FDA) in mid 1999. This lens (formerly Storz Surgical) is a one-piece IOL design with PMMA haptics fused to an 18% water content hydrogel polymer optic material. This lens is not yet available in our USA autopsy database. This is a manufacturer's illustration and diagram with dimensions (Figure 6-12B).

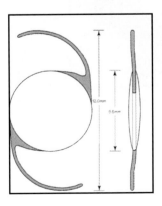

Figure 6-12B. Bausch and Lomb Surgical, Inc. manufactures a hydrophilic hydrogel design, the Hydroview H-55S and H60M series. This was approved by the Food and Drug Administration (FDA) in mid 1999. This lens (formerly Storz Surgical) is a one-piece IOL design with PMMA haptics fused to an 18% water content hydrogel polymer optic material. This lens is not yet available in our USA autopsy database. This is a manufacturer's illustration (Figure 6-12A) and diagram with dimensions.

Figure 6-13A. Gross photograph of an eye obtained postmortem (Miyake-Apple posterior photographic technique) showing a well-centered Bausch and Lomb Surgical Hydroview IOL with good clarity of the media. Note complete cortical cleanup. (Courtesy of Dr. G. Ravalico Trieste, Italy).

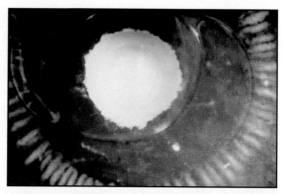

Figure 6-13B. Gross photograph of an eye obtained postmortem (Miyake-Apple posterior photographic technique) showing a well-centered Bausch and Lomb Surgical Hydroview IOL with good clarity of the media (courtesy Dr. G. Ravalico Trieste, Italy). Note complete cortical cleanup and miminal Soemmering's ring. (Courtesy of Dr. G. Ravalico Trieste, Italy).

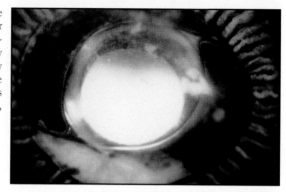

Figure 6-14A. Gross photograph of a bisected and explanted Bausch and Lomb Surgical, Inc., Hydroview H55/H60M hydrogel IOL showing surface deposits composed of calcuim. (This figure shows an unstained specimen with diffuse white deposit.)

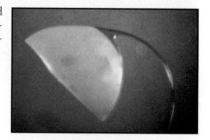

Figure 6-14B. Gross photograph of a bisected and explanted Bausch and Lomb Surgical, Inc., Hydroview H55/H60M hydrogel IOL showing surface deposits composed of calcuim. (This figure shows an alizeran red stain. The red color is positive for calicum.)

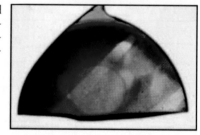

Table 6-8. *Hydroview* Bausch and Lomb Surgical, Inc.	
Design	3-piece-IOL
Model	Hydroview H55S/H60M
Manufacturer	Bausch and Lomb Surgical, Inc. (previously Storz Surgical)
Overall diameter [mm]	12.0
Optic diameter [mm]	Biconvex 5.5/6.0
Optic material	Hydrogel polymer
Water content	18%
Refractive index	1.474
Haptic material	Hydrogel polymer
Haptic angulation	5.7° and 6.5°
A-constant	118.3
ACD [mm]	5.14
Diopter [range]	+15.0 to +30.0
Incision [mm]	3.2 to 3.8

study is warranted to determine whether this will be an isolated occurance or if it may become more evidenced over time. We cannot comment from our database on PCO rates, although relatively high rates of both anterior capsule opacification (ACO) and posterior capsule opacification (PCO) have been noted in investigational clinical studies in Europe.[2]

Examples of two other IOL designs manufactured by Bausch and Lomb Surgical that are categorized as hydrophilic acrylics are the EasAcryl 1 design (Figure 6-15 and Table 6-9) and the HE 26 C design (Figure 6-16 and Table 6-10).

Mentor MemoryLens Intraocular Lens

This unique design (Figures 6-17 to 6-18) was first developed in the late 1980s. It is a wet packed IOL with polypropylene haptic that must be kept refrigerated. Manufacturer's specifications are listed in Table 6-11. Upon insertion into the eye, with heating in the aqueous to 37°, the lens gradually unfolds. We have not had the opportunity to examine this IOL in a human autopsy series, but we have studied it experimentally with insertions into eyes obtained postmortem using the Miyake-Apple posterior photographic technique. These experimental implantations documented good centration and a good "fit" in the capsular bag. This has been confirmed in clinical investigational implantations, including one in our facility (Figure 6-18). This IOL has a square-truncated optic edge similar to that seen with the elastimide-polyimide lens (Chapter 4) and the Alcon AcrySof IOL (Chapter

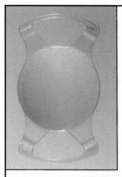
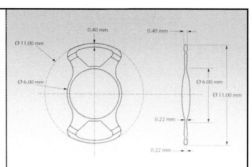
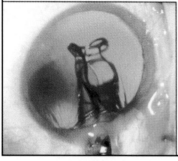
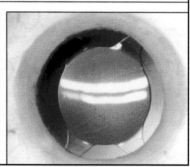

Figure 6-15. Manufacturer's illustration and design of the Bausch and Lomb Surgical EasAcryl hydrophobic acrylic IOL (see Table 6-9).

Table 6-9.
EasAcryl
Bausch and Lomb Surgical, Inc.

Design	1-piece-acrylic-IOL
Model	EasAcryl 1
Manufacturer	Bausch and Lomb Surgical, Inc. (previously DomiLens)
Overall diameter [mm]	11.0
Optic diameter [mm]	Biconvex 6.0
Optic material	Acrylic polymer
Water content	26%
Refractive index	1.465
Haptic material	Acrylic
Haptic angulation	0°
A-constant	119.0
ACD [mm]	4.9
Diopter [range]	+10.0 to +30.0
Incision [mm]	2.3

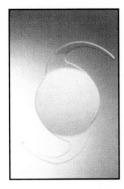

Figure 6-16A. Manufacturer's illustration and diagram (Figure 6-16B) of the Bausch and Lomb Surgical HE26C IOL. (see Table 6-10)

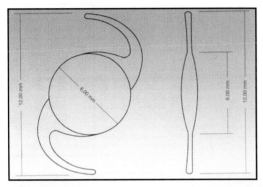

Figure 6-16B. Manufacturer's illustration (Figure 6-16A) and diagram of the Bausch and Lomb Surgical HE26C IOL. (see Table 6-10)

Table 6-10. *HE 26 C* Bausch and Lomb Surgical, Inc.	
Design	1-piece-acrylic-IOL
Model	HE 26 C
Manufacturer	Bausch and Lomb Surgical, Inc. (previously DomiLens)
Overall diameter [mm]	12.0
Optic diameter [mm]	Biconvex 6.0
Optic material	Acrylic polymer
Water content	(26%)
Refractive index	1.465
Haptic material	Acrylic
Haptic angulation	0°
A-constant	119
ACD [mm]	5.3
Diopter [range]	+10 to +30
Incision [mm]	N/A

Figure 6-17A. Mentor MemoryLens, manufacturer's illustration of the IOL and wet pack container for delivery (Figure 6-17B) (see Table 6-11).

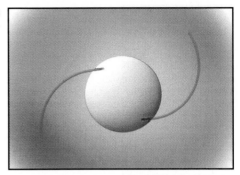

Figure 6-17B. Mentor MemoryLens, manufacturer's illustration of the IOL (Figure 6-17A) and wet pack container for delivery (see Table 6-11).

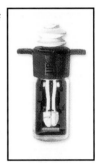

Figure 6-18. In vitro and investigational studies on the Mentor MemoryLens have been carried out in our facility. This is a clinical photograph of a patient with a MemoryLens showing good centration and clarity of the media. Note the square truncated optic edge best viewed on the right. The folds that course obliquely across the center of the optic were preexisting folds in the posterior capsule and unrelated to the lens. (Surgery by Kerry Solomon, MD, Charleston, SC.)

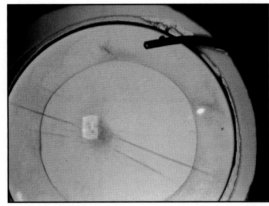

Table 6-11. *MemoryLens* Ciba Vision, Inc.	
Design	3-piece-hydrogel-IOL
Model	MemoryLens U940A
Manufacturer	Ciba Vision, Inc.
Overall diameter [mm]	13.0
Optic diameter [mm]	6.0
Optic material	Hydrogel polymer
Water content	20 %
Refractive index	1.47
Haptic material	Polypropylene
Haptic angulation	10°
A-constant	119
ACD [mm]	5.6
Diopter [range]	N/A
Incision [mm]	N/A

5, see also Chapter 7).Therefore, it is probable, but yet to be proved, that this would provide a favorably low PCO rate.

To date, some clinical studies have been favorable, but we cannot yet comment on these from the viewpoint of clinicopathologic correlation.

European Hydrophilic Acrylic Intraocular Lens

Hydrophobic plate IOL designs have been implanted for 2 decades (Figures 6-19 and 6-20) and several very interesting modern hydrophilic designs are illustrated in Figures 6-21 to 6-25. European hydrophobic acrylic IOL that we are familiar with included models of Corneal, France (Figures 6-21 to 6-25 and Tables 6-12 to 6-16) and Rayner, Ltd., United Kingdom. With the exception of the IOL illustrated in Figure 6-23B, submitted to our laboratory by Prof. Reudiger Welt of Ludwigshafen, Germany, we have not received specimens for clinicopathologic correlation.

A hydrophilic acrylic IOL design manufactured in the United States but marketed overseas is produced by Medical Developmental Research, Inc. (Formerly DRG IOLs Corp.), Clearwater, Florida. It has not been submitted for USA Food and Drug Administration (FDA) approval so it is of course not available for our US autopsy database.

Figure 6-19. Gross photograph from behind of a human eye obtained postmortem (Miyake-Apple posterior photographic technique) showing an example of an early hydrogel plate lens from the early 1980s. This lens was implanted with one haptic in the capsular bag (left), with the other haptic forward into the ciliary sulcus (right). Note the exuberant Soemmering's ring with capsular opacification over a part of the optical zone on the right. Total in-the-bag fixation is one of the important criteria in preventing PCO (see Chapter 7).

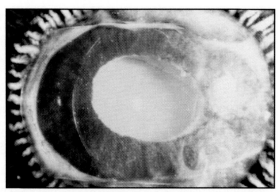

Figure 6-20. Another example of an early hydrogel plate design was the Alcon IOGel Lens, late 1980s. This is a gross photograph from behind of a human eye obtained postmortem (Miyake-Apple posterior photographic technique), showing excellent centration with moderate peripheral Soemmering's ring formation. Although this lens was very biocompatible and in general provided excellent results, it was removed from the market following reports of several cases of dislocation into the vitreous after Nd:YAG laser posterior capsulotomy.

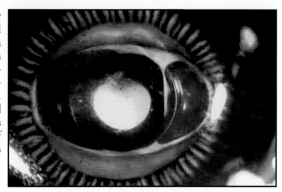

Figure 6-21A. A modern plate IOL fabricated from a hydrophilic material, the one-piece AC 55, manufactured by Corneal, France (see Table 6-12). It is composed of a hydrophilic, acrylic polymer, with a water content of 26%. (Manufacturer's illustration.) (Courtesy of Dr. G. Ravolico, Trieste, Italy.)

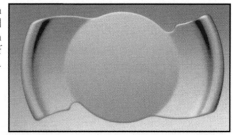

Figure 6-21B. A modern plate IOL fabricated from a hydrophilic material, the one-piece AC 55, manufactured by Corneal, France (see Table 6-12). It is composed of a hydrophilic, acrylic polymer, with a water content of 26%. This is a gross photograph from behind of a human eye obtained postmortem (Miyake-Apple posterior photographic technique) showing the Corneal AC-55 lens well-centered in the capsular bag. (see also Table 6-12). (Courtesy of Dr. G. Ravolico, Trieste, Italy.)

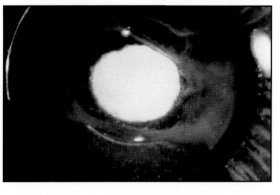

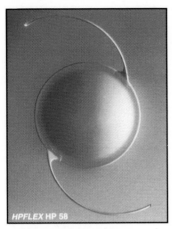

Figure 6-22. Corneal, France manufactures a lens with features of a one-piece IOL, a fusion of a hydrophilic acrylic optic with PMMA haptics, the HP58 design. This is the manufacturer's illustration (see also Table 6-13).

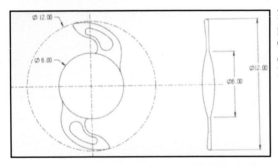

Figure 6-23A. The ACR6D design is also a one-piece, hydrophilic acrylic IOL manufactured by Corneal, France. (Manufacturer's diagram with dimensions.) (Table 6-14.) (Courtesy of Prof. Ruediger Welt, Ludwigshafen, Germany.)

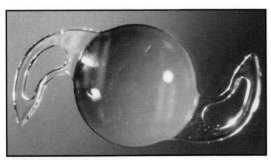

Figure 6-23B. The ACR6D design is also a one-piece, hydrophilic acrylic IOL manufactured by Corneal, France. This is a gross photograph of an explanted AC60 IOL from Corneal, removed because of problems with the surgical technique (Table 6-14). (Courtesy of Prof. Ruediger Welt, Ludwigshafen, Germany.)

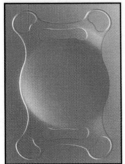

Figure 6-24A. The Quattro design manufactured by Corneal, France, is a four-point fixation IOL composed of hydrophilic acrylic material. This lens is not available in the United States. This is a manufacturer's illustration and diagram with dimensions (Figure 6-24B) (see Table 6-15).

Figure 6-24B. The Quattro design manufactured by Corneal, France, is a four-point fixation IOL composed of hydrophilic acrylic material. This lens is not available in the United States. This is a manufacturer's illustration (Figure 6-24A) and diagram with dimensions (see Table 6-15).

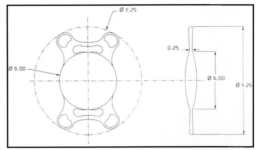

Figure 6-25A. Corneal, France also manufactures the model M1050, a four-point fixation PC IOL design manufactured from hydrophilic acrylic material. This is not available in the United States. Figures 6-25 A through C are manufacturer's illustrations with dimensions (see Table 6-16).

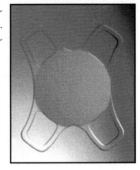

Figure 6-25B. Corneal, France also manufactures the model M1050, a four-point fixation PC IOL design manufactured from hydrophilic acrylic material. This is not available in the United States. Figures 6-25 A through C are manufacturer's illustrations with dimensions (see Table 6-16).

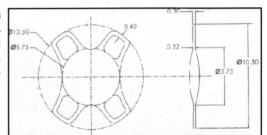

Figure 6-25C. Corneal, France also manufactures the model M1050, a four-point fixation PC IOL design manufactured from hydrophilic acrylic material. This is not available in the United States. Figures 6-25 A through C are manufacturer's illustrations with dimensions (see Table 6-16).

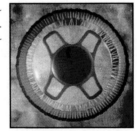

Table 6-12.
AC.55
Corneal, Inc.

Design	1-piece-Acrylic-IOL
Model	AC.55
Manufacturer	Corneal, Inc., France
Overall diameter [mm]	10.5
Optic diameter [mm]	Biconvex 5.5 and 6.0
Optic material	Acrylic polymer
Water content	26 %
Refractive index	1.465
Haptic material	Acrylic
Haptic angulation	0°
A-constant	119
ACD [mm]	5.3
Diopter [range]	+0.0 to +30.0
Incision [mm]	(Company rec.) N/A

Table 6-13.
HP Flex
Corneal, Inc.

Design	1-piece-Acrylic-IOL
Model	HP Flex HP 58
Manufacturer	Corneal, Inc., France
Overall diameter [mm]	11.5 to 13.0
Optic diameter [mm]	Biconvex 5.8 to 6.0
Optic material	Acrylic polymer
Water content	26 %
Refractive index	1.465
Haptic material	PMMA
Haptic angulation	5°
A-constant	118.5
ACD [mm]	4.9
Diopter [range]	+10 to +30
Incision [mm]	N/A

Table 6-14.
ACR 6D
Corneal, Inc.

Design	1-piece-Acrylic-IOL
Model	ACR 6D
Manufacturer	Corneal, Inc., France
Overall diameter [mm]	12.0
Optic diameter [mm]	Biconvex 6.0
Optic material	Acrylic polymer
Water content	26 %
Refractive index	1.465
Haptic material	Acrylic
Haptic angulation	0°
A-constant	119
ACD [mm]	5.3
Diopter [range]	+10.0 to +30.0
Incision [mm]	(Company rec.) 3.5 to 4.0

Table 6-15.
Quattro
Corneal, Inc.

Design	1-piece-Acrylic-IOL
Model	Quattro
Manufacturer	Corneal, Inc., France
Overall diameter [mm]	11.25
Optic diameter [mm]	Biconvex 6.0
Optic material	Acrylic polymer
Water content	26 %
Refractive index	1.465
Haptic material	Acrylic
Haptic angulation	0°
A-constant	119
ACD [mm]	5.3
Diopter [range]	+10 to +30
Incision [mm]	N/A

Table 6-16.
M.10 50
Corneal, Inc.

Design	1-piece-Acrylic-IOL
Model	M.10 50
Manufacturer	Corneal, Inc., France
Overall diameter [mm]	10.5
Optic diameter [mm]	Biconvex 5.75
Optic material	Acrylic polymer
Water content	26 %
Refractive index	1.465
Haptic material	Acrylic
Haptic angulation	0°
A-constant	119
ACD [mm]	5.3
Diopter [range]	+10 to +30
Incision [mm]	N/A

REFERENCES

Barrett G. A new hydrogel intraocular lens design. *J Cataract Refract Surg.* 1994;20(1):18-25.

Bucher PJ, de Courten C, Faggioni R. 3 years' clinical experience with IOGel lenses. *Klinische Monatsblatter fur Augenheilkunde.* 1990;196:320-321.

Faschinger C, Haller EM, Reich M. Superficial damage to the MemoryLens in implantation. Klinische *Monatsblatter fur Augenheilkunde.* 1996;209:37-39.

Kohnen T, Magdowski G, Koch DD. Scanning electron microscopic analysis of foldable acrylic and hydrogel intraocular lenses. *J Cataract Refract Surg.* 1996;22(suppl 2):1342-1350.

Levy JH, Pisacano AM, Anello RD. Displacement of bag-placed hydrogel lenses into the vitreous following neodymium:YAG laser capsulotomy. *J Cataract Refract Surg.* 1990;16:563-566.

Lowe KJ, Easty DL. A comparison of 141 polymacon (IOGel) and 140 poly(methyl methacrylate) intraocular lens implants. *Br J Ophthalmol.* 1992;76:88-90.

Menapace R, Amon M, Radax U. Evaluation of 200 consecutive IOGel 1103 capsular-bag lenses implanted through a small incision. *J Cataract Refract Surg.* 1992;18:252-264.

Menapace R, Papapanos P, Radax U, Amon M. Evaluation of 100 consecutive IOGEL 1003 foldable bag-style lenses implanted through a self-sealing tunnel incision. *J Cataract Refract Surg.* 1994;20:432-439.

Menapace R, Skorpik C, Juchem M, Scheidel W, Schranz R. Evaluation of the first 60 cases of poly HEMA posterior chamber lenses implanted in the sulcus. *J Cataract Refract Surg.* 1989;15:264-271.

Menapace R, Skorpik C. Technic and initial results of capsule sack implantation of hydrogen lenses using a small incision. *Klin Monatsb Augenheikunde.* 1989;195:349-352.

Menapace R, Yalon M. Exchange of IOGEL hydrogel one-piece foldable intraocular lens for bag-fixated J-loop poly(methyl methacrylate) intraocular lens. *J Cataract Refract Surg.* 1993;19:425-430.

Menapace R. Posterior capsule opacification and capsulotomy rates with taco-style hydrogel intraocular lenses. *J Cataract Refract Surg.* 1996;22(suppl 2):1318-1330.

Menapace R, Amon M, Radax U. Evaluation of 200 consecutive IOGEL 1103 capsular-bag lenses implanted through a small incision. *J Cataract Refract Surg.* 1992;18:252-264.

Menapace R, Papapanos P, Radax U, Amon M. Evaluation of 100 consecutive IOGEL 1003 foldable bag-style lenses implanted through a self-sealing tunnel incision. *J Cataract Refract Surg.* 1994;20:432-439.

Menapace R, Skorpik C, Wedrich A. Evaluation of 150 consecutive cases of poly HEMA posterior chamber lenses implanted in the bag using a small-incision technique [published erratum appears in J Cataract Refract Surg. 1991 Jan;17(1):111]. *J Cataract Refract Surg.* 1990;16:567-577.

Packard RB, Garner A, Arnott EJ. Poly-hema as a material for intraocular lens implantation: a preliminary report. *Br J Ophthalmol.* 1981;65:585-587.

Percival P. Prospective study comparing hydrogel with PMMA lens implants. *Ophthalmic Surg.* 1989;20:255-261.

Percival SP. Comparing like with like: A prospective study of hydrogel and polymethylmethacrylate lenses. *Dev Ophthalmol.* 1989;18:111-113.

Percival SP, Jafree AJ. Preliminary results with a new hydrogel intraocular lens. *Eye.* 1994;8:672-675.

Percival P. Prospective study comparing hydrogel with PMMA lens implants. *Ophthalmic Surgery.* 1989;20:255-261.

Percival SP, Jafree AJ. Preliminary results with a new hydrogel intraocular lens. *Eye.* 1994;8:672-675.

Percival SP. Comparing like with like: A prospective study of hydrogel and polymethylmethacrylate lenses. *Developments in Ophthalmology.* 1989;18:111-113.

Pham DT, Wollensak J, Welzl-Hinterkorner E. Experiences with the phema posterior chamber lens]. *Fortschritte der Ophthalmologie.* 1990;87:144-146.

Pham DT, Wollensak J, Welzl-Hinterkorner E. Experiences with the p-hema posterior chamber lens. *Fortschritte der Ophthalmologie.* 1990;87:144-146.

Potzsch DK, Losch-Potzsch CM. Four year follow-up of the MemoryLens. *J Cataract Refract Surg.* 1996;22(suppl 2):1336-1341.

Potzsch DK, Losch-Potzsch CM. Four year follow-up of the MemoryLens. *J Cataract Refract Surg.* 1996;22(suppl 2):1336-1341.

Ravalico G, Baccara F, Vajente S. Long-term results with Iogel IOLs. *Ophthalmologica.* 1993;207:202-207.

Sanchez E, Artaria L. Evaluation of the first 50 ACR360 acrylic intraocular lens implantations. *J Cataract Refract Surg.* 1996;22(suppl 2):1373-1378.

Complications

Section

4

Complications

Chapter 7

Posterior Capsule Opacification

INTRODUCTION

Posterior capsule opacification (PCO, secondary cataract) has existed since the beginning of ECCE (Harold Ridley documented this complication in his very first cases.[1] It was particularly common and severe in the early days of PC IOL surgery (late 1970s, early 1980s), when the importance of cell and cortex removal was much less understood than it is today (Figures 7-1 to 7-3). This nagging and expensive (Table 7-1) complication of ECCE PC IOL surgery occurred at an incidence of between 30 and 50% through the 1980s and early 1990s. It has been a major hindrance to implementation of pediatric IOLs (Figure 7-3).

As we enter the new millennium, we are pleased that we can now report a gradual—almost unnoticed—decrease in the incidence of PCO. This has paralleled the move into what we have designated as Generation VI, capsular surgery (see Chapter 2, Figure 2-19 and Table 2-2). Our current data show that with modern techniques and IOLs the expected rate of PCO and the need for subsequent Nd:YAG laser posterior capsulotomy is decreasing down towards a rate of single digits.

In this chapter, we discuss the pathogenesis of PCO and present results that support this optimistic prediction. We devote an entire chapter to this topic for three reasons: 1) the specific surgical tools and appropriate IOLs for eradication of PCO are now available and warrant a detailed discussion (Tables 7-2 and 7-3); 2) a reduced incidence of PCO and hence a decrease need for Nd:YAG posterior capsulotomy will alleviate a major financial burden to our Healthcare system (see Table 7-1); and 3) successful expansion of ECCE in the developing world can be expedited. This is highly dependent on eradication or at least diminishing of PCO. Patient follow-up in a developing world setting is difficult and access to the Nd:YAG laser is not widely available. Reduction in incidence of PCO is now regularly occurring in the industrialized world and hopefully this discussion will provide new information and guidance regarding this condition that will help surgeons prevent it in the developing world.

Figure 7-1. Clinical photograph of a case of PCO with extensive "pearl" formation behind an injection-molded optic of a three-piece PMMA IOL (late 1980s).

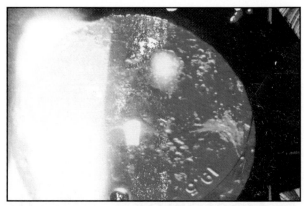

Figure 7-2A. Gross photograph from behind (Miyake-Apple posterior photographic technique) of a human eye obtained postmortem showing the "fibrous" form of PCO. Notice the dense fibrous strands and areas of white discoloration behind the optic.

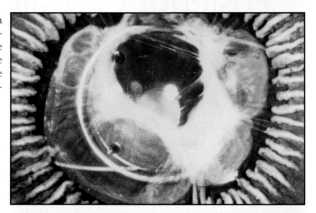

Figure 7-2B. Gross photograph from behind (Miyake-Apple posterior photographic technique) of a human eye obtained postmortem showing massive overgrowth of a Soemmering's ring over the lens optic. This has created a "pearl form" of total PCO. This lens was asymmetrically fixated. The left haptic is in the capsular bag. The right haptic (not visible) is in the ciliary sulcus.

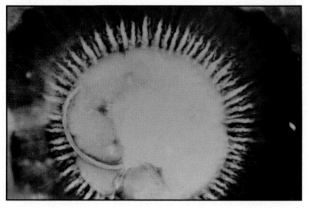

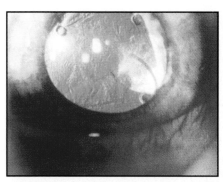

Figure 7-3. PCO in a child treated for pediatric cataract. In addition to extensive "pearl" formation, note the severe crimping of one of the polypropylene haptics of this IOL onto the IOL optic. (photograph courtesy M. Edward Wilson, MD.)

Table 7-1.
Relative Cost to U.S. Medicare System of Major Surgical Procedures (4 of 10 are eye procedures)*

1. Primary cataract operation (removal of opaque lens and insertion of an IOL.)
2. Secondary cataract (PCO) treatment of Nd:YAG laser posterior capsulotomy
3. Prostatectomy
4. Knee replacement
5. Coronary artery bypass (3 vessels)
6. Hip joint replacement
7. Coronary artery bypass (4 vessels)
8. Femur fracture
9. Panretinal photocoagulation (Diabetic retinopathy)
10. Laser trabeculoplasty (Glaucoma)

* U.S. Health Care Finance Administration (HCFA), 1997.

Table 7-2.
Six Factors to Reduce PCO

3 Surgery-Related Factors
"Capsular" Surgery

1. Hydrodissection-enhanced cortical clean-up.

2. In-the-bag fixation.

3. CCC diameter slightly smaller than that of IOL optic. This places the CCC edge on the anterior surface of the optic and help sequester the capsular bag. This creates a "shrink wrap" of the capsule around the IOL optic.

Table 7-3.
Six Factors to Reduce PCO

3 IOL-Related Factors
("Ideal" IOL)

1. Biocompatible IOL to reduce stimulation of cellular proliferation.

2. Maximal IOL optic-posterior capsule contact, angulated haptic, "bio-adhesive" biomaterial to create a "shrink wrap".

3. IOL optic geometry square, truncated edge.

Secondary cataract disease needs to be eliminated for many reasons, including these important five:

1. The main treatment of PCO is Nd:YAG laser secondary posterior capsulotomy (Figure 7-4), a sometimes dangerous procedure (Figure 7-5).

2. PCO has been a significant cost burden to the US health care system (see Table 7-1). Until recently, Nd:YAG laser treatments of almost 1 million PCO-afflicted patients per year have cost the US health care system up to $0.25 billion ($250 million) annually.

3. Modern cataract surgery is now approaching the realm of refractive surgery. Patients expect almost perfect results, often with emmetropia. Satisfactory use of multifocal IOLs and "piggyback IOLs" (see Chapter 8) will require a low PCO rate. Furthermore, any hope of safe genuinely clear lens extraction for myopic eyes that many surgeons are researching requires avoidance of Nd:YAG laser secondary posterior capsulotomy. If such a capsulotomy is required, there is an unacceptable increased risk of retinal detachment.

4. Because PCO is a common complication of pediatric IOL implantation (see Figure 7-3), control of this condition will help improve the safety and efficacy of IOL implantation in childhood (see Chapter 5, Figures 5-14 to 5-17).

5. This complication has greatly impeded the spread of successful cataract surgery/IOL implantation to the 25 million people worldwide blind from cataract (visual acuity <20/400), not to mention 110 million individuals with cataract-induced visual disability (visual acuity <20/200). Cataract is by far the most common cause of visual impairment in the developing world. It is important that high rates of PCO do not compromise the results of increased numbers of ECCE surgeries now being conducted in underprivileged regions.

PATHOGENESIS

The epithelium of the crystalline lens (Figures 7-6A through C) consists of a sheet of anterior epithelial cells (A cells) that are in continuity with the cells of the equatorial lens bow (E cells). The latter cells comprise the germinal cells that undergo mitosis as they peel

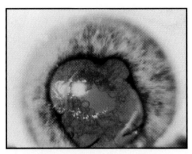

Figure 7-4A. The treatment of PCO is a posterior capsulotomy, either surgical or with Nd:YAG laser. This is a clinical photograph of a laser-treated "pearl"-type PCO with the central orifice created by the laser. A reduction of the overall incidence of PCO will help diminish the need for this expensive and potentially dangerous procedure.

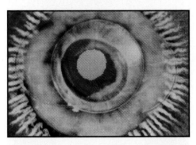

Figure 7-4B. Gross photograph from behind (Miyake-Apple posterior photographic technique) of a human eye obtained postmortem showing a case in which PCO required treatment with the Nd:YAG laser. The central orifice created by the laser is the clear area in the middle roughly concentric with the pupil. This should not be confused with the capsulorhexis, which has a larger diameter and a smoother round edge.

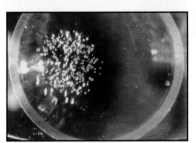

Figure 7-5. Multiple defects ("pitting") on the surface of an IOL optic secondary to Nd:YAG laser treatment.

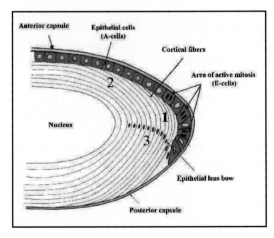

Figure 7-6A. The primary cells of origin for PCO are the mitotic germinal cells of the epithelial lens bow. These cells normally migrate centrally from the lens equator and contribute to formation of the nucleus, epinucleus, and cortex throughout life. In pathologic states, they tend to migrate posteriorly to form such lesions as a posterior subcapsular cataract, as well as post-ECCE PCO. This figure is a schematic illustration of the microscopic anatomy of the lens, showing the important germinal epithelial cells of the equatorial lens bow. Proliferation of cells potentially lead to classic PCO (#1). Anterior epithelial proliferation creates anterior subcapsular plaques (#2). There is a newly described syndrome of cell proliferation in the central area between "piggyback" IOLs (#3) (see Chapter 8).

Figure 7-6B. The primary cells of origin for PCO are the mitotic germinal cells of the epithelial lens bow. These cells normally migrate centrally from the lens equator and contribute to formation of the nucleus, epinucleus. and cortex throughout life. In pathologic states, they tend to migrate posteriorly to form such lesions as a posterior subcapsular cataract, as well as post-ECCE PCO. This figure is a photomicrograph of the equatorial region of the human lens, showing the cellular elements and fibers as described in Figure 7-6A (hematoxylin and eosin stain; original magnification x200).

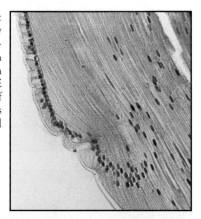

Figure 7-6C. The primary cells of origin for PCO are the mitotic germinal cells of the epithelial lens bow. These cells normally migrate centrally from the lens equator and contribute to formation of the nucleus, epinucleus. and cortex throughout life. In pathologic states, they tend to migrate posteriorly to form such lesions as a posterior subcapsular cataract, as well as post-ECCE PCO. Functionally, one can differentiate the cells of the lens into two functional groups: the cells lining the anterior capsule and those of the epithelial lens bow. The "A" cells of the anterior epithelium tend to undergo a pseudofibrous metaplasia and remain in situ (do not tend to migrate). They are responsible for fibrotic phenomena, such as fibrotic anterior subcapsular cataracts or anterior polar congenital cataracts. The "E" cells, from the equatorial lens bow, are the primary cells that may proliferate and migrate, creating a postoperative Soemmering's ring and PCO.

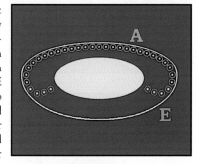

off from the equator (Figure 7-6A). They constantly form new lens fibers during normal lens growth. Although both the anterior and equatorial lens epithelial cells stem from a continuous cell line and remain in continuity, it is useful to divide these into two discrete functional groups (A cells and E cells). They differ in terms of function, growth patterns, and pathologic processes. The anterior cells, or A cells (#2 in Figure 7-6C), when disturbed, tend to remain in place and not migrate. They are prone to a transformation into fibrous-like tissue (pseudofibrous metaplasia).

In sharp contrast, in pathologic states, the E cells of the equatorial lens bow (#1 in Figure 7-6A and Figure 7-6C) tend to migrate posteriorly along the posterior capsule; e.g., in posterior subcapsular cataracts, and the pearl form of PCO (see Figures 7-1, 7-2A, and 7-3). In general, instead of undergoing a fibrotic transformation, they tend to form large, balloon-like bladder cells (the cells of Wedl). These are the cells that are clinically visible as "pearls." These equatorial cells are the primary source of classic secondary cataract, especially the pearl form of PCO. The E cells have also been implicated in the pathogenesis of opacification between piggyback IOLs (Figure 7-6A), also termed interlenticular opacification (IOL) (see Chapter 8, Figures 8-10 to 8-17).

Figure 7-7 exemplifies the type of fibrous plaque formation that typically occurs with disruption of the anterior capsule. This is a photomicrograph of a post-uveitis anterior sub-

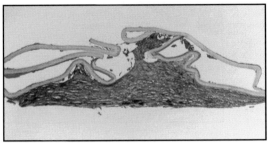

Figure 7-7. An anterior subcapsular cataract is an example of proliferation and pseudofibrous metaplasia of anterior cells ("A" cells; see Figure 7-6). This is a photomicrograph of an anterior subcapsular cataract that occurred secondarily to uveitis removed during continuous curvilinear capsulorhexis (CCC). It is composed of dense fibrous tissue and stains positive for fibrous tissue (blue) with the Masson trichrome stain. Note coiled remnants of anterior lens capsule above the plaque. (Masson's trichrome stain; original magnification x200).

capsular cataract, removed via capsulorhexis (CCC). Note that the anterior capsule overlies a dense fibrous plaque, which is derived from the transformed epithelium. The A cells are the cell of origin of any form of anterior capsular cataract—eg, congenital, post-traumatic, and post-uveitis as seen here (Figure 7-7).

Recently, a new potential complication of A-cell proliferation has emerged in the field of refractive IOL surgery. The anterior subcapsular opacities that have been described with various phakic PC IOLs (see Chapter 8, Figure 8-20) are based on A-cell proliferation. The fibrotic response of the anterior lens epithelium (A cell) is what determines the degree of anterior capsular thickening following implantation of a phakic PC IOL in close proximity (or on) the anterior surface of the crystalline lens.

We have now confirmed the various rigid and foldable IOL biomaterials now in use cause varying degrees of reaction of A cells (Figures 7-8 to 7-12; see also Chapter 3, Figures 3-8A to 3-14).[2] Figure 7-8A displays an anterior capsule at the edge of the capsulorhexis showing not only an absence of fibrous metaplasia but also an actual dropout of A cells. This pattern is most commonly seen with the Alcon AcrySof foldable IOL (see Figure 7-9). On a scale of 0 to 3 (0 = none, 3 = maximum) (Figure 7-9), an intermediate amount of fibrous proliferation (+1 to +2) occurs on average with PMMA IOLs, as noted in Figure 7-8B. In general, there is on average more fibrous reaction and anterior capsular thickening and opacification with silicone material, especially with the plate IOL designs (Figures 7-8C, 7-9, and 7-10A and B; see also Chapter 3, Figures 3-8 and 3-14).

In addition to anterior subcapsular opacity, important complications related to fibrous proliferation of the anterior capsule are IOL decentration and luxation, especially into the plate IOL design (see Figures 3-15A through C) related to capsular fibrosis (contractile cicitrization [Figure 7-11]) and the capsulorhexis contraction syndrome (capsular phimosis [Figures 7-12A through D]). In general, this complication can be avoided by not making the CCC diameter too small; e.g., keeping it at least 4 to 4.5 mm in diameter.

Returning to the E cells of the equatorial lens bow (Figures 7-6A through C), recall that these are the cellular elements that form "pearls" (bladder cells) and cortical material. These are the cells that are responsible for formation of a Soemmering's ring (Figures 7-13 to 7-16), a lesion that residents learn about in basic ophthalmic pathology training, but heretofore, has rarely been accorded its importance in the pathogenesis of PCO. A Soemmering's ring is a donut-shaped lesion composed of retained/regenerate cortex and cells that may form following any type of disruption of the anterior lens capsule. This lesion was initially

Figure 7-8A. The amount of ACO can be graded from 0 (none) to 3 (maximum). This figure shows an anterior capsule in an eye with an Alcon AcrySof IOL, showing virtually no anterior capsular fibrosis (grade 0) (Masson's trichrome stain, original magnification x400).

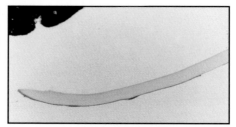

Figure 7-8B. The amount of ACO can be graded from 0 (none) to 3 (maximum). This figure shows 2+ proliferation of the subcapsular epithelium in a case with a classic PMMA IOL (Masson's trichrome stain, original magnification x400).

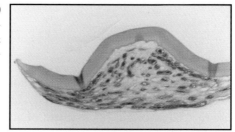

Figure 7-8C. The amount of ACO can be graded from 0 (none) to 3 (maximum). This figure shows 3+ proliferation of the subcapsular epithelium in a case with a silicone plate IOL (Masson's trichrome stain, original magnification x400).

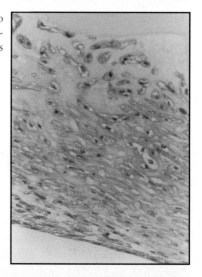

Figure 7-9. This table summarizes ACO scores for all eight IOL types present in our database. The score range is from 0-3. The Alcon AcrySof IOL has the lowest mean score (0.51). The AcrySof shows very low capsular reactivity both in terms of anterior subcapsular proliferation (Figure 7-8A), as well as PCO (see below Figures 7-79 and 7-80). (Courtesy of Dr. Liliana Werner.)

January 1988 thru January 1999 Anterior Capsule Opacification Scores (Apple and associates, 1999)		
IOL Group	**Sample Size**	**Mean**
1 PC Silicone Plate, Large Hole	40	1.77
1 PC Silicone Plate, Small Hole	67	1.28
3 PC Silicone-PMMA (Allergan SI 40)	14	1.21
3 PC Silicone-Prolene	92	1.09
3 PC PMMA (Rigid)	51	1.07
1 PC All-PMMA (Rigid)	50	.94
3 PC Silicone-Polyimide	40	.92
3 PC Acrylic-PMMA (Acrysof)	96	.51

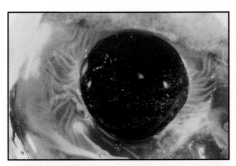

Figure 7-10A. Gross photograph of an eye obtained postmortem with a silicone plate IOL showing grade 3 ACO. (Anterior, or surgeon's view, with cornea and iris removed. Note the folds created by contractile fibrous tissue.) (Courtesy of Dr. Liliana Werner.)

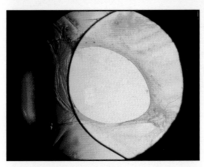

Figure 7-10B. Gross photograph of an eye obtained postmortem with a silicone plate IOL showing grade 3 ACO. (View from behind with the Miyake-Apple posterior photographic technique.) (Courtesy of Dr. Liliana Werner.)

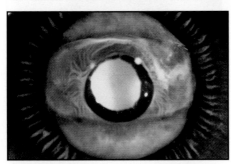

Figure 7-11. Clinical photograph showing IOL optic decentration caused by anterior capsular fibrosis with cicatrization and capsulorhexis contraction. (Courtesy of Alan Carlson, MD.)

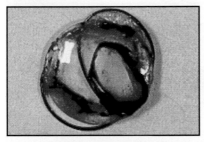

Figure 7-12A. An example of capsulorhexis (CCC) contraction syndrome (phimosis), a condition that occurs as a result of fibrosis of anterior cells (A cells), which occurs most often when a very small capsulorhexis of 4.5 mm or less is performed. A small CCC tends to constrict or narrow. This figure shows a gross photograph of an explanted IOL from the 1980s with severe crimping of the haptics caused by the contractile process.

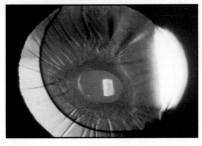

Figure 7-12B. An example of capsulorhexis (CCC) contraction syndrome (phimosis), a condition that occurs as a result of fibrosis of anterior cells (A cells), which occurs most often when a very small capsulorhexis of 4.5 mm or less is performed. A small CCC tends to constrict or narrow. This figure shows a clinical photograph of a capsulorhexis contraction, syndrome (Courtesy of Alan Carlson, MD.)

Figure 7-12C. An example of capsulorhexis (CCC) contraction syndrome (phimosis), a condition that occurs as a result of fibrosis of anterior cells (A cells), which occurs most often when a very small capsulorhexis of 4.5 mm or less is performed. A small CCC tends to constrict or narrow. This figure shows a gross photograph anterior view of a human eye obtained postmortem showing another case with capsulorhexis contraction (phimosis).

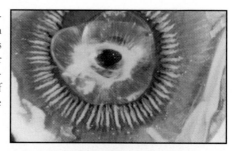

Figure 7-12D. An example of capsulorhexis (CCC) contraction syndrome (phimosis), a condition that occurs as a result of fibrosis of anterior cells (A cells), which occurs most often when a very small capsulorhexis of 4.5 mm or less is performed. A small CCC tends to constrict or narrow. This figure shows a gross photograph from behind (Miyake-Apple posterior photographic technique) of an eye containing a foldable silicone three-piece IOL showing marked CCC contraction, with eccentric position. Note marked fibrosis of anterior epithelial cells entirely surrounding the CCC orifice, especially toward the left.

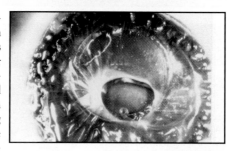

Figure 7-13A. A sketch from the early part of this century showing an example of post-traumatic Soemmering's ring formation. These typically follow ocular penetration and rupture of the anterior capsule. Note in the extensive Elschnig pearl formation as lens cells extrude out through the broken capsule (arrow).

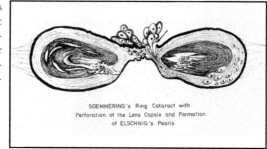

Figure 7-13B. A photomicrograph from the early part of this century showing an example of post-traumatic Soemmering's ring formation. These typically follow ocular penetration and rupture of the anterior capsule. Note the central perforation of the cornea (see wound tract or leukocoria adhesion) has coursed lens capsule rupture.

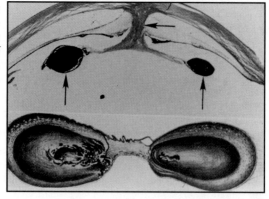

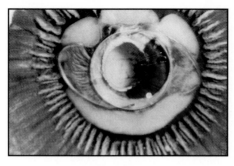

Figure 7-14A. It is not widely appreciated that a Soemmering's ring occurs after every ECCE procedure. A classic Soemmering's ring is a doughnut-shaped lesion, the basic pathogenic factor being any traumatic or surgical rupture of the anterior lens capsule with extrusion of central lens material. It was classically described as a post-traumatic lesion, and generally is associated with Elschnig pearls. The equatorial remnants of a Soemmering's ring are composed of cortical material and proliferating E cells. Figures 7-14A through C are human eyes obtained postmortem with marked Soemmering's ring formation around PC IOLs (Miyake-Apple posterior photographic technique).

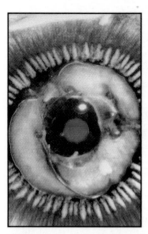

Figure 7-14B. It is not widely appreciated that a Soemmering's ring occurs after every ECCE procedure. A classic Soemmering's ring is a doughnut-shaped lesion, the basic pathogenic factor being any traumatic or surgical rupture of the anterior lens capsule with extrusion of central lens material. It was classically described as a post-traumatic lesion, and generally is associated with Elschnig pearls. The equatorial remnants of a Soemmering's ring are composed of cortical material and proliferating E cells. Figures 7-14A through C are human eyes obtained postmortem with marked Soemmering's ring formation around PC IOLs (Miyake-Apple posterior photographic technique).

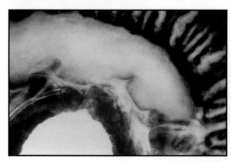

Figure 7-14C. It is not widely appreciated that a Soemmering's ring occurs after every ECCE procedure. A classic Soemmering's ring is a doughnut-shaped lesion, the basic pathogenic factor being any traumatic or surgical rupture of the anterior lens capsule with extrusion of central lens material. It was classically described as a post-traumatic lesion, and generally is associated with Elschnig pearls. The equatorial remnants of a Soemmering's ring are composed of cortical material and proliferating E cells. Figures 7-14A through C are human eyes obtained postmortem with marked Soemmering's ring formation around PC IOLs (Miyake-Apple posterior photographic technique).

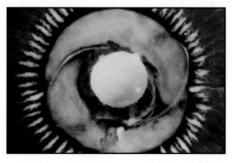

Figure 7-15A. Gross photograph from behind of a human eye obtained postmortem (Miyake-Apple posterior photographic technique) showing an extensive Soemmering's ring.

Figure 7-15B. Photomicrograph through the equatorial region of the capsular bag showing the haptic of the PC IOL on the left (clear circular space within the equatorial fornix) and a large mass of cortical/cellular material (right) forming the body of the Soemmering's ring. (Hematoxylin and Eosin stain, original magnification X150).

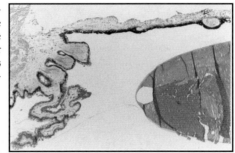

Figure 7-16. The E cells within a Soemmering's ring are the precursors of PCO in most cases. This is a gross photograph from behind of a human eye obtained postmortem (Miyake-Apple posterior photographic technique) showing growth of a PCO, membrane derived neutral from the Soemmering's ring across the visual axis.

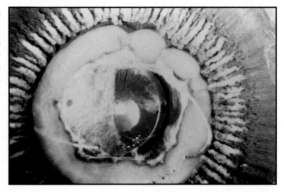

described in connection with ocular trauma (see Figures 7-13A and B). The basic pathogenic factor of the Soemmering's ring is the anterior capsular break, which may then allow exit of central nuclear and cortical material out of the lens, with subsequent Elschnig pearl formation. It is not widely appreciated that a Soemmering's ring forms virtually every time any form of ECCE is done, whether manually, automated, or with phacoemulsification. Examples are seen in Figures 7-14 to 7-16. The characteristic white material forming the donut peripheral to the IOL's optic component stems from the E cells of the equatorial lens bow (see Figure 7-6C). Most significantly, these cells have the capability to proliferate and migrate posteriorly across the visual axis, creating PCO (Figure 7-16). For practical purposes it is useful to consider this lesion as the basic precursor of classic PCO, especially the "pearl" form (see Figures 7-1, 7-2A, 7-3, 7-4A and B, and 7-14 to 7-16).

FACTORS TO REDUCE THE INCIDENCE OF POSTERIOR CAPSULAR OPACIFICATION

Since 1982, beginning in Salt Lake City, Utah, continuing since 1988 in Charleston, South Carolina, we have been doing active laboratory research regarding the persistent problem of PCO. Much of this was summarized in a 1992 review article.[3] Our analyses have increased in intensity over the last 3 years, largely stimulated by the regularly increasing accession of eyes with PC IOLs obtained postmortem (see Figures 1-1 and 1-2). Studies in our laboratory and other centers have provided insight into the essential mechanisms and factors important in eradicating this complication. After analyzing Nd:YAG posterior capsulotomy rates in the databases of eyes obtained postmortem and after compiling information derived from laboratory[4] and clinical studies from several centers worldwide, we have come to the very positive conclusion that surgeons now have the sufficient tools and appropriate IOLs to help reduce the incidence of PCO.

Coherent principles of prevention of PCO can be formulated on what we now know regarding the pathogenesis and cellular origin of PCO. We have defined two major principles that may be applied to prevention of PCO. These are categorized as follows: 1) One should strive to minimize the number of retained/regenerated lens epithelial cells (especially equatorial cells) and cortex following cortical cleanup. This is the first line of defense against this complication. 2) If unwanted, proliferative cells remain, one can create a secondary line of defense by erecting a barrier to block growth of cells from the equatorial region (Soemmering's ring) toward the center of the visual axis.

Although all steps of the cataract operation are, of course, important in reducing any complication, we have identified six factors that stand out as particularly important in relation to preventing or at least delaying this complication (see Tables 7-2 and 7-3).

There are two basic means of reducing formation of the postoperative Soemmering's ring: 1) remove as much cellular-cortical material as possible using hydrodissection-enhanced cortical removal techniques (see Table 7-2); and 2) attempt to identify an appropriately biocompatible IOL that may help reduce stimulation of cellular proliferation (see Table 7-3). The advantages obtained by such a biocompatible IOL can probably be enhanced by tightly sequestering the pseudophakos within the capsular bag (the "shrink wrap" phenomenon), which is best achieved by creating a relatively small diameter CCC. The important second line of defense in reducing growth of cells across the visual axis, the barrier effect, is created by the edge of the IOL's optic. We will detail several factors that enhance this barrier effect: 1) in-the-bag fixation; 2) creation of maximal IOL optic-capsular contact, which in turn appears to be enhanced by highly adherent (bioadhesive) biomaterial to the posterior capsule; and 3) the geometry of the IOL optic.

We now briefly describe each of the six factors listed in Tables 7-2 and 7-3 and show the role of each in helping reduce PCO. All of these factors as a unit are key to achieving this goal.

HYDRODISSECTION-ENHANCED CORTICAL CLEANUP

Hydrodissection (see Table 7-2, #1) has been used for many years by many surgeons, including pioneers such as Cornelius Binkhorst, Henry Claymon, Aziz Anis, and many others. The first formal literature documentation and the naming of this procedure was published by Dr. Kenneth Faust of Leesburg, Fla in 1984 (Figure 7-17).[5] Note from Faust's diagram that this publication occurred during the era of can-opener anterior capsulotomy. Successful hydrodissection is difficult with this capsulotomy technique because the jagged edges of the capsular edge formed after the can-opener cut would often tear radially because of the pressure of the fluid entering the eye during injection). However, the principles of direct subcapsular injection as illustrated by Faust (Figure 7-17), in which he showed the movement of fluid along the posterior subcapsular region, define the principle

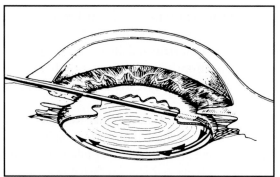

Figure 7-17. The term hydrodissection was coined in the literature by Dr. Kenneth Faust, Leesburg, Fla. This is a diagram from his original publication. This article was published in the mid 1980s at a time when the can opener capsulectomy was still prominent. Therefore, as hydrodissection does not work well with can opener capsulectomy (because of increased incidence of radial tears of the capsule), this technique did not become popular until much later, especially when Howard Fine, MD, improved and modified it, and coined the term "cortical cleaving hydrodissection."

of today's hydrodissection. We have studied the mechanisms of this technique in our laboratory (Figures 7-18 to 7-20).[6] Most importantly, Dr. Howard Fine of Eugene, Oregon, has discovered and popularized the technique he terms cortical cleaving hydrodissection.[7] Many surgeons use the hydrodissection procedure with special focus on of freeing and rotating the lens nucleus in order to facilitate lens substance removal and thus enhance the overall safety of the operation. In addition to these important intraoperative considerations, we emphasize here an important additional long-term advantage of hydrodissection; namely, a much more efficient removal of cortex and cells that in turn is essential in reducing PCO (Figures 7-20 to 7-22). With careful, copious hydrodissection, the operation is much easier and faster, and cortex/cell removal is much more thorough formation of unwanted Soemmering's ring (Figures 7-14 to 7-16) is minimized. The entire lens can actually be extracted using variations of hydrodissection—eg, hydroexpression (Figure 7-19)—or with injection of viscoelastics, a viscoexpression.

Until fairly recently, most surgeons have had a rather fatalistic attitude regarding removal of lens cortex and cells during ECCE. It was commonly assumed that removing all or even most cells from the bag was impossible (Figure 7-22). PCO was therefore considered to be an inevitable complication. This negative conclusion was partly based on the fact that PCO occurred in up to 50% of cases. We now know from autopsy and experimental studies (Figures 7-21A through C) that good cortical and cellular cleanup can be accomplished in a much more efficient fashion in a majority of cases than had previous been believed.[8] Figures 7-21A through C show capsular bags of human eyes in which experimental surgery done with copious hydrodissection was performed. Note that cleanup of equatorial cells and cortex was virtually complete in each case, leaving a clean interior to the bag. In contrast, Figure 7-22 is an example of a human cadaver eye operated on experimentally without hydrodissection. Note that cortical cleanup, especially the critical removal of E cells at the lens equator, was incomplete. This figure clearly shows that retained cortical material is not just amorphous material, but consists of viable cells with their nuclei within the retained cortex. These have the ability to proliferate and migrate, causing PCO.

One other significant finding regarding the A cells in Figure 7-22 requires mention. Note that virtually all anterior epithelial A cells in this section are present adjacent to the anterior capsule, albeit vacuolated. It is theoretically desirable and efficacious to also

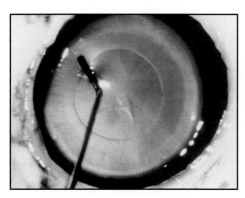

Figure 7-18. Gross photograph of experimental surgery on a human cadaver eye from our laboratory showing the technique of subcapsular hydrodissection (cortical cleaving hydrodissection). This is an anterior (surgeon's) view showing injection via a 27-gauge bent cannula.

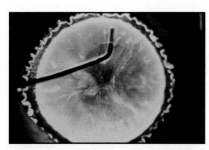

Figure 7-19. Assia and associates have shown that lens substance can be removed by subcapsular injection of fluid (hydroexpression).

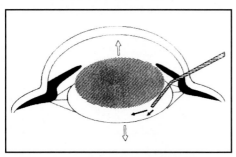

Figure 7-20A. Illustration of experimental subcapsular (cortical cleaving) hydrodissection in human cadaver eyes. (Anterior, or surgeon's, view with cornea and iris removed. Note that the bent cannula is immediately under the edge of the capsulorhexis.)

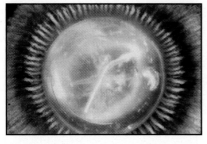

Figure 7-20B. Illustration of experimental subcapsular (cortical cleaving) hydrodissection in human cadaver eyes. (Miyake-Apple posterior photographic technique.)

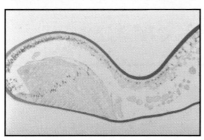

Figure 7-20C. Illustration of experimental subcapsular (cortical cleaving) hydrodissection in human cadaver eyes. This figure shows a photomicrograph of a sagittal view of a crystalline lens after an unsuccessful hydrosection. Note residual cortical material and equatorial lens epithelial cells. (Periodic acid-Schiff stain, original magnification 250x)

Figure 7-21A. Microphotograph demonstrating thorough removal of lens substances. In our laboratory studies on human eyes obtained postmortem, we were pleasantly surprised that with copious hydrodissection and meticulous cortical cleanup, most cortex and most if not all lens epithelial cells from the equator (E cells) could be removed. This photomicrograph of a lens capsular bag of an eye that underwent experimental cataract surgery associated with copious hydrodissection. Note excellent removal of lens material and E cells—a very clear capsular bag in each case. (Periodic acid-Schiff stain, original magnification x750).

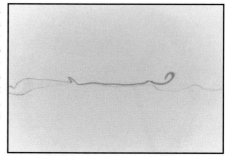

Figure 7-21B. Microphotograph demonstrating thorough removal of lens substances. In our laboratory studies on human eyes obtained postmortem, we were pleasantly surprised that with copious hydrodissection and meticulous cortical cleanup, most cortex and most if not all lens epithelial cells from the equator (E cells) could be removed. This photomicrograph of a lens capsular bag of an eye that underwent experimental cataract surgery associated with copious hydrodissection. Note excellent removal of lens material and E cells—a very clear capsular bag in each case. (Periodic acid-Schiff stain, original magnification x750).

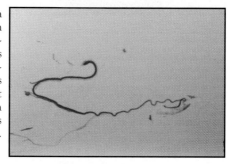

Figure 7-21C. Microphotograph demonstrating thorough removal of lens substances. In our laboratory studies on human eyes obtained postmortem, we were pleasantly surprised that with copious hydrodissection and meticulous cortical cleanup, most cortex and most if not all lens epithelial cells from the equator (E cells) could be removed. This photomicrograph of a lens capsular bag of an eye that underwent experimental cataract surgery associated with copious hydrodissection. Note excellent removal of lens material and E cells—a very clear capsular bag in each case. (Periodic acid-Schiff stain, original magnification x750).

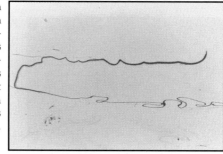

Figure 7-22. Photomicrograph showing an example of poor cortical cleanup in an eye where hydrodissection was not performed. Note that the retained cortical material is not just composed of amorphous or acellular strands, but contains cells (note the multiple cellular nuclei in the mass of retained cortex), which are precisely those that undergo proliferation toward PCO. Note also the presence of residual anterior epithelial cells (top), which in most cases are left at surgery. These do not contribute nearly as often to PCO, but occasionally provide problems associated with A cells (see Figures 7-7 to 7-12) (periodic acid-Schiff stain, original magnification x200).

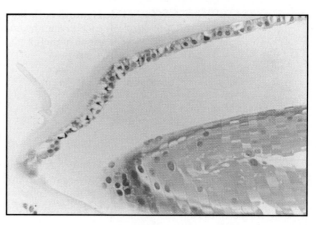

remove as many of these A cells as possible,[9] but it is not mandatory and not practical in terms of time. Remembering that the A cells of the anterior capsule tend to undergo fibrous metaplasia in situ and are not prone to migrate, it is logical that they are not the major factor in the pathogenesis of classic PCO. It should therefore be clear that the goal of hydrodissection is to remove equatorial E cells and cortex, as opposed to the cells comprising the single layer of anterior epithelium. There is a form of fibrous PCO (see Figure 7-2A). From our laboratory observations, we believe that most cases are derived from a metabolic transformation of posteriorly migrated E cells into fibrocysts as opposed to migration of A cells onto the posterior capsule. The formation of a posterior subcapsular cataract composed of a fibrous plaque is a common occurrence in many cataracts seen in the rural developing world.[10] This is because there are often long waiting periods for cataract surgery in these regions and the classic E-cell-derived pearl forms of cataract tend to transform into fibrous elements over a long period of time.

IN-THE-BAG (CAPSULAR) FIXATION

As has been shown in detail in Chapter 2 (see Table 2-2 and Figure 2-19), the hallmark of modern cataract surgery is the achievement of consistent and secure in-the-bag fixation (capsular fixation) (see Table 7-2, #2). Indeed, Generation VI (see Figure 2-19) is designated as the era of capsular surgery.[11] The most obvious advantage of in-the-bag fixation is the accomplishment of good optic centration. However, an equally important advantage is often overlooked.[12] In-the-bag placement is extremely important, indeed mandatory, in reducing the incidence of PCO.

Recalling that the pathogenesis of PCO is multifactorial, it is clear that the two most important surgical factors in reducing PCO are the previously described hydrodissection-enhanced cortical cleanup and in-the-bag fixation. In-the-bag fixation functions primarily to enhance the IOL-optic barrier effect (Figure 7-23). The barrier effect is functional and maximal (see Figure 6-23A) when the lens optic is fully in the bag with direct contact with the posterior capsule. When one or both haptics are out of the bag (Figure 7-23B), a potential space exists that allows an avenue for ingrowth of cells toward the visual axis. The reader may recall the barrier ridge IOL design devised by Kenneth Hoffer in the 1980s (see Figure 7-49). This did not function well at that time, not because of a problem with the concept or the IOLs themselves, but because in those days only one-third of implanted IOLs were truly in the bag (Figure 7-24).

Figure 7-24 charts data obtained from our autopsy series regarding PC IOL haptic fixation since the early 1980s.[12] Note that the incidence of in-the-bag fixation (red line) has grown steadily over the years, after having stabilized at a range of about 30% in the late 1980s. The growth, although steady and positive, has reached what appears to be a limit today of about 60%. This is best explained by the fact that many cases over the years had been done with classic large-incision extracapsular surgery, often with can-opener anterior capsulotomy. This curve coincides with the movement into modern capsular surgery (Generation VI) (Figure 2-19 and Figure 7-25). We therefore note that secure and permanent in-the-bag fixation only occurred in a maximum of about 60% of cases, probably the best achievable with these early techniques. However, when considering modern foldable lens implantation (blue line), the number surges to 90% (see Figure 7-24). It is not the

Figure 7-23A. In addition to hydrodissection-enhanced cortical removal, it is essential that an IOL be placed in the capsular bag to reduce PCO. The barrier effect of the IOL optic is generally negated when the lens is not in the capsular bag. This figure shows a schematic illustration of an in-the-bag IOL with complete blockage of cells by the optic's barrier effect (arrows).

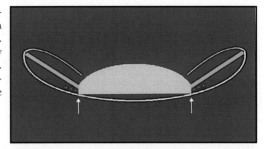

Figure 7-23B. In addition to hydrodissection-enhanced cortical removal, it is essential that an IOL be placed in the capsular bag to reduce PCO. The barrier effect of the IOL optic is generally negated when the lens is not in the capsular bag. This figure shows a schematic illustration of an IOL with one haptic in the bag (left) and one haptic out of the bag (right). This leads to diminution or loss of the barrier effect and ingrowth of cells behind the IOL optic occurs.

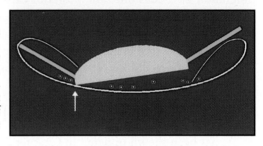

Figure 7-24. Regarding in-the-bag fixation, our analysis of the autopsy database from 1984 to the present shows evidence that the best capsular fixation achievable with classic extracapsular large-incision surgery occurs in approximately 60% of cases (red line). Most noteworthy, however, we have noted that with modern foldable lenses, which require meticulous in-the-bag fixation for proper functioning, the rate of secure capsular fixation has soared to 90% in recent years (see asterisk).

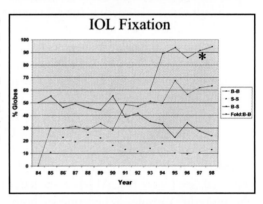

Figure 7-25. The transition to modern capsular surgery, especially small-incision phacoemulsification techniques, occurred in the early 1990s. (Courtesy of David Leaming, MD, Palm Springs, Calif.)

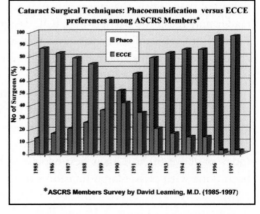

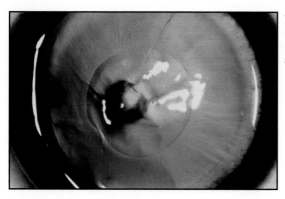

Figure 7-26. Gross photograph from in front (surgeon's view) of the anterior lens surface (cornea and iris removed), showing a relatively small CCC.

foldable IOL itself, or even the small incision in and of itself that provides this positive result, but rather the fact that successful foldable IOL insertion generally requires very precise surgery for success, which includes good in-the-bag placement of haptics.

CAPSULORHEXIS EDGE ON INTRAOCULAR LENS SURFACE

By far the most important surgical factors in reducing PCO are the above mentioned hydrodissection-enhanced cortical cleanup and attainment of secure in-the-bag fixation. A less obvious but significant addition is the move away from the often very large diameter can opener anterior capsulotomies of the past to the modern continuous curvilinear capsulorhexis or tear CCC (Figures 7-26 and 7-27) (see Table 7-2, #3). This has measurably helped reduce the incidence of anterior capsular tears and thus helps prevent unwanted exit of IOL haptics from the capsular bag (pea-podding, see Figure 2-33 for the historical correlate for this).[13] We now believe a CCC with a diameter slightly smaller than that of the IOL optic, so that the anterior CCC edge rests on the IOL optic (Figure 7-28), is efficacious. For example, if the IOL optic were 6.0 mm, the capsulorhexis diameter would ideally be slightly smaller, perhaps 5.0-5.5 mm. Figures 7-29A through C show three eyes implanted with the Alcon AcrySof foldable IOL showing the phenomenon of a CCC size smaller than the diameter of the IOL optic. The CCC cut edge rests on the optic surface (Figure 7-30). The same phenomenon is shown with an Allergan SI-30 three-piece silicone IOL design (Figure 7-31), a silicone plate IOL design (Figure 7-32), and the CeeOn Edge 911 lens of Pharmacia-Upjohn, a three-piece silicone IOL design (Figure 7-33). Placing the capsulorhexis edge over the optic helps provide a tight fit (analogous to a "shrink wrap") of the capsule around the optic and also helps sequester the interior compartment of the capsule containing the IOL optic from the surrounding aqueous humor. This may help protect the milieu within the capsule from at least some potentially deleterious factors within the aqueous, especially in some macro molecules, and some inflammatory mediators. The concept of capsular sequestration is subtle (see Table 7-2), but more and more surgeons appear to be applying this principle and seeing its advantages.

Figure 7-27A. Morphology of a capsulorhexis. Low power scanning electron micrograph of a human eye obtained postmortem, anterior or surgeon's view, showing the placement of a CCC (original magnification x15).

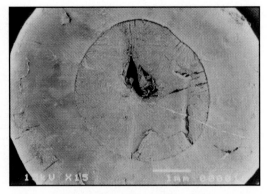

Figure 7-27B. Scanning electron micrograph of an edge of the capsulorhexis tear done experimentally on the same human lens shown in Figure 7-27A. Note the extremely smooth edge of the tear (right, original magnification x50).

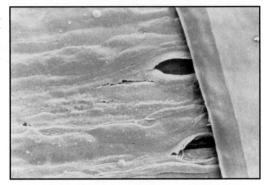

Figure 7-27C. High-power photomicrograph of the scanning electron micrograph seen in Figure 7-27B showing a detailed view of the capsulorhexis edge, which is extremely smooth. This type of edge is ideal to avoid radial tears of the anterior capsule (Original magnification is x500).

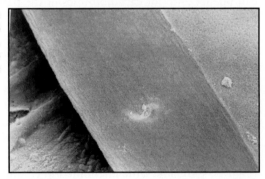

Figure 7-28. Schematic illustration showing contact of the CCC edge to the anterior lateral surface of the IOL optic (E = equatorial capsules).

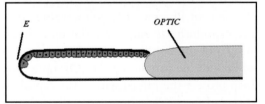

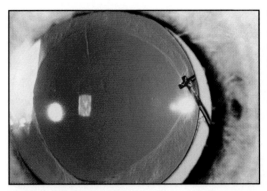

Figure 7-29A. Clinicopathologic studies on human eyes obtained postmortem have shown that a CCC diameter slightly smaller than the IOL optic helps sequester the optic within the capsular bag, which helps reduce the chance of PCO. This figure shows a clinical photograph of a case in which an Alcon Acrysof IOL was implanted in the capsular bag after creating a CCC orifice smaller than the IOL optic.

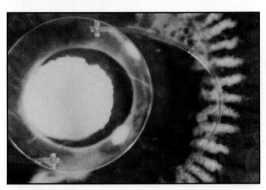

Figure 7-29B. Clinicopathologic studies on human eyes obtained postmortem have shown that a CCC diameter slightly smaller than the IOL optic helps sequester the optic within the capsular bag, which helps reduce the chance of PCO. This figure shows a clinical photograph of a case in which an Alcon Acrysof IOL was implanted in the capsular bag after creating a CCC orifice smaller than the IOL optic.

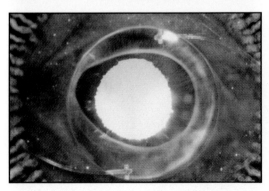

Figure 7-29C. Clinicopathologic studies on human eyes obtained postmortem have shown that a CCC diameter slightly smaller than the IOL optic helps sequester the optic within the capsular bag, which helps reduce the chance of PCO. This figure shows a clinical photograph of a case in which an Alcon Acrysof IOL was implanted in the capsular bag after creating a CCC orifice smaller than the IOL optic.

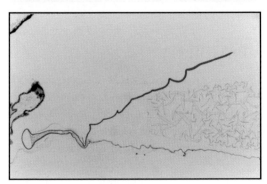

Figure 7-30. Photomicrograph of the anterior segment of an eye containing an Alcon AcrySof IOL implanted in the capsular bag with a CCC diameter smaller than that of the IOL optic. The IOL optic acrylic biomaterial has partially dissolved out of the section during processing. The haptic site is the small round empty space (left) in the equatorial fornix. The anterior and posterior capsule are fused together near the haptic, signifying good cortical removal. Note that the anterior capsule and CCC edge extend to the right over the IOL optic's anterior surface (periodic acid-Schiff stain, original magnification x400).

Figure 7-31. Gross photograph from behind of a human eye obtained postmortem (Miyake-Apple posterior photographic technique) showing an Allergan SI-30 IOL implanted well within the capsular bag, with the capsulorhexis orifice smaller than the IOL optic.

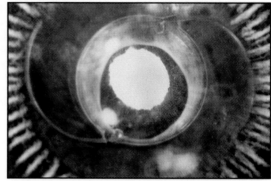

Figure 7-32. Clinical photomicrograph of a Staar Surgical/Bausch and Lomb Surgical plate style 1-piece silicone IOL well-implanted in the capsular bag. The relatively small capsulorhexis allows the posterior surface of the anterior capsule around the CCC to hug the anterior surface of the optic closely. We believe that this helps create a closed system. This helps sequester ("shrink wrap," see Table 7-2) the lens in the capsular bag, and also enhances the IOL optic's barrier effect.

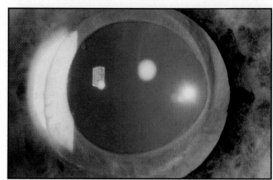

Figure 7-33. Clinical photomicrograph of a Pharmacia-Upjohn 911 CeeOn edge silicone IOL well-implanted in the capsular bag. The relatively small capsulorhexis allows the posterior surface of the anterior capsule around the CCC to hug the anterior surface of the optic closely. We believe that this helps create a closed system. This helps sequester the lens in the capsular bag, and also enhances the IOL optic's barrier effect.

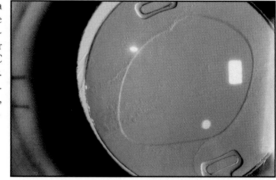

INTRAOCULAR LENS BIOCOMPATIBILITY

In a discussion of PCO, one might define biocompatibility of an IOL biomaterial with a narrow focus and in a simplified way as follows: "the ability to neutralize or inhibit postoperative stimulation of lens epithelial cell proliferation" (see Table 7-3, #1). We have studied and graded the amount of lens epithelial cell proliferation on cadaver eyes in our laboratory database, evaluating both peripheral and central opacification (Figures 7-34 and 7-35)[14]

The tabulated results of this scoring are listed in Figure 7-36. The amount of cell proliferation is multifactorial, depending on such factors as quality of surgery, duration of the

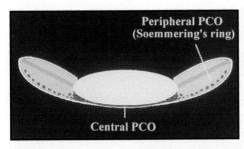

Figure 7-34. IOL material biocompatibility can be assayed by evaluating and scoring peripheral PCO (Soemmering's ring) and central PCO. Using these techniques we have been able to note apparent differences in cellular reactivity of various materials in terms of inhibiting both central and peripheral PCO. This is a schematic sagittal section.

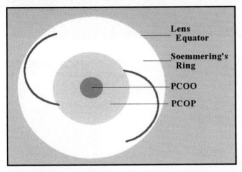

Figure 7-35. In a biocompatibility assay, we were able to score amount of Soemmering's ring in each eye. These include the intensity (SRI) and area covered (SRA) of cortical material within the Soemmering's ring, as well as the opacification behind the center of the optic (PCOO) and behind the periphery of the optic (PCOP). This is a schematic frontal section showing zones of peripheral central PCO.

Biocompatibility Scores January 1988 to January 1999 (From Apple and assoc., 1999)					
Piece	PCOO	PCOP	SRI	SRA	SRA X SRI
3PC PMMA (Rigid)	0.141	1.226	2.586	3.003	7.766
1 PC All-PMMA (Rigid)	0.132	1.189	2.022	3.006	6.078
1 PC Silicone Plate, Small Hole	0.111	1.394	2.010	2.657	5.341
1 PC Silicone Plate, Large Hole	0.122	1.146	1.634	3.244	5.301
3PC Silicone-Prolene	0.142	1.183	1.775	2.773	4.922
3 PC Silicone-Polyimide	0.104	0.979	1.708	2.651	4.528
3 PC Silicone-PMMA (Allergan SI 40)	0.045	1.000	1.091	2.545	2.777
3 PC Acrylic-PMMA (Acrysof)	0.052	0.461	0.957	1.948	1.864
All Lenses since 1/88	0.106	1.072	1.723	2.728	4.7
Foldable lenses	0.096	1.027	1.529	2.636	4.03
Rigid Lenses	0.136	1.208	2.304	3.005	6.924

Figure 7-36. Analysis of the IOL database as of January 1, 1999, provided the following scores. The lenses with the least cellular proliferation are listed above and those with the most listed below. The best way to measure the relative scores of the Soemmering's ring is to multiply Soemmering's ring area (SRA) x Soemmering's ring intensity (SRI). Note that the Alcon AcrySof IOL has the lowest score in all categories. Note also that foldable lenses as a whole had a lower score (SRA x SRI = 5.864) than did the rigid lenses (SRA x SRI = 8.082). Three factors appear to be large responsible for variations in scores, namely, less than perfect cortical cleanup, long duration of the IOL in the eye, post-implantation, and basic biocompatibility factors.

implant in the eye, and biomaterial factors. Note that the Alcon AcrySof IOL showed the lowest mean biocompatibility score, translated as the amount of cell proliferation. This was measured according to Soemmering's ring formation (Soemmering's ring intensity and Soemmering's ring area [SRI and SRA, Figure 7-36]). These scores ranged from 0 (no Soemmering's ring) to +4 (maximum Soemmering's ring area and Soemmering's ring intensity [SRI x SRA]).

Figures 7-37 through 7-44 show examples of comparing low and high scores of all the lenses studied in Figure 7-36. These are illustrated in descending order as tabulated in Figure 7-36, beginning with the Alcon AcrySof IOL (lowest score, Figure 7-37A and B),

Figures 7-37A. Gross photograph from behind (Miyake-Apple posterior photographic technique) of a human eye obtained postmortem showing an example of a variation of biocompatibility scores of the Alcon AcrySof IOL (PMMA haptics and a hydrophobic acrylic optic.) The mean score (SRI x SRA) was 3.5891; Figure 7-36. This IOL design had the lowest mean biocompatibility score; ie, least cellular proliferation reactivity (see Figure 7-36).

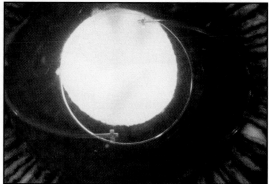

Figures 7-37B. Gross photograph from behind (Miyake-Apple posterior photographic technique) of a human eye obtained postmortem showing an example of a variation of biocompatibility scores of the Alcon AcrySof IOL (PMMA haptics and a hydrophobic acrylic optic.) The mean score (SRI x SRA) was 3.5891; Figure 7-36. This IOL design had the lowest mean biocompatibility score; ie, least cellular proliferation reactivity (see Figure 7-36).

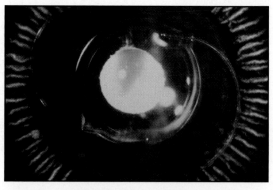

Figures 7-38A. Gross photograph from behind (Miyake-Apple posterior photographic technique) of a human eye obtained postmortem showing an example of a variation of biocompatibility scores of the Allergan SI-40 silicone IOL design, (PMMA haptics and a silicone optic). The mean score (SRI x SRA) was 6.024, (see Figure 7-36).

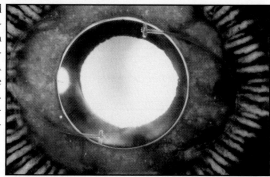

Figures 7-38B. Gross photograph from behind (Miyake-Apple posterior photographic technique) of a human eye obtained postmortem showing an example of a variation of biocompatibility scores of the Allergan SI-40 silicone IOL design, (PMMA haptics and a silicone optic). The mean score (SRI x SRA) was 6.024, (see Figure 7-36).

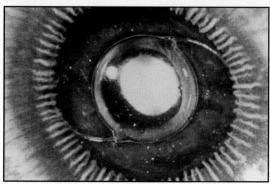

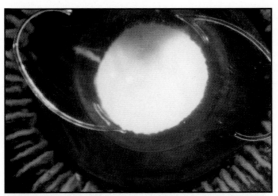

Figures 7-39A. Gross photograph from behind (Miyake-Apple posterior photographic technique) of a human eye obtained postmortem showing an example of variations of biocompatibility scores of an elastimide optic-polyimide haptic IOL. The mean score (SRI x SRA) was 6.5000; (see Figure 7-36).

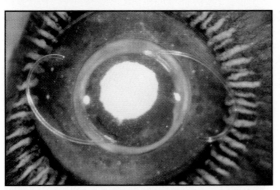

Figures 7-39B. Gross photograph from behind (Miyake-Apple posterior photographic technique) of a human eye obtained postmortem showing an example of variations of biocompatibility scores of an elastimide optic-polyimide haptic IOL. The mean score (SRI x SRA) was 6.5000 (see Figure 7-36).

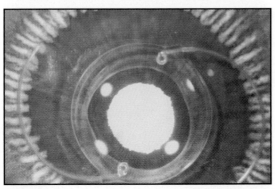

Figure 7-40A. Gross photograph from behind (Miyake-Apple posterior photographic technique) of a human eye obtained postmortem showing an example of variations extremes of biocompatibility scores of a SI-30 prolene-haptic silicone-optic IOL. The mean score (SRI x SRA) was 6.613 (see Figure 7-36).

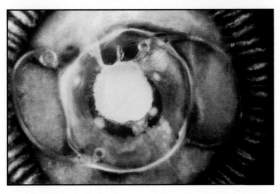

Figure 7-40B. Gross photograph from behind (Miyake-Apple posterior photographic technique) of a human eye obtained postmortem showing an example of variations extremes of biocompatibility scores of a SI-30 prolene-haptic silicone-optic IOL. The mean score (SRI x SRA) was 6.613 (see Figure 7-36).

Figures 7-41A. Gross photograph from behind (Miyake-Apple posterior photographic technique) of a human eye obtained postmortem showing an example of variations of biocompatibility scores with a large hole silicone plate IOL. The mean score (SRI x SRA) was 6.592 (see Figure 7-36).

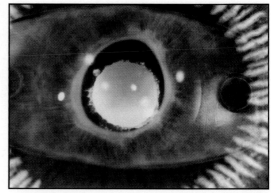

Figures 7-41B. Gross photograph from behind (Miyake-Apple posterior photographic technique) of a human eye obtained postmortem showing an example of variations of biocompatibility scores with a large hole silicone plate IOL. The mean score (SRI x SRA) was 6.592 (see Figure 7-36).

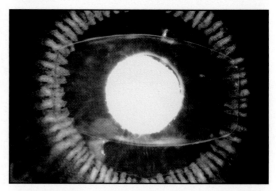

Figure 7-42A. Gross photograph from behind (Miyake-Apple posterior photographic technique) of a human eye obtained postmortem showing an example of varieties of biocompatibility scores with a small-hole silicone plate IOL. The mean score (SRI x SRA) was 6.748 (see Figure 7-36).

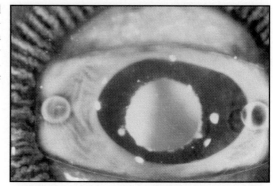

Figure 7-42B. Gross photograph from behind (Miyake-Apple posterior photographic technique) of a human eye obtained postmortem showing an example of varieties of biocompatibility scores with a small-hole silicone plate IOL. The mean score (SRI x SRA) was 6.748 (see Figure 7-36).

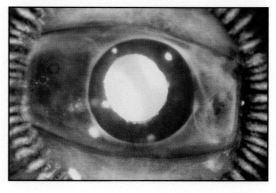

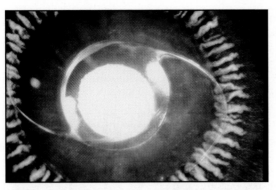

Figure 7-43A. Gross photograph from behind (Miyake-Apple posterior photographic technique) of a human eye obtained postmortem showing an example of variations of biocompatibility scores with a one-piece all-PMMA IOL. The mean score (SRI x SRA) was 7.463 (see Figure 7-36).

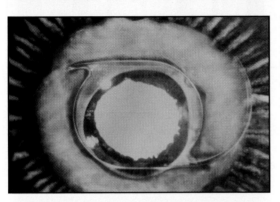

Figure 7-43B. Gross photograph from behind (Miyake-Apple posterior photographic technique) of a human eye obtained postmortem showing an example of variations of biocompatibility scores with a one-piece all-PMMA IOL. The mean score (SRI x SRA) was 7.463 (see Figure 7-36).

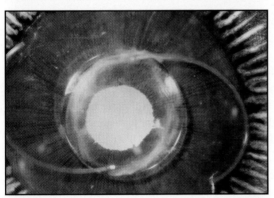

Figure 7-44A. Gross photograph from behind (Miyake-Apple posterior photographic technique) of a human eye obtained postmortem showing an example of variations of cell proliferation (biocompatibility scores) with a three-piece IOL with rigid PMMA optic. The mean score was 8.583 (see Figure 7-36).

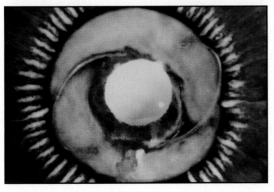

Figure 7-44B. Gross photograph from behind (Miyake-Apple posterior photographic technique) of a human eye obtained postmortem showing an example of variations of cell proliferation (biocompatibility scores) with a three-piece IOL with rigid PMMA optic. The mean score was 8.583 (see Figure 7-36).

Figure 7-45. In a 1999 study comparing various IOL biomaterials, Ram and associates confirmed that the Alcon AcrySof IOL showed a very low rate of PCO and Nd:YAG laser capsulotomy as compared with several other rigid and foldable IOL designs.[13]

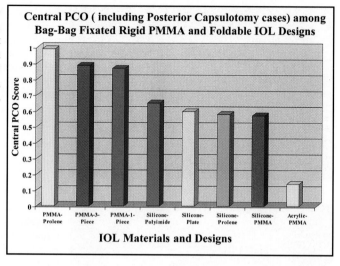

concluding with the three-piece PMMA design (highest score, Figure 7-44). The low score achieved by the Alcon AcrySof IOL is statistically significant when compared to all other designs (Figure 7-36 and 7-45), but further long-term studies are required to assess further the clinical significance of this IOL in retarding PCO.

MAXIMAL INTRAOCULAR LENS OPTIC-POSTERIOR CAPSULE CONTACT

The best means of attaining a tight contact between the IOL optic and posterior capsule (see Table 7-3, #2), a state required to inhibit ingrowth of cells across the visual axis (the "no space, no cells" concept), is to achieve in-the-bag fixation. Posterior angulation of the IOL haptics (demonstrated schematically in Figure 7-23A) and posterior convexity of the optic (already present in Sir Harold Ridley's first IOL design [1950], Figure 7-46) also assist in this. The creation of a small CCC, as mentioned above (see Table 7-2, #3), helps create a "shrink wrap" fit of the posterior capsule against the back of the IOL optic. A final factor appears to be related to the "stickiness" of the IOL biomaterial that in turn might create an adhesion of the capsule and IOL optic. There is preliminary evidence that the Alcon AcrySof IOL biomaterial provides enhanced adhesion of the bioadhesive factor binding capsule to the IOL optic (see Chapter 5 for detailed references by Linnola and associates in this field). Confirmation of this will require further study.

BARRIER EFFECT OF THE INTRAOCULAR LENS OPTIC

As noted above, the IOL optic barrier effect (see Table 7-3, #3) comes into play as a second line of defense against PCO in cases where retained cortex and cells are left following ECCE. The concept of the barrier effect is not new. In fact, the original Ridley lens, when actually implanted in the capsular bag (Figure 7-46), provided an excellent barrier effect,

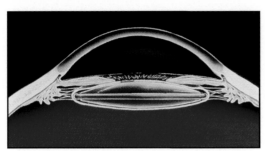

Figure 7-46. The barrier effect of an IOL optic has been an effective retardant of PCO since the time of Ridley's invention 50 years ago. This schematic illustration of Ridley's biconvex disc IOL totally filling the capsular bag demonstrates the concept of the barrier effect. This is sometimes termed the "no space, no cells" concept.

with almost complete filling of the capsular bag and contact of the posterior IOL optic to the posterior capsule ("no space, no cells"). In sharp contrast, a lens with one or both haptics "out-of-the-bag" has much less chance to produce a barrier effect (schematically illustrated in Figures 7-23A and B and 7-47). In retrospect, it is now clear that the IOL optic's barrier function has been one of the main reasons that PC IOLs implanted after ECCE throughout the decades have avoided a thoroughly unacceptably high incidence of florid PCO (Figure 7-48). The barrier effect of IOLs has helped PC IOL implants post-ECCE during the past two decades achieve their success. Notice in Figure 7-48 that, although a large mass of cortex surrounds the lens optic forming an extreme Soemmering's ring, the central optic remains relatively cell free because the presence of the optic has blocked central migration of cells from the substance of Soemmering's ring.

In the 1980s there were various attempts to modify the IOL optic to enhance its barrier effect against cell growth. The Hoffer barrier ridge design (Figure 7-49) in essence created a square edge not dissimilar to those advocated today (see Figures 7-57 to 7-63A later in this chapter). These early ridges were only partially effective because in-the-bag fixation was only achieved in about 30% of cases at that time (see Figure 7-24). Now that in-the-bag placement is successful in approximately 90% of cases with foldable IOLs (see Figure 7-24), the square or truncated optic edge is achieving a comeback as a physical barrier against PCO.

In the early 1980s, many IOLs were often poorly polished and their optics had square, sharp edges (see Chapter 2 and Figure 7-50). In these days, especially with the high incidence of uveal fixation (sulcus-sulcus, or bag sulcus) (see Figure 7-24), in which contact with delicate iris or ciliary body tissues occurred, there was a high incidence of deleterious sequelae secondary to tissue contact (chafe) with the sharp edges. For this reason a major push toward better rounding of optic edges occurred (Figure 7-51). Studies in rabbits by Nishi in Japan,[15] similar rabbit studies in our laboratory, and studies of human eyes obtained postmortem in our laboratory (see Figure 7-58)[8] have shown that IOL optics with rounded edges, when placed in the capsular bag, may allow some ingrowth of cells onto the posterior capsule as they migrate under the tapered, peripheral-posterior edge of the optic (Figures 7-52 to 7-56). However, several currently implanted foldable IOLs have a more squared, truncated edge, e.g., the Alcon AcrySof IOL (Figures 7-57 to 7-59), and studies have shown that this sharp bend appears to provide a good barrier to ingrowth of cells onto the visual axis (Figures 7-57 to 7-59). Even in cases where cortical cleanup has been incomplete, a truncated optic edge appears to create an effective block to cells growing onto the posterior capsule (Figures 7-60 to 7-62). Other IOLs that have truncated optic designs include the Pharmacia-Upjohn CeeOn Edge 911 design (Figure 7-63), some PMMA designs (Figure 7-64), the Staar Surgical and Bausch and Lomb Surgical elastimide-polyimide design (see Figures 4-4 to 4-51), and the CibaVision-Mentor MemoryLens IOL.

Figure 7-47. As opposed to in-the-bag fixation, implantation of one or both haptics outside of the bag is not conducive to formation of good barrier effect. This schematic illustration of ciliary sulcus fixation exaggerates displacement of the bulk of the IOL optic away from the central capsular bag, but illustrates this principle (see also Figures 7-23A and B).

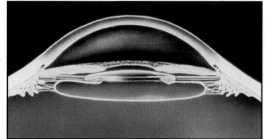

Figure 7-48. Gross photograph from behind (Miyake-Apple posterior photographic technique) of a human eye obtained postmortem showing the principle of the barrier effect. This rigid PMMA optic PC IOL was implanted in the 1980s. Even though the lens optic is bathed in a massive pool of cortex and cells (Soemmering's ring), the barrier effect created by the edge of the optic has retarded a significant growth of cells toward the central visual axis.

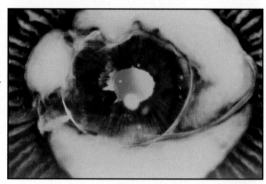

Figure 7-49. In the 1980s, Kenneth Hoffer, MD, of Santa Monica, Calif, developed an IOL with a 360° peripheral ridge this in effect that created a square optic edge which functioned to provide a barrier to the ingrowth of cells. The only reason that this did not gain popularity at that time was because in-the-bag fixation was not consistent, being successfully accomplished in less than 30% of cases (see Figures. 7-23 and 7-24) The posterior aspect of the optic is above in this photomicrograph. However, the principle of the square edge barrier effect is now achieving a renaissance (scanning electron micrograph, original magnification x10).

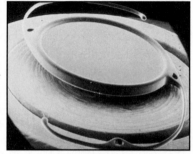

Figure 7-50. Early PMMA IOLs had relatively square-edged optics, primarily because of lesser or poor quality polishing than is performed today. Lenses like this one in the 1980s could cause complications due to chafing if uveal contact occurred (see Figure 2-28). With modern in-the-bag fixation, this is now rare. However, in retrospect, we now know that such an edge is efficacious against PCO. (scanning electron micrograph, original magnification x50).

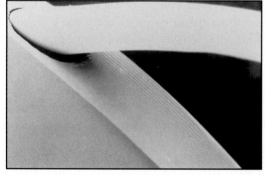

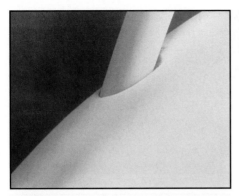

Figure 7-51. Because earlier IOLs often had uveal contact, better polishing and rounding of the optic edge to help alleviate complications due to tissue chafing became the standard, as is shown here (scanning electron micrograph, original magnification x50).

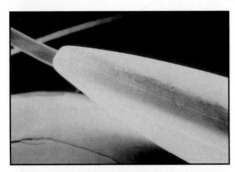

Figure 7-52. An IOL optic of a modern foldable design with a classic tapered or rounded edge (scanning electron micrograph, original magnification x30).

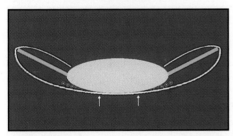

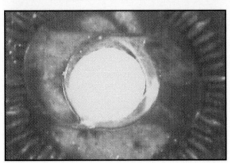

Figure 7-53. Schematic illustration showing the subtle differences that Dr. O. Nishi of Japan has noted in the rabbit model and Dr. David Apple and associates have noted in human cadaver eyes regarding the barrier effect of an IOL optic with a rounded edge versus a square truncated edge. With a round edge, some cells may squeeze behind the posterior peripheral aspect of the optic, creating a paracentral rim (arrows) of opacification. It is important to emphasize that this usually spares the visual axis.

Figure 7-54. Gross photograph from behind (Miyake-Apple posterior photographic technique) of a human eye obtained postmortem showing a one-piece all-PMMA PC IOL with a round-edged optic. Some cells of the Soemmering's ring have grown in behind the periphery of the optic.

Figure 7-55. Gross photograph from behind (Miyake-Apple posterior photographic technique) of a human eye obtained postmortem showing an Allergan SI-30 silicone IOL well centered in the capsular bag. Note the ingrowth of some cortical and cellular elements of the Soemmering's ring around the far peripheral edge of the rounded lens optic. The material has barely gained entrance to the periphery of the optical component, but has not reached the central visual axis.

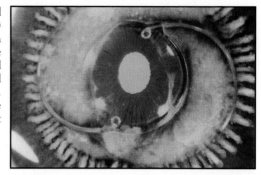

Figure 7-56A. Photomicrograph illustrating the histopathologic profile of cortex and cell growth around the posterior peripheral aspect of a round-edged IOL optic (see Figure. 7-53). Migration of pearls (red material in posterior capsule; lower right) derived from the large Soemmering's ring mass (also red color, left). The IOL optic is the empty space between the capsules on the right. (Masson's trichrome, original magnification x25).

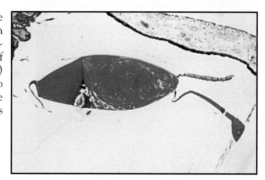

Figure 7-56B. Photomicrograph illustrating the histopathologic profile of cortex and cell growth around the posterior peripheral aspect of a round-edged IOL optic (see Figure. 7-53). A round-edged optic showing posterior peripheral migration, but clear central capsules over the visual axis. Note in Figures 7-56B and C the posteriorly migrated cells have undergone a pseudofibrous metaplasia with wrinkling of the posterior capsule secondary to fibrosis. Note also significant anterior capsule fibrosis (ACO) in both figures (also see Figures 7-6 to 7-10). (Periodic acid-Schiff stain, original magnification x25.)

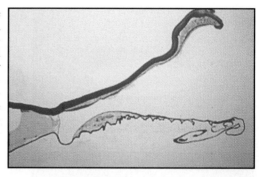

Figure 7-56C. Photomicrograph illustrating the histopathologic profile of cortex and cell growth around the posterior peripheral aspect of a round-edged IOL optic (see Figure. 7-53). A round-edged optic showing posterior peripheral migration, but clear central capsules over the visual axis. Note in Figures 7-56B and C the posteriorly migrated cells have undergone a pseudofibrous metaplasia with wrinkling of the posterior capsule secondary to fibrosis. Note also significant anterior capsule fibrosis (ACO) in both figures (also see Figures 7-6 to 7-10). (Periodic acid-Schiff stain, original magnification x25.)

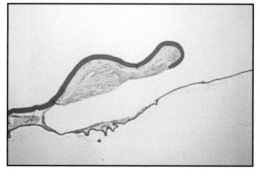

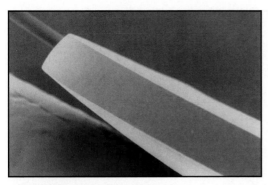

Figure 7-57. Sagittal (side) view showing the truncated edge (left) of the acrylic optic of the Alcon AcrySof IOL (scanning electron micrograph, original magnification x20).

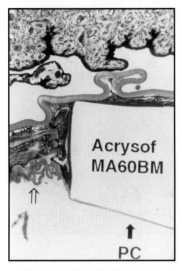

Figure 7-58. Photomicrograph of the anterior segment of a rabbit eye experimentally implanted with an Alcon AcrySof IOL by Dr. Okiro Nishi and associates in Japan. This clearly demonstrates the effective block of retained epithelial cells and cortex (arrows, left) created by the square edge of the lens, with complete blockage of growth onto the posterior capsule (PC). (photograph courtesy of Dr. O. Nishi, Osauka, Japan.)

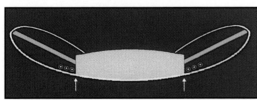

Figure 7-59. Schematic illustration demonstrating how square, truncated IOL optic edge provides an abrupt barrier (arrows), leaving the entire region behind the optical zone free of cells. This barrier effect is predicated on a tight contact between the optic biomaterial and the posterior capsule.

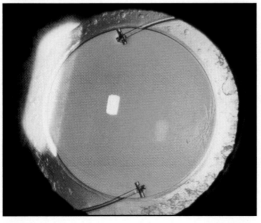

Figure 7-60. Clinical photograph illustrating the barrier effect of the Alcon AcrySof IOL. Despite the fact that numerous pearls are seen within the Soemmering's ring surrounding the IOL optic, the region behind the optic is free of pearls.

Figure 7-61A. Even when a significant Soemmering's ring remains in the eye, a square truncated edge such as what exists on the AcrySof IOL provides a second line of defense against cortical ingrowth. Other IOLs with square or truncated optic edges include the Ciba Mentor MemoryLens, the Staar Surgical/Bausch and Lomb Surgical elastimide-polyimide silicone design, the Pharmacia-Upjohn CeeOn Edge 911 silicone IOL, and plate haptic IOLs. Gross photograph from behind (Miyake-Apple posterior photographic technique) of a human eye obtained postmortem containing an AcrySof IOL. Some cortical remnants (a Soemmering's ring) remain peripherally but the optical zone remains totally cell free, with no encroachment of cells past the edge of the IOL optic.

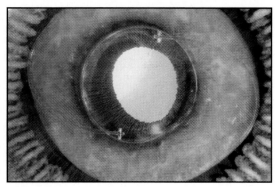

Figure 7-61B. Even when a significant Soemmering's ring remains in the eye, a square truncated edge such as what exists on the AcrySof IOL provides a second line of defense against cortical ingrowth. Other IOLs with square or truncated optic edges include the Ciba Mentor MemoryLens, the Staar Surgical/Bausch and Lomb Surgical elastimide-polyimide silicone design, the Pharmacia-Upjohn CeeOn Edge 911 silicone IOL, and plate haptic IOLs. Gross photograph from behind (Miyake-Apple posterior photographic technique) of a human eye obtained postmortem showing another Alcon AcrySof IOL implanted into the capsular bag. Cortical removal was incomplete and a moderate size Soemmering's ring is present. However, growth is totally blocked by the optic barrier effect of the edge of the square truncated optic. Therefore, the optical zone remains clear. The crescent-shaped area of opacity over the upper aspect of the optic is actually the anterior capsule, not PCO.

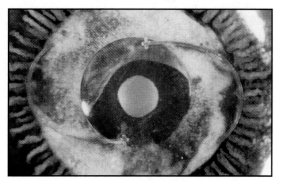

Figure 7-62A. Photomicrograph of an eye in which a Alcon AcrySof IOL was implanted. Cleanup was not complete and a Soemmering's ring resulted. However, the Soemmering's ring remnants (red) remain confined to the left of the square optic edge, leaving the posterior capsule (lower right) cell-free. (Masson's trichrome stain, original magnification x 100.)

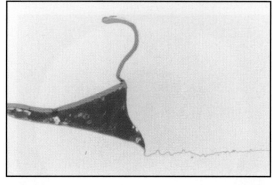

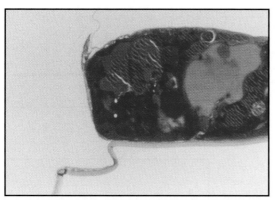

Figure 7-62B. Photomicrograph of an eye in which a Alcon AcrySof IOL was implanted. Cleanup was not complete and a Soemmering's ring resulted. However, the Soemmering's ring remnants (red) remain confined to the left of the square optic edge, leaving the posterior capsule (lower right) cell-free. (Masson's trichrome stain, original magnification x 100.)

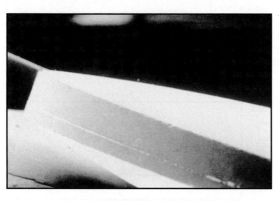

Figure 7-63A. Scanning electron micrograph of another IOL with a square-truncated optic edge; namely, the Pharmacia-Upjohn CeeOn edge 911 (original magnification x50).

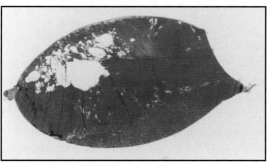

Figure 7-63B. Photomicrograph of a capsular bag with a Pharmacia-Upjohn CeeOn edge 911 IOL (see Figure 7-63A) experimentally implanted into a rabbit eye. Note the site of the square-edge optic to the right of the Soemmering's ring, where the lens material abutted against the optic. The silicone optic has dissolved out during processing. There is a total blockade of cells and cortex (red mass to the left), so that the posterior capsule (far right) remains clear in the direction of the visual axis+. (Masson's trichrome stain, original magnification x100.)

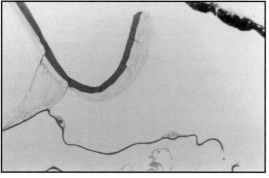

Figure 7-64. Photomicrograph of the capsular bag from a case of an early one-piece all-PMMA design, which was unpolished and had a square edge (see Figure 7-50). The imprint of the square-edged optic is noted here and the posterior capsule in the direction of the visual axis (lower right) is clear except for one or two minute cell deposits (Periodic acid-Schiff stain, x100).

Figure 7-65. Figures 7-65 to 7-69 show schematic illustration of various scenarios of the histopathology of the capsular bag after in-the-bag IOL implantation of various optic styles in the scenario in this figure, cortical cleanup was complete and the capsulorhexis diameter was larger than the IOL optic. There is total fusion of the anterior and posterior capsules (E = equator). No barrier effect is required with this scenario so the type of optic, round or truncated, is not operative in terms of blocking PCO.

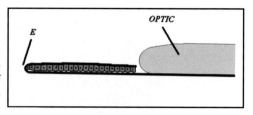

Figure 7-66. In this scenario, the capsulorhexis diameter was smaller than that of the lens optic. Since cortical clean-up was incomplete in this scenario, the space between the anterior and posterior capsule is largely cell-free and no barrier effect is required (E=equator).

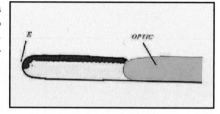

Figure 7-67. In this scenario, the capsulorhexis diameter is larger than the optic diameter so the cut edge fuses with the posterior capsule. This may help sequester the Soemmering's ring (SR) from the posterior capsule and thus block PCO.

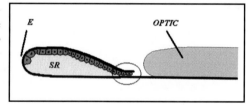

Figures 7-65 to 7-70 are schematic illustrations showing the variety of in-the-bag fixation scenarios seen with rigid and foldable IOL implantation. Figures 7-65 and 7-66 are scenarios in which cortical cleanup is complete or almost complete. Figures 7-67 to 7-69 represent a scenario in which cortical cleanup is incomplete. Figures 7-68 and 7-69 are scenarios requiring the second line of defense provided by the IOL optic.

To summarize the concept of the barrier effect, there is a subtle difference between classic optics with a round tapered edge (Figures 7-53 and 7-68) and optics with a square truncated edge (Figures 7-59 and 7-68). Figures 7-53 and 7-68 (top) show a common scenario seen with an IOL optic with a rounded, tapered edge. There is some growth of cells behind the posterior-lateral aspect of the optic toward the paracentral region of the lens (peripheral orange haze). However, the central axis is usually not involved. The drawings in Figures 7-59, 7-68 (bottom), and 7-69 show the scenario often obtained when there is a truncated, square-edged optic, in which a complete blockade of cells at the optic edge leaves the posterior capsule free of cells. This provides the clinical appearance of a "clear capsule" that has often been observed by surgeons when following patients with the AcrySof IOL. The enhanced barrier effect provided by this optic geometry probably functions as an "icing on the cake" by providing an additional reserve factor (in addition to the basic cortical cleanup (Table 7-2, #1) that has been proven to be of the utmost importance in helping reduce the overall incidence of visually significant PCO).

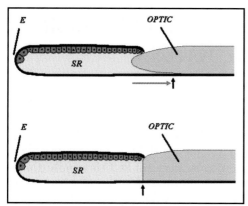

Figure 7-68. The scenario when significant cortical retention/regeneration occurs. Top: When the Soemmering's ring is blocked by the tapered, round edge of a biconvex optic, ingrowth behind lens periphery may occur (horizontal arrow). Bottom: When the Soemmering's ring cell ingrowth is blocked by a square, truncated optical edge, ingrowth behind the optic is abruptly blocked at the outer edge of the optic.

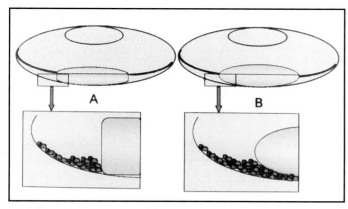

Figure 7-69. In this scenario, the capsulorhexis diameter is slightly smaller than the lens optic, so its edge rests on the anterior surface. The IOL optic shown on the left has a square edge, which blocks cells from the posterior capsule. The optic on the right has a round edge, which in some cases can allow ingrowth of Soemme-ring's ring (SR) onto the posterior surface of the optic (arrow). This ingrowth usually does not encroach upon the visual axis.

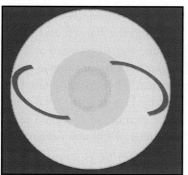

Figure 7-70A. Optic design showing the barrier effect of a classic biconvex IOL with a round, tapered edge. There is some potential of cell growth around the posterior peripheral edge of the optic into the area of posterior capsule behind the periphery of the optic. This frontal view shows the pattern of ingrowth of cells and cortex that may occur behind the outer periphery of the optic.

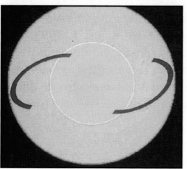

Figure 7-70B. Optic design demonstrating the barrier effect of a classic biconvex IOL with a thicker square or truncated edge. With the square edge abrupt blockage of cell growth at the optic edge is more likely. This frontal view shows that ingrowth over the optic may be completely retarded as a result of the abrupt blockage of cells by the truncated, square edge, leaving a totally clear capsule.

ANALYSIS OF ND:YAG LASER POSTERIOR CAPSULOTOMY RATES

We recently published results of an ongoing study[4] that has increased our overall understanding of PCO and has helped us develop the above mentioned six factors (see Tables 7-2 and 7-3) that we believe greatly contribute to the reduction of PCO. This study, an analysis of Nd:YAG laser posterior capsulotomy rates among eight commonly used IOL models, has led us to the optimistic conclusion that the incidence of PCO is rapidly diminishing, particularly in the industrialized world.

Using both the anterior (surgeon's) view and the Miyake-Apple posterior photographic technique, it is easy to determine whether an eye has had an Nd:YAG laser posterior capsulotomy. We applied this to our database of IOL-related specimens accessioned between 1982 and 2000 (see Figure 1-1). As of August 1999, there were over 15,000 IOL-related specimens accessioned, almost 7000 eyes obtained postmortem containing IOLs. Five thousand and seventy-nine eyes with PC IOLs were accessioned between January 1988 and August 1999-the time period of this analysis. Six hundred and eighty-one were foldable designs (as of August 1, 1999). Only eyes operated on in the United States were available for this analysis.

The lenses analyzed included the two most commonly implanted rigid designs prevalent over the last decade, one- and three-piece PMMA-optic IOLs, as well as six modern foldable designs (Figures 7-71 to 7-80). These eight IOL designs were available in postmortem eyes in the United States, but several important foldable lens designs not yet available for analysis in postmortem eyes in the United States could not be included in this study. These included, among others: 1) all non-US manufactured lenses; 2) Pharmacia-Upjohn CeeOn Edge 911 IOL; 3) all hydrogel designs, including the Bausch and Lomb Hydroview; and 4) CibaVision Mentor Memory Lens. Each globe was accessioned and categorized according to the presence or absence of a Nd:YAG posterior capsulotomy as determined using the Miyake-Apple posterior photographic technique. The Nd:YAG rate seen with each IOL design (Figures 7-71 to 7-78A) was determined by 1) noting the total number of accessions of the IOL style and then 2) determining the number of Nd:YAG lasers performed on the IOLs in each group. The rate (%) as of August 1, 1999 was determined by dividing these two numbers (Figures 7-71 to 7-78, figure A in each).

In addition to noting the Nd:YAG laser capsulotomy rate (in percentages) as of August 1, 1999 (Figures 7-71 to 7-80), we created a "timeline" curve for each IOL analyzed (Figures 7-71 to 7-78, (figure B in each). We plotted the percentage of Nd:YAG rates at monthly intervals during the entire period from January 1988 to August 1, 1999. This allows documentation of a trend for each lens. Determination of past and future Nd:YAG rates over an ever increasing time helps compensate for the fact that the implantation date for each case was not always known. As the number of eyes and duration of time during which the eyes were studied increases, the important factor of postoperative time (implant duration) is less a factor as a major variable.

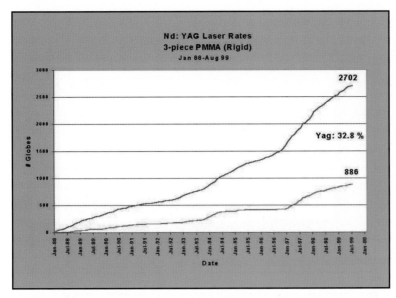

Figure 7-71A. (The series of graphs in Figures 7-71 through 7-78 demonstrate how the data on the eight IOLs were accumulated in order to tabulate a rank of Nd:YAG laser rates (see Figures 7-79 and 7-80). In figure A of each group, we show the Nd:YAG laser rates of each IOL as of August 1, 1999, and, in figure B of each group, Nd:YAG laser trends or time-lines to determine trends over time of Nd:YAG rates for each model. In other words, for each lens, we show both the basic Nd:YAG laser capsulotomy data (%) (as of August 1, 1999), as well as a time-line documenting Nd:YAG laser capsulotomy percentages obtained at 6-month intervals for the duration of each IOLs' existence.) Three-piece rigid PMMA optic IOL. The IOL had an Nd:YAG laser rate of 32.8% as of August 1, 1999.

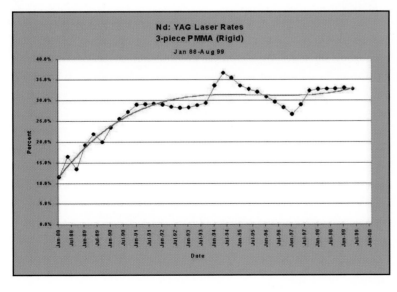

Figure 7-71B. The trend line of the three-piece PMMA-optic IOL appears to have stabilized over time.

Figure 7-72A. One-piece all-PMMA rigid IOL design. This IOL style shows an Nd:YAG laser rate of 26.2% as of August 1, 1999.

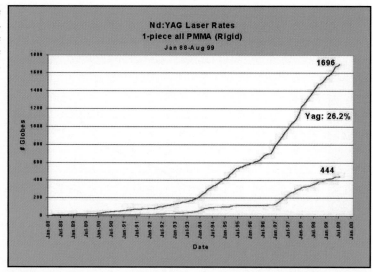

Figure 7-72B. One-piece all-PMMA rigid IOL design. The trend line shows a slight increase. One-piece all PMMA rigid IOLs showed a slight increase.

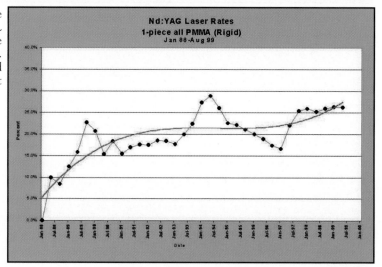

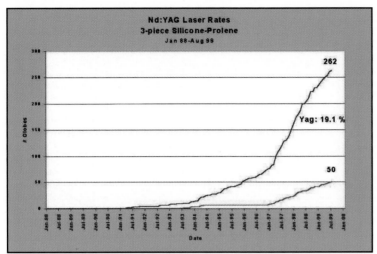

Figure 7-73A. Three-piece silicone optic-prolene haptic IOL (Allergan SI-30 design). This IOL shows an Nd:YAG laser rate of 19.1% as of August 1, 1999.

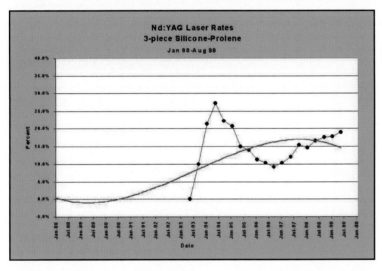

Figure 7-73B. Three-piece silicone optic-prolene haptic IOL (Allergan SI-30 design). The trend line of this IOL is decreasing slightly.

Figure 7-74A. Three-piece silicone (elastimide-polyimide) IOL. This IOL shows an Nd:YAG laser rate of 11.1% as of August 1, 1999.

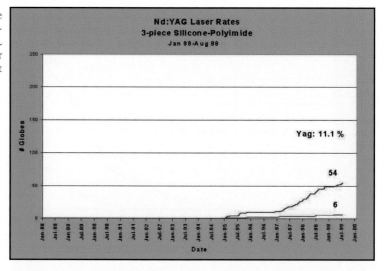

Figure 7-74B. Three-piece silicone (elastimide-polyimide) IOL. Trend line of this IOL is decreasing.

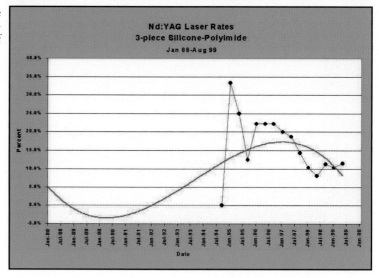

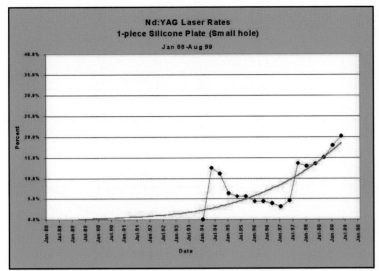

Figure 7-75B. Small hole silicone plate IOL. Trend line of this IOL is decreasing.

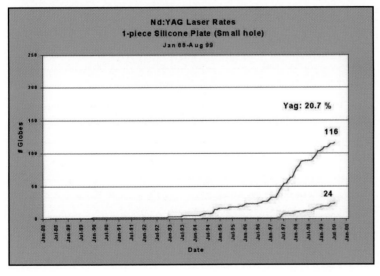

Figure 7-75A. Small hole silicone plate IOL. This IOL showed an Nd:YAG laser rate of 20.7% as of August 1, 1999.

Figure 7-76A. Large hole 1-piece silicone plate IOL. This IOL shows an Nd:YAG laser rate of 8.2% as of August 1, 1999.

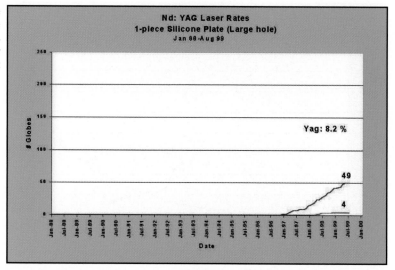

Figure 7-76B. Large hole 1-piece silicone plate IOL. Trend line of this IOL appears to be increasing.

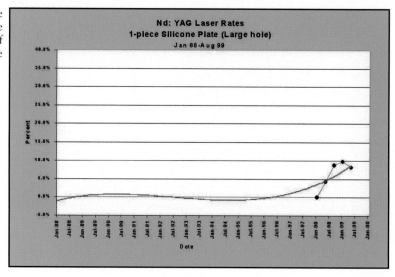

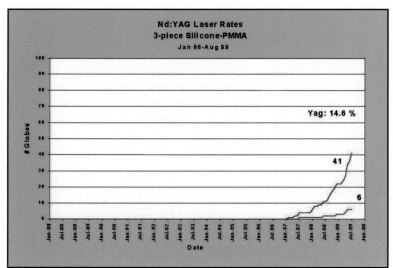

Figure 7-77A. Allergan SI-40 silicone optic PMMA haptic foldable IOL. This IOL showed an Nd:YAG laser rate of 14.6% as of August 1, 1999.

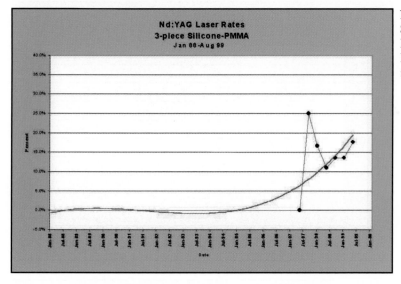

Figure 7-77B. Allergan SI-40 silicone optic PMMA haptic foldable IOL. The trend line is increasing.

Figure 7-78A. Alcon AcrySof IOL, hydrophobic optic-PMMA haptics. This design showed the lowest Nd:YAG laser rate of all lenses studied,1.7%.

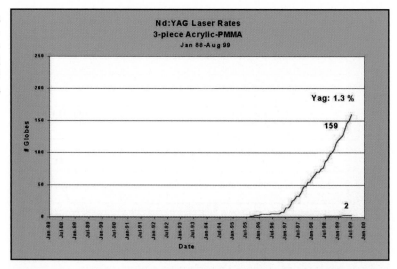

Figure 7-78B. Alcon AcrySof IOL, hydrophobic optic-PMMA haptics. Trend line of the AcrySof is a flat curve that is almost immeasurable.

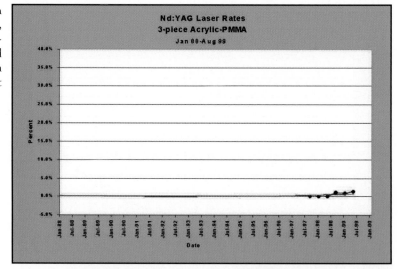

Figure 7-79. Tabulation of Nd:YAG laser capsulotomy rates on eight different rigid and foldable IOL types available in our United States autopsy database, accessioned between January 1988 and August, 1999. These are listed with the lowest capsulotomy rates above. The Alcon Acrysof IOL had the lowest rate and the two rigid PMMA optic IOL designs had the highest rates.

Nd:YAG Rate (%) January 88 thru August 99 (Apple and associates, 1999)			
Lens	**Total**	**Nd:YAG**	**YAG %**
3 PC Acrylic-PMMA (Acrysof)	159	2	1.3%
1 PC Silicone Plate, Large Hole	49	4	8.2%
3 PC Silicone-Polyimide	54	6	11.1%
3 PC Silicone-PMMA (Allergan SI 40)	41	6	14.6%
3 PC Silicone-Prolene	262	50	19.1%
1 PC Silicone Plate, Small Hole	116	24	20.7%
1 PC All-PMMA (Rigid)	1696	444	26.2%
3 PC PMMA (Rigid)	2702	886	32.8%
All Lenses since 1/88	5079	1422	28.0%
Foldable lenses	681	92	13.5%
Rigid Lenses	4398	1330	30.2%

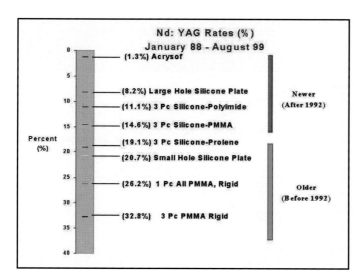

Figure 7-80. This figure summarizes the Nd:YAG laser capsulotomy data that were tabulated in Figure 7-79. Note that the lenses with the relatively low Nd:YAG laser capsulotomy rates (15% or less) are relatively new, mostly implanted after 1992. This suggests that the rate of PCO is a delicate balance between surgical quality and IOL quality. After 1992, much better capsular surgical techniques (Generation VI-a and b) were available (see Chapter 2, Figures 2-19 and 7-25, and Table 2-2).

The data for all eight lenses are shown in the curves illustrated in Figures 7-71 to 7-78 and in tabulation forms in Figures 7-79 and 7-80. These are listed in increasing order according to the percentage Nd:YAG rate of each IOL as of August 1, 1999. The IOL with the lowest Nd:YAG laser posterior capsulotomy rate was the Alcon AcrySof IOL (Figure 7-71A). As of August 1, 1999, 154 AcrySof IOLs had been accessioned and only two Nd:YAG lasers were noted, a low rate of 1.3% (Figure 7-71A). Trend line analysis of this IOL showed an almost immeasurable value (Figure 7-78B). Note that the three-piece rigid optic IOL designs, which have the longest history of implantation, had the highest PCO Nd:YAG rate of 36.8% (Figure 7-78A). The trend or "time-line" of this lens design shows that this rate appears to have stabilized (Figure 7-78B). The one-piece all-PMMA design, which still represents the gold standard among rigid IOLs, had an Nd:YAG rate of 26.2% (Figure 7-72A), also with a relatively stable trend line (Figure 7-77).

Figure 7-80 summarizes the Nd:YAG laser posterior capsulotomy data that were tabulated in Figure 7-79. Note that the 4 IOLs with the lowest Nd:YAG laser posterior capsulotomy rate (circa 15% or less) were the relatively new designs, mostly implanted after 1992. This is about the time that modern capsular surgery, Generation VI, became the procedure of choice in the industrialized world (Figure 7-81, see also Figure 7-25) . The lenses with a relatively high PCO rate were older designs. The information tabulated here must therefore be viewed considering the age and duration of each implant. Figure 7-81 demonstrates the transition from precapsular to capsular surgical techniques that really began to occur around 1992 and Figure 7-82 emphasizes that the PCO and Nd:YAG laser posterior capsulotomy rate represents a delicate balance between the quality of the IOL and the quality of the surgery (Figure 7-83).

Figure 7-84 is noteworthy, showing a very low Nd:YAG laser posterior capsulotomy rate of around 13.5% with modern foldable lenses, as opposed to 30.2% with rigid lenses. Again, the major factor here is not so much in the type of lens, but rests with the fact that many of the rigid lenses were implanted over several generations of ECCE PC IOL, for example in Generations V-a and V-b (see Chapter 2). The foldable lenses are now being

Figure 7-81. Implementation of improved capsular surgical techniques, including small-incision phacoemulsification techniques, increased rapidly in the early 1990s (see also Figure 7-25), especially after 1992. (Precapsular= prehydrodissection, CCC and in-the-bag fixation.)

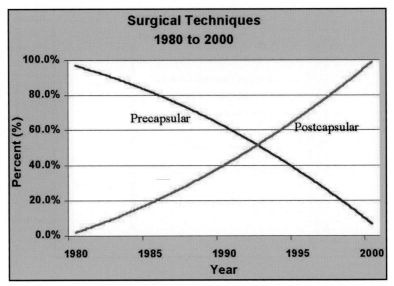

Figure 7-82. The incidence of PCO and the Nd:YAG laser rate of each lens type depend on several factors, including a balance between of IOL quality and utilization of modern capsular surgery.

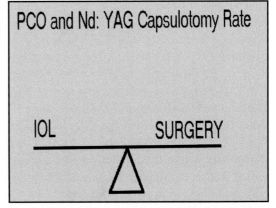

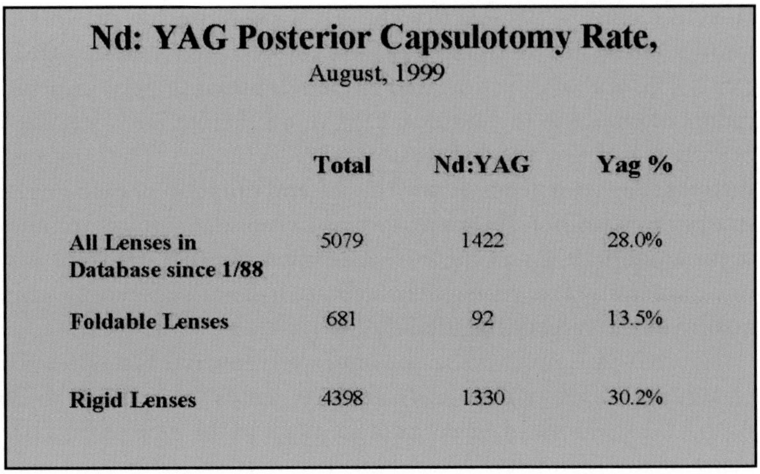

Figure 7-83. Our series shows clearly that the PCO rate and the Nd:YAG laser capsulotomy rate is much lower with modern foldable lenses in Generation VIb (see Figure 2-19 and Table 2-2)-13.5% as opposed to 30.2% of all the rigid optic IOLs in this series. This reflects a balance between the modern high-quality IOLs and the high-quality capsular surgical techniques required for insertion of foldable lenses that are now available.

Nd: YAG Posterior Capsulotomy Rate, August, 1999

	Total	Nd:YAG	Yag %
All Lenses in Database since 1/88	5079	1422	28.0%
Foldable Lenses	681	92	13.5%
Rigid Lenses	4398	1330	30.2%

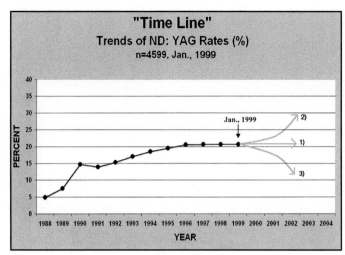

Figure 7-84. As we continue studies on eyes obtained postmortem with PC IOLs, it is important to continue creation of a trend or timeline of Nd:YAG percentage rates for each IOL design as determined over time at 6-month intervals. We began this proliferative study on January 1, 1999. This will help determine whether each individual lens design: 1) maintains a stable rate, 2) increases, or 3) decreases. This will help differentiate whether the results seen with each lens are based more on changes in surgical quality, duration of the implant, or quality of the IOL itself.

implanted in Generation VI-b (Chapter 2, see Figure 2-19), and therefore undoubtedly have the advantages of being implanted with much better technique. To evaluate a difference in lens quality in relation to PCO Nd:YAG laser posterior capsulotomy rates, a timeline must be followed over the long term (Figure 7-84). If, for example, the generic curve shown in Figure 7-84 is followed over a 6-month interval with a tracing of each IOL's Nd:YAG rate, one can determine if a given lens rate has stabilized (#1), is increasing over time (#2), or is decreasing over time (#3). This should help provide a definitive comparison between each IOL style. This will be necessary to help rule on other factors such as quality of surgery and the duration of the implant in the eye to assess differences between the IOLs properly. We began this study as of January 1999 (Figure 7-84) and are currently performing an ongoing study of our database. We will report on this every 6 months for the next several years.

In summary, we now observe that there is a clear and rapid decrease in the incidence of PCO and hence the need for Nd:YAG laser posterior capsulotomy—occurring at least in the industrialized world. We have identified several important factors accounting for this (see Tables 7-2 and 7-3), and have noted that success rates depend on a balance between the quality of surgery and the quality of the IOL. The Alcon AcrySof has shown excellent performance in reducing PCO, especially in terms of general biocompatibility, generally low rates of intracapsular cellular reactivity and low Nd:YAG laser capsulotomy rates (Figure 7-85). We now document that the incidence of Nd:YAG laser posterior capsulotomy for secondary cataract has diminished to a level of 15% or less (Figure 7-86). This is in sharp contrast to the earlier Nd:YAG laser rates of 30 to 50% of the 1980s and early 1990s. The latter is no longer an acceptable standard as we enter the new millennium.

The decrease in PCO incidence noted in this study and confirmed in recent experimental and clinical studies is important for several reasons:
1. Financially, health care system costs for laser treatment and PCO are being reduced from hundreds of millions of dollars per year to a fraction of that amount.
2. A lower PCO rate is now allowing better pediatric and refractive IOL surgery, including multifocal IOLs and clear lens extraction.

Figure 7-85. In this tabulation, we summarize the Nd:YAG laser rates and biocompatibility scores of each IOL design studied in our series. Note that the Alcon AcrySof IOL fares extremely well and is associated with low epithelial cell reactivity in the capsular bag and hence has a low rate of PCO. Note also the favorable scores at all levels of the modern foldable lenses as opposed to the earlier rigid lenses (two top lines).

Biocompatibility Scores
January 1988 thru August 1999
(From Apple and associates, 1999)

Piece	PCOO	PCOP	SRI	SRA	SRA X SRI
3 PC Acrylic-PMMA (Acrysof)	0.044	0.494	1.158	2.184	3.589
3 PC Silicone-PMMA (Allergan SI 40)	0.146	1.171	1.707	3.049	6.024
3 PC Silicone-Polyimide	0.259	1.056	1.870	2.833	6.500
1 PC Silicone Plate, Large Hole	0.245	1.204	1.816	3.327	6.592
3PC Silicone-Prolene	0.388	1.168	1.820	2.823	6.613
1 PC Silicone Plate, Small Hole	0.450	1.360	2.108	2.739	6.748
1 PC All-PMMA (Rigid)	0.451	1.200	2.118	3.067	7.463
3 PC PMMA (Rigid)	0.548	1.226	2.624	3.033	8.583
All Lenses since 1/94	0.467	1.184	2.282	2.992	7.712
Foldable lenses	0.280	1.032	1.706	2.708	5.864
Rigid Lenses	0.505	1.214	2.397	3.048	8.082

Figure 7-86. Our analyses of eyes obtained postmortem over the last 10 years have led us to the optimistic conclusion that, using the above mentioned six factors (Tables 7-2 and 7-3), the rate of PCO, ranging from 30 to 50% in the 1980s, is now beginning to decrease to less than 10% as we begin the new century. The tools and lenses necessary to implement these six factors are available in the industrialized world. It is important that these soon be implemented in the developing world.

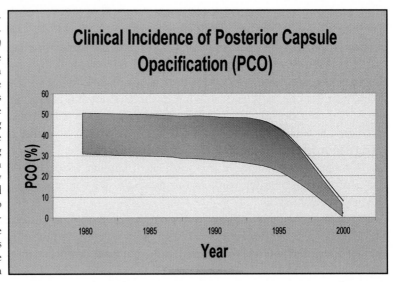

3. Control of PCO gives us confidence that modern cataract-IOL surgery can be done successfully worldwide—including not only the industrialized and former communist countries, but also developing countries—without fear of the blinding complications of secondary cataract. Now that tools, techniques, and lenses are available to reduce the PCO rate drastically, a major effort must be made to transfer this technology to the rural developing world to expedite further the success of the ECCE PC IOL procedure in these regions.

REFERENCES

1. Apple DJ, Peng Q, Ram J. The fiftieth anniversary of the intraocular lens and a quiet revolution. *Ophthalmology*. 1999;106(10):1-2.

2. Werner L, Pandey SK, Escobar-Gomez M, et al. Anterior capsule opacification: A histological study comparing different IOL styles. *Ophthalmology*. 2000;107(3):463-471.

3. Apple DJ, Solomon KD, Tetz MR, et al. Posterior capsular opacification, a review (Monograph). *Surv Ophthalmol*. 1992;37(2):73-116.

4. Apple DJ, Peng Q, Visessook N, et al. Comparison of Nd:YAG posterior capsulotomy rates of rigid and foldable intraocular lenses. An analysis of 5079 eyes with PC IOLs obtained postmortem accessioned between January 1988 and January 1999. *J Cataract Refract Surg*. 2000. [In press]

5. Faust KJ. Hydrodissection of soft nuclei. *J Am Intraocular Imp Soc*. 1984;10(1):75-77.

6. Peng Q, Apple DJ, Visessook N, Schoderbek R. Surgical Prevention of Posterior Capsule Opacification. Part II. Enhancement of cortical clean up by increased emphasis and focus on the hydrodissection procedure. *J Cataract Refract Surg*. 2000;26(2):188-197.

7. Fine IH. Cortical cleaving hydrodissection. *J Cataract Refract Surg*. 1992;18:508-512.

8. Peng Q, Visessook N, Apple DJ, et al. Surgical prevention of posterior capsule opacification. Part III. The IOL barrier effect functions as a second line of defense. *J Cataract Refract Surg*. 2000;26(2):198-213.

9. Apple DJ, Peng Q, Visessook N, et al. Surgical prevention of posterior capsule opacification. Part I. How are we progressing in eliminating this complication of cataract surgery? *J Cataract Refract Surg*. 2000;26(2):180-187.

10. Peng Q, Hennig A, Vasavada AR, Apple DJ. Posterior capsular plaque, a common complication of cataract surgery in the Developing World; Pathogenesis and clinical significance. *Am J Ophthalmol*. 1998;125:621-626.

11. Apple DJ, Reidy J, Googe J, et al. A comparison of ciliary sulcus and capsular bag fixation of posterior chamber intraocular lenses. *J Am Intraocular Implant Soc*. 1985;11:44-63.

12. Ram J, Apple DJ, Peng Q, et al. Update on fixation of rigid and foldable posterior chamber intraocular lenses (IOLs). Part I. Elimination of decentration to achieve precise optical correction and visual rehabilitation. *Ophthalmology*. 1999;106:883-890.

13. Assia EI, Apple DJ, Barden A, et al. An experimental study comparing various anterior capsulectomy techniques. *Arch Ophthalmol*. 1991;109:642-647.

14. Visessook N, Apple DJ, Peng Q, et al. Soemmering's ring formation evaluation in a series of 4599 eyes with PC IOLs obtained postmortem. An assay of IOL biocompatibility. *J Cataract Refract Surg*. 1999.

15. Nishi O, Nishi K, Sakanishi K. Inhibition of migrating lens epithelial cells at the capsular bend created by the rectangular optic edge of a posterior chamber intraocular lens. *Ophthalmic Surg & Lasers*. 1998;29:587-594.

BIBLIOGRAPHY

Apple DJ, Assia EI, Wasserman D, et al. Evidence in support of the continuous tear anterior capsulectomy (capsulorhexis technique). In: Cangelosi GC, ed. *Advances in Cataract Surgery*. Thorofare, NJ: SLACK Incorporated; 1991;21-47.

Apple DJ, Auffarth GU, Wesendahl TA. Pathophysiology of Modern Capsular Surgery. In: Steinert, Auffarth GU, Wesendahl TA, Assia EI, Apple DJ. *Textbook of Modern Cataract Surgery: Technique, Complications, & Management*. Philadelphia, Pa: W. B. Saunders Company; 1995;314-324.

Apple DJ, Brems RN, Ellis GW, et al. Posterior Chamber Intraocular Lens Fixation. In: Buratto L, ed. *Extracapsular Cataract Microsurgery and Posterior Chamber Intraocular Lenses*. Vol 2. Milano, Italy: Centro Ambrosiano Microchirurgia Oculare; 1989:473-478.

Apple DJ, Davison JA, Nordan LT, Maxwell WA. Capsulorhexis, PC IOL centration, and trans-scleral PC IOL fixation. In: Nordan LT, Maxwell WA, Davison JA, eds. *The Surgical Rehabilitation of Vision: An Integrated Approach to Anterior Segment Surgery*. London, New York: Gower Medical Publishing; 1992:9.1-9.12.

Apple DJ, Hansen S, Richard S, Tetz M. Histopathological and experimental aspects of modern lens implant surgery. In: Rosen E, Kalb I, eds. *Intercapsular Cataract Extraction*. Oxford, England: Pergamon Press; 1988;1-11.

Apple DJ, Kincaid MC, Mamalis N, Olson RJ. *Intraocular Lenses. Evolution, Designs, Complications, and Pathology*. Baltimore, Md: Williams & Wilkins, 1989.

Apple DJ, Mamalis N, Loftfield K, et al. Complications of intraocular lenses. A historical and histopathological review. *Surv Ophthalmol*. 1984;29:1-54.

Apple DJ, Morgan RC, Tsai JC, Lim ES. Update on implantation of posterior chamber intraocular lenses. In: Weinstock FJ, ed. *Management and Care of the Cataract Patient*. Boston, Ma: Blackwell Scientific Publications; 1992; 128-134.

Apple DJ, Rabb MF. Lens and Pathology of Intraocular Lenses. In: *Ocular Pathology. Clinical Applications and Self-Assessment*. 5th ed. St. Louis, Mo: Mosby Year-Book, Inc., 1998; 117-204.

Apple DJ, Tetz MR, Hansen SO. Use of Viscoelastics in Intraocular Lens Removal. In: Rosen E, ed., *Viscoelastic Materials*. Oxford, England: Pergamon Press; 1988.

Apple DJ. Capsulorhexis. *Proceedings of The Third International, Implant, Microsurgical & Refractive Keratoplasty Meeting*. Fukuoka, Japan: 1989.

Apple DJ. How we can Stamp out posterior capsular opacification? *Review of Ophthalmol*. 1997;10:170-171.

Apple DJ. Pathological Aspects of Capsular Surgery. *Eur J Implant Ref Surg*. 1994;6:

Apple, DJ, Casanova R, Davison J. Technique of PC IOL implantation using a small smooth circular continuous tear capsulotomy (capsulorhexis). A demonstration using the posterior video technique of human cadaver eyes. *Video presentation at the Annual Meeting of the American Academy of Ophthalmology*, New Orleans, 1989.

Aron-Rosa D, Aron J-J, Griesemann M, et al. Use of the neodymium-YAG laser to open the posterior capsule after lens implant surgery: A preliminary report. *J Am Intraocul Implant Soc*. 1980;6:352-354.

Arshinoff S. Classifying capsulorhexis complications. *J Cataract Refract Surg*. 1994;20:475.

Arshinoff SA. Dispersive-cohesive viscoelastic soft shell technique. *J Cataract Refract Surg*. 1999;25:167-173.

Assia EI, Apple DJ, Lim ES, Morgan RC, Tsai JC. Removal of viscoelastic material after experimental cataract surgery in vitro. *J Cataract Refract Surg*. 1992;18:3-6.

Assia EI, Apple DJ, Morgan RC, Legler UFC, Brown SJ. The relationship between the stretching capability of the anterior capsule and zonules. Invest *Ophthalmol Vis Sci*. 1991;32:2835-2839.

Assia EI, Apple DJ, Tsai JC, Lim ES. The elastic properties of the lens capsule in capsulorhexis. *Am J Ophthalmol*. 1991;111:628-632.

Assia EI, Apple DJ, Tsai JC, Lim ES. The elastic properties of the lens capsule in capsulorhexis. *Am J Ophthalmol*. 1991;112(4):474-475.

Assia EI, Apple DJ, Tsai JC, Lim ES. The elastic properties of the lens capsule in capsulorhexis. *Am J Ophthalmol*. 1991;112:355.

Assia EI, Apple DJ, Tsai JC, Morgan RC. Mechanism of radial tear formation and extension after anterior capsulotomy. *Ophthalmology*. 1991;98:432-437.

Assia EI, Apple DJ. Side-view analysis of the lens. Part I. The crystalline lens and the evacuated capsular bag. *Arch Ophthalmol*. 1992;110:89-93.

Assia EI, Apple DJ. Side-view analysis of the lens. Part II. Positioning of intraocular lenses. *Arch Ophthalmol.* 1992;110:94-97.

Assia EI, Blumenthal M, Apple DJ. Effect of expandable full-size intraocular lenses on lens centration and capsule opacification in rabbits. *J Cataract Refract Surg.* 1999;25:347-356.

Assia EI, Blumenthal M, Apple DJ. Hydrodissection and visco extraction of the nucleus in planned extracapsular cataract extraction. *Eur J Implant Refract Surg.* 1992;4:3-8.

Assia EI, Blumenthal M, Legler UFC, Apple DJ. Photoanalysis of fixation of posterior chamber intraocular lenses. *Eur J Implant Refract Surg,* 1993.

Assia EI, Castaneda VE, Legler UFC, et al. Studies on cataract surgery and intraocular lenses at the Center for Intraocular Lens Research. *Ophthalmol Clin N Am.* 1991;4:251-266.

Assia EI, Hoggatt J, Apple DJ. Experimental nucleus extraction through a capsulorhexis in an eye with pseudoexfoliation syndrome. *Am J Ophthalmol.* 1991;111:645-647.

Assia EI, Legler UFC, Apple DJ. The Capsular Bag After Short- and Long-Term Fixation of Intraocular Lenses. *Ophthalmology.* 1995;102(8):1151-1157.(RPB)

Assia EI, Legler UFC, Castaneda VE, Apple DJ. Loop Memory of Posterior Chamber Intraocular Lenses Of Various Sizes, Designs and Loop Materials. *J Cataract Refract Surg.* 1992;18:541-546.

Assia EI, Legler UFC, Castaneda VE, et al. Clinicopathologic study on the effect of radial tears and loop fixation on intraocular lens decentration. *Ophthalmology.* 1993;100:153-158.

Assia EI, Legler UFC, Libby C, et al: Size and configuration of the capsular bag after short and long term fixation of posterior chamber intraocular lenses in-the-bag. Invest *Ophthalmol Vis Sci.* 1991;32(4):747.

Auer C, Gonvers M. Silicone one piece intraocular implant and anterior capsule fibrosis. *Klin Monatsbl Augenheilkund.* 1995;206:293-295.

Auffarth GU, Apple DJ. Einflub von Intraokularlinsendesign und operativen Techniken auf die Nachstarentwicklung1. In: Ohroloff C, et al., eds. *Transactions of the 11th Congress of the German Intraocular Lens Implant Society (DGII).* Berlin, Germany: Springer-Verlag (Publ), 1997: Berlin-Heidelberg, New York; 1998:241-249.

Auffarth GU, Beischel CJ, Wesendahl TA, Apple DJ. Soemmerring's Ring Bildung nach Kataraktoperation und HKL Implantation: Eine Studie von 827 Autopsieaugen. In: Rochels R, Dunker G, Hartmann Ch, eds., *Transactions of the 9th Congress of the German Intraocular Lens Implant Society,* Kiel, Germany. Heidelberg, Berlin, New York: Springer (Publ); 1995.

Bath P, Hoffer K, Aron-Rosa D, et al: Glare disability secondary to YAG laser intraocular lens damage. *J Cataract Refract Surg.* 1987;13:309-313.

Bath PE, Romberger A, Brown P, Quon D. Quantitative concepts in avoiding intraocular lens damage from the Nd:YAG laser in posterior capsulotomy. *J Cataract Refract Surg.* 1986;12:262-266.

Bath PE, Romberger AB, Brown P. A comparison of Nd:YAG laser damage thresholds for PMMA and silicone intraocular lenses. *Inv Ophthalmol Vis Sci.* 1986;27:795-798.

Blomstedt G, Fagerholm P, Gallo J, Philipson B. After-cataract in the rabbit eye following extracapsular cataract extraction-a wound healing reaction. *Acta Ophthalmologica.* 1987;65 (suppl 182): 93-99.

Blumenthal M, Assia E, Schochot Y: Lens anatomical principles and their technical implications in cataract surgery. Part I. The lens capsule. *J Cataract Refract Surg.* 1991;17(2):205-210.

Carlson AN, Tetz MR, Apple DJ. Infectious complications of modern cataract surgery and intraocular lens implantation. *Infect Dis Clin North Am.* 1989;3:339.

Dahlhauser KF, Wroblewski KJ, Mader TH. Anterior capsule contraction with foldable silicone intraocular lenses. *J Cataract Refract Surg.* 1998;24:1216-1219.

Dana MR, Chatzistefanou K, Schaumberg DA, Foster CS. Posterior capsule opacification after cataract surgery in patients with uveitis. *Ophthalmology.* 1997;104:1387-1394.

Davison J. A short haptic diameter mod-J-loop PC-IOL for improved bag performance. *J Cataract Refract Surg.* 1988;14:161-166.

Davison JA. Analysis of capsular bag defects and intraocular lens positions for consistent centration. *J Cataract Refract Surg.* 1986;12:124-129.

Davison JA. Capsule contraction syndrome. *J Cataract Refract Surg.* 1993;19:582-589.

Dick B, Schwenn O, Eisenmann D. Reflections on Nd:YAG capsulotomy in lens opacity after multifocal lens implantation. *Klin Monatsbl Augenheilkund.* 1997;211:363-368.

Dick B, Schwenn O, Pfeiffer N. Extent of damage to different intraocular lenses by neodymium:YAG laser treatment--an experimental study. *Klin Monatsbl Augenheilkund.* 1997;211:263-271.

Downing J. Long-term discission rates after placing posterior chamber lenses with the convex surface posterior. *J Cataract Refract Surg.* 1986;12:651-654.

Elschnig A. Klinisch-anatomischer Beitrag zur Kenntnis des Nachstares. *Klin Monatsbl Augenheilkd.* 1911;49:444-451.

Eshaghian J, Streeten B. Human posterior subcapsular cataract: An ultrastructural study of the posteriorly migrating cells. *Arch Ophthalmol.* 98:134-143, 1980.

Fagerholm P. On the formation of Elschnig's pearls: A tissue culture study of regenerating rat lens epithelium. *Acta Ophthalmol.* 1980;58:963-970.

Fine IH, Hoffman RS. Clear corneal cataract surgery. *Ophthalmic Surg Lasers.* 1998;29:822-831.

Fine IH, Hoffman RS. Late reopening of fibrosed capsular bags to reposition decentered intraocular lenses. *J Cataract Refract Surg.* 1997;23:990-994.

Font R, Brownstein S. A light and electron microscopic study of anterior subcapsular cataracts. *Am J Ophthalmol.* 1974;78:972-984.

Frezzotti R, Caporossi A, Mastrangelo D, et al. Pathogenesis of posterior capsule opacification: Part II. Histopathological and in vitro culture findings. *J Cataract Refract Surg.* 1990;16:353-360.

Gimbel HV, Neuhann T. Development, advantages, and methods of the continuous circular capsulorhexis technique. *J Cataract Refract Surg.* 1990;16:31-37.

Gimbel HV. Hydrodissection and hydrodelineation. *Int Ophthalmol Clin.* 1994;34:73-90.

Gimbel HV. Posterior capsulorhexis with optic capture in pediatric cataract and intraocular lens surgery. *Ophthalmology.* 1996;103:1871-1875.

Gimbel HV. Posterior continuous curvilinear capsulorhexis and optic capture of the intraocular lens to prevent secondary opacification in pediatric cataract surgery. *J Cataract Refract Surg.* 1997;23(suppl 1):652-656.

Gonvers M, Sickenberg M, van Melle G. Change in capsulorhexis size after implantation of three types of intraocular lenses. *J Cataract Refract Surg.* 1997;23:231-238.

Green W, Boase D. How clean is your capsule? *Eye.* 1989;3:678-684.

Green W, McDonnell P. Opacification of the posterior capsule. *Trans Ophthalmol Soc UK.* 1985;104:727-739.

Guthoff R, Abramo F, Draeger J, et al. Forces on intraocular lens haptics induced by capsular fibrosis; an experimental study. Graefes *Arch Clin Exp Ophthalmol.* 1990;228:363-368.

Guthoff R, Abramo F, Draeger J. Flexibility of intraocular lens haptics of various geometry and materials. *Klin Monatsbl Augenheilkund.* 1990;197:27-32.

Hansen S, Tetz M, Solomon K, et al: Decentration of flexible loop posterior chamber intraocular lenses in a series of 222 postmortem eyes. *Ophthalmology.* 1988;95:344-349.

Hansen SO, Apple DJ, Tetz MR, et al. Comparative Histopathologic Study of Various Lens Biomaterials in Primates After Nd:YAG Laser Treatment. *J Cataract Refract Surg.* 1987;13:657-661.

Hansen SO, Crandall AS, Olson RJ. Progressive constriction of the anterior capsule opening following intact capsulorhexis. *J Cataract Refract Surg.* 1993;19:77-82.

Hansen SO, Solomon KD, McKnight GT, et al. Posterior capsular opacification and intraocular lens decentration. Part I: Comparison of various posterior chamber lens designs implanted in the rabbit model. *J Cataract Refract Surg.* 1988;14:605-614.

Hara T, Hara T, and Yamada Y. "Equator ring" for maintenance of the completely circular contour of the capsular bag equator after cataract removal. *Ophthalmic Surg.* 1991;22(6):358-359.

Hara T, Hara T. Clinical results of endocapsular phacoemulsification and complete in-the-bag intraocular lens fixation. *J Cataract Refract Surg.* 1987;13:279-286.

Hara T, Hara T: Observations on lens epithelial cells and their removal in anterior capsule specimens. *Arch Ophthalmol.* 1988;106:1683-1687.

Hara T, Sakanishi K, Yamada Y. Efficacy of equator rings in an experimental rabbit study. *Arch Ophthalmol.* 1995;113:1060-1065.

Harfstrand A, Stenevi U, Schenholm M, et al. Sodium hyaluronate is naturally occurring on corneal endothelial cells of various species including man. *3rd Int Symp Ocular Microsurgery.* 1990;41-46.

Hayashi H, Hayashi K, Nakao F, Hayashi F. Quantitative comparison of posterior capsule opacification after polymethylmethacrylate, silicone, and soft acrylic intraocular lens implantation. *Arch Ophthalmol.*1998;116:1579-1582.

Hayashi K, Hayashi H, Nakao F, Hayashi F. In vivo quantitative measurement of posterior capsule opacification after extracapsular cataract surgery. *Am J Ophthalmol* 1998;125:837-843.

Hayashi K, Hayashi H, Nakao F, Hayashi F. Reduction in the area of the anterior capsule opening after polymethylmethacrylate, silicone, and soft acrylic intraocular lens implantation. *Am J Ophthalmol* 1997;123:441-447.

Hayashi K, Hayashi H, Nakao F, Hayashi F. Reproducibility of posterior capsule opacification measurement using Scheimpflug video-photography. *J Cataract Refract Surg.* 1998;24:1632-1635.

Hoffer K. Five year's experience with the ridged laser lens implant. In: Emery JM, Jacobson AC, eds., *Current Concepts in Cataract Surgery.* [Selected Proceedings of the Sixth Biennial Cataract Surgical Congress.] Norwalk, Appleton-Century-Crofts, 1980, pp 296-299.

Hollick EJ, Spalton DJ, Ursell PG, et al. The effect of polymethylmethacrylate, silicone, and polyacrylic intraocular lenses on posterior capsular opacification 3 years after cataract surgery. *Ophthalmology* 1999;106:49-54.

Hollick EJ, Spalton DJ, Ursell PG, Pande MV. Biocompatibility of poly(methyl methacrylate), silicone, and AcrySof intraocular lenses: randomized comparison of the cellular reaction on the anterior lens surface. *J Cataract Refract Surg.* 1998;24:361-366.

Hollick EJ, Spalton DJ, Ursell PG, Pande MV. Lens epithelial cell regression on the posterior capsule with different intraocular lens materials. *Br J Ophthalmol.* 1998;82:1182-1188.

Holweger RR, Marefat B. Intraocular pressure change after neodymium:YAG capsulotomy. *J Cataract Refract Surg.* 1997,23:115-121.

Hunold W, Wirtz M, Kaden P, Kreiner CF. Protektiver Effekt viskoelastischer Lösungen bei der Anwendung eines Nekrosefaktors zur Nachstarverhütung. In: Wenzel M, Reim M, Freyler H, Hartmann C, eds. *Kongress der Deutschen Gesellschaft für Intraokularlinsen Implantation.* Berlin, Heidelberg, New York: Springer; 1991:711-723.

Hütz W, Küstermann R, Hessemer V. Prospektive Studie über die Häufigkeit des Nachstares bei verschiedenen Linsentypen mit und ohne Laserridge. *Fortschr Ophthalmol.* 1990;87(6):583-587.

Javitt JC, Tielsch JM, Canner JK, et al. National outcomes of cataract extraction. Increased risk of retinal complications associated with Nd:YAG laser capsulotomy. *Ophthalmology.* 1992;99:1487-1498.

Javitt JC, Vitale S, Canner JK, et al. National outcomes of cataract extractions: Retinal detachment after inpatient surgery. *Ophthalmology.* 1991;98:895-902.

Joo CK, Shin JA, Kim JH. Capsular opening contraction after continuous curvilinear capsulorhexis and intraocular lens implantation. *J Cataract Refract Surg.* 1996;22:585-590.

Juechter K. Histopathology of capsule-fixated intraocular lenses. In: Emery JM, ed., *Current Concepts in Cataract Surgery. Selected Proceedings of the Fifth Biennial Cataract Surgical Congress.* St. Louis, Mo: CV Mosby;1978;165-172.

Kappelhof J, Vrensen G, Vester C, et al. The ring of Soemmerring in the rabbit: A scanning electron microscopic study. *Graefes Arch Clin Exp Ophthalmol.* 1985;223:111-120.

Kappelhof JP, Vrensen GF. The pathology of after-cataract. A mini review. *Acta Ophthalmologica.* 1992;(Suppl):13-24.

Kato K, Kurosaka D, Bissen-Miyajima H, et al. Elschnig pearl formation along the posterior capsulotomy margin after neodymium:YAG capsulotomy. *J Cataract Refract Surg.* 1997;23:1556-1560.

Kershner R. Capsular rupture at hydrodissection. *J Cataract Refract Surg.* 1992;18:423.

Kershner RM. Sutureless one-handed intercapsular phacoemulsification. The keyhole technique. *J Cataract Refract Surg.* 1991;17:Suppl:719-725.

Kim MJ, Lee HY, Joo CK. Posterior capsule opacification in eyes with a silicone or poly(methyl methacrylate) intraocular lens. *J Cataract Refract Surg.* 1999;25:251-255.

Koch DD, Kohnen T. Retrospective comparison of techniques to prevent secondary cataract formation after posterior chamber intraocular lens implantation in infants and children [published erratum appears in *J Cataract Refract Surg.* 1997 Sep;23(7):974]. *J Cataract Refract Surg.* 1997;23:Suppl 1:657-63.

Koch DD, Liu JF. Multilamellar hydrodissection in phacoemulsification and planned extracapsular surgery. *J Cataract Refract Surg.* 1990;16:559-562.

Legler UFC, Apple DJ, Assia EI, et al. Inhibition Of Posterior Capsular Opacification: The Effect of Colchicine In A Sustained Drug Delivery System. *J Cataract Refract Surg.* 1993;19:462-470.

Legler UFC, Assia EI, Castaneda VE, Hoggatt JP, Apple DJ. A prospective experimental study on factors related to posterior chamber intraocular lens decentration. *J Cataract Refract Surg.* 1992;18:449-455.

Lim SJ, Kang SJ, Kim HB, Kurata Y, Sakabe I, Apple DJ. Analysis of zonular-free zone and lens size in relation to axial length of eye with age, *J Cataract Refract Surg.* 1998;24:390-396.

Linnola RJ. Sandwich theory: Bioactivity-based explanation for posterior capsule opacification. *J Cataract Refract Surg.* 1997;23:1539-1542.

Maltzman B, Haupt E, Cucci P. Effect of the laser ridge on posterior capsule opacification. *J Cataract Refract Surg.* 1989;15:644-646.

Mamalis N, Craig M, Price F. Spectrum of Nd:YAG laser-induced intraocular lens damage in explanted lenses. *J Cataract Refract Surg.* 1990;16:495-500.

Mamalis N, Phillips B, Kopp CH, Crandall AS, Olson RJ. Neodymium: YAG capsulotomy rates after phacoemulsification with silicone posterior chamber intraocular lenses. *J Cataract Refract Surg.* 1996;22:Suppl 2:1296-1302.

Masket S. Postoperative complications of capsulorhexis. *J Cataract Refract Surg.* 1993;19:721-724.

Menapace R. Posterior capsule opacification and capsulotomy rates with taco-style hydrogel intraocular lenses. *J Cataract Refract Surg.* 1996;22:Suppl 2:1318-1330.

Milauskas AT. Posterior capsule opacification after silicone lens implantation and its management. *J Cataract Refract Surg.* 1987;13:644-648.

Miyake K, Ota I, Miyake S, Maekubo K. Correlation between intraocular lens hydrophilicity and anterior capsule opacification and aqueous flare. *J Cataract Refract Surg.* 1996;22:Suppl 1:764-769.

Nagamoto T, Eguchi G. Effect of intraocular lens design on migration of lens epithelial cells onto the posterior capsule. *J Cataract Refract Surg.* 1997;23:866-872.

Nagamoto T, Eguchi G. Morphologic compatibility of intraocular lens haptics and the lens capsule. *J Cataract Refract Surg.* 1997;23:1254-1259.

Nagata T, Minakata A, Watanabe I. Adhesiveness of a soft acrylic intraocular lens to a collagen film. *J Cataract Refract Surg.* 1998;24:367-370.

Nagata T, Watanabe I. Optic sharp edge or convexity: comparison of effects on posterior capsular opacification. *Jpn J Ophthalmol.* 1996;40:397-403.

Nasisse MP, Dykstra MJ, Cobo LM. Lens capsule opacification in aphakic and pseudophakic eyes. *Graefes Arch Ophthalmol Clin Exper Ophthalmol.* 1995;233:63-70.

Neuhann TH. Intraocular folding of an acrylic lens for explantation through a small incision cataract wound. *J Cataract Refract Surg.* 1996;22:Suppl 2:1383-1386.

Newland TJ, Auffarth GU, Wesendahl TA, Apple DJ.: Neodymium: YAG laser damage on silicone intraocular lenses. A comparison of lesions on explanted lenses and experimentally produced lesions. *J Cataract Refract Surg.* 1994;20:527-533.

Newland TJ, McDermott ML, Eliott D, et al. Experimental Neodymium:YAG Laser Damage to Acrylic, PMMA, and Silicone Intraocular Lens Materials, *J Cataract Refract Surg.* 1999;25:72-76.

Nishi O, Nakai Y, Mizumoto Y, Yamada Y. Capsule opacification after refilling the capsule with an inflatable endocapsular balloon. *J Cataract Refract Surg.* 1997;23:1548-1555.

Nishi O, Nishi K, Mano C, Ichihara M, Honda T. The inhibition of lens epithelial cell migration by a discontinuous capsular bend created by a band-shaped circular loop or a capsule-bending ring. *Ophthalmic Surg & Lasers* .1998;29:119-125.

Nishi O, Nishi K, Menapace R. Capsule-bending ring for the prevention of capsular opacification: a preliminary report. *Ophthalmic Surg & Lasers.* 1998;29:749-753.

Nishi O, Nishi K, Takahashi E. Capsular bag distention syndrome noted 5 years after intraocular lens implantation. *Am J Ophthalmol.* 1998;125:545-547.

Nishi O, Nishi K. Intraocular lens encapsulation by shrinkage of the capsulorhexis opening. *J Cataract Refract Surg.* 1993;19:544-545.

Nishi O, Nishi K. Intercapsular cataract surgery with lens epithelial cell removal. Part II. Long-term follow-up of posterior capsular opacification. *J Cataract Refract Surg.* 1991;17(2):218-220.

Nishi O. Posterior capsule opacification. Part 1. Experimental investigations. *J Cataract Refract Surg.* 1999;25:106-117.

Obstbaum SA. Clear lens extraction for high myopia and high hyperopia editorial; comment. *J Cataract Refract Surg.* 1994;20:271

Obstbaum SA. The anterior capsulotomy revisited. *J Cataract Refract Surg.* 1998;24:143-144.

Ohmi S, Uenoyama K, Apple DJ. Implantation of IOLs with different diameters. *Acta Soc Ophthalmol Jpn.* 1992;96(9):1093-1098.

Olson RJ, Crandall AS. Silicone versus poly(methyl methacrylate) intraocular lenses with regard to capsular opacification. *Ophthalmic Surg & Lasers.* 1998;29:55-58.

Osher RH. Clear lens extraction. *J Cataract Refract Surg.* 1994;20:674.

Oshika T, Nagata T, Ishii Y. Adhesion of lens capsule to intraocular lenses of poly(methyl methacrylate), silicone, and acrylic foldable materials: an experimental study [see comments]. *Br J Ophthalmol.* 1998;82:549-553.

Pande M, Spalton DJ, Marshall J. Continuous curvilinear capsulorhexis and intraocular lens biocompatibility. *J Cataract Refract Surg.* 1996;22:89-97.

Pande MV, Spalton DJ, Kerr-Muir MG, Marshall J. Postoperative inflammatory response to phacoemulsification and extracapsular cataract surgery: Aqueous flare and cells. *J Cataract Refract Surg.* 1996;22(suppl 1):770-774.

Pande MV, Ursell PG, Spalton DJ, Heath G, Kundaiker S. High-resolution digital retroillumination imaging of the posterior -004 capsule after cataract surgery. *J Cataract Refract Surg.* 1997;23:1521-1527.

Peng Q, Visessook N, Schoderbek R, Whiteside SB, Apple DJ. Comparison of modern foldable IOLs with respect to decreasing the incidence of posterior capsular opacification: an experimental study in rabbits. Abstract. *Symposium on Cataract, IOL and Refractive Surgery, American Society of Cataract and Refractive Surgery*; 1998:6.

Piest K, Kincaid M, Tetz M, et al. Localized endoph-thalmitis: A newly described cause of the so-called toxic lens syndrome. *J Cataract Refract Surg*. 1987;13:498-510.

Pisella PJ, Pietrini D, Limon S. Anterior cellular proliferation and silicone implant. Apropos of a case. *J Fran Ophtalmologie*. 1996;19:615-618.

Ram J, Apple DJ, Peng Q, et al. Update on fixation of rigid and foldable posterior chamber intraocular lenses (IOLs). Part II. Choosing the correct IOL designs to help eradicate posterior capsule opacification. *Ophthalmology*. 1999;106:891-900.

Ravalico G, Tognetto D, Palomba M, Busatto P, Baccara F. Capsulorhexis size and posterior capsule opacification. *J Cataract Refract Surg*. 1996;22:98-103.

Saika S, Ohmi S, Tanaka S, et al. Light and scanning electron microscopy of rabbit lens capsules with intraocular lenses. *J Cataract Refract Surg*. 1997;23:787-794.

Saxby L, Rosen E, Boulton M. Lens epithelial cell proliferation, migration, and metaplasia following capsulorhexis. *Br J Ophthalmol*. 1998;82:945-952.

Schaumberg DA, Dana MR, Christen WG, Glynn RJ. A systematic overview of the incidence of posterior capsular opacification. *Ophthalmology*. 1998; 105:1213-1221.

Sellman T, Lindstrom R. Effect of plano-convex posterior chamber lens on capsular opacification from Elschnig pearl formation. *J Cataract Refract Surg*. 1988;14:68-72.

Shah SM, Spalton DJ. Natural history of cellular deposits on the anterior intraocular lens surface. *J Cataract Refract Surg*. 1995; 21:466-471.

Sheperd J. Capsular opacification associated with silicone implants. *J Cataract Refract Surg*. 1989;15:448-450.

Soemmerring D. *Beobachtungen ueber die organischen Veraenderungen des Auges nach Staaroperationen*. Frankfurt/a/M, Wesche, 1828.

Solomon K, Apple D, Mamalis N, et al. Complications of intraocular lenses with special reference to an analysis of 2500 explanted intraocular lenses (IOLs). *Eur J Implant Refract Surg*. 1991;3:196-200.

Sourdille P. Overview of posterior capsule opacification. *J Cataract Refract Surg*. 1997;23:1431-1432.

Spencer M. The 1.97 cent solution: Low tech capsulorhexis and hydrodissection. *J Cataract Refract Surg*. 1991;17:372-373.

Steinert RF, Puliafito CA, Kumar SR, Dudak SD, Patel S. Cystoid macular edema, retinal detachment, and glaucoma after Nd: YAG laser posterior capsulotomy. *Am J Ophthalmol*. 1991;112:373-380.

Sterling S, Wood T. Effect of intraocular lens convexity on posterior capsule opacification. *J Cataract Refract Surg*. 1986;12(6):655-657.

Streeten B, Eshaghian J. Human posterior subcapsular cataract. A gross and flat preparation study. *Arch Ophthalmol*. 1987;96:1653-1658.

Strenn K, Menapace R, Vass C. Capsular bag shrinkage after implantation of an open-loop silicone lens and a poly(methyl methacrylate) capsule tension ring. *J Cataract Refract Surg*. 1997;23:1543-1547.

Sun R, Gimbel HV. In vitro evaluation of the efficacy of the capsular tension ring for managing zonular dialysis in cataract surgery. *Ophthalmic Surg & Lasers*. 1998;29:502-505.

Sveinsson O. The ultrastructure of Elschnig's pearls in a pseudophakic eye. *Acta Ophthalmologica*. 1993;71:95-98.

Tan JC, Spalton DJ, Arden GB. Comparison of methods to assess visual impairment from glare and light scattering with posterior capsule opacification. *J Cataract Refract Surg*. 1998;24:1626-1631.

Tassignon MJ, De Groot V, Smets RM, Tawab B, Vervecken F. Secondary closure of posterior continuous circular capsulorhexis. *Bulletin de la Societe Belge d Ophtalmologie* 1996;261:87-91.

Tawab BM, Tassignon MJ. Ocular and systemic factors associated with posterior capsule opacification. *Bulletin de la Societe Belge d Ophtalmologie.* 1995;259:21-25.

Tetz M, Apple D, Hansen S, et al. Localized endophthalmitis. A complication of extracapsular cataract extraction. *Imp Ophthalmol.* 1987;1(3):93-97.

Tetz M, Sperker M, Blum M, Auffarth GU, Volcker HE. Clinical evaluation of secondary cataract in pseudophakic eyes. Method and reproducibility. *Ophthalmologe.* 1996;93:33-37.

Tetz MR, Apple DJ, Price FW Jr, et al. A newly described complication of Neodymium-YAG laser capsulotomy: Exacerbation of an intraocular infection. *Arch Ophthalmol.* 1987;105:1324-1325.

Tetz MR, Auffarth GU, Sperker M, Blum M, Volcker HE. Photographic image analysis system of posterior capsule opacification. *J Cataract Refract Surg.* 1997;23:1515-1520.

Tetz MR, O'Morchoe DJC, Gwin TD, et al. Posterior capsular opacification and intraocular lens decentration. Part II: Experimental findings on a prototype circular IOL design. *J Cataract Refract Surg.* 1988;14:614-623.

Tu KL, Gaskell A. Capsular bag distension syndrome. *Br J Ophthalmol.* 1997;81:610.

Ursell PG, Spalton DJ, Pande MV, et al. Relationship between intraocular lens biomaterials and posterior capsule opacification. *J Cataract Refract Surg.* 1998;24:352-360.

Ursell PG, Spalton DJ, Pande MV. Anterior capsule stability in eyes with intraocular lenses made of poly(methyl methacrylate), silicone, and AcrySof. *J Cataract Refract Surg.* 1997;23:1532-1538.

Wasserman D, Apple DJ, Castaneda VE, et al. Anterior capsular tears and loop fixation of posterior chamber intraocular lenses. *Ophthalmology.* 1991;98:425-431.

Wedl C. *Altas der pathologischen Histologie des Auges.* Leipzig, Germany: George Wigan Verlag; 1860.

Wesendahl T, Auffarth G, Brown S, Apple D. IOL surface texturing a new concept for PCO prevention. Abstract. *Ger J Ophthalmol.* 1993;2(4/5):365.

Wesendahl TA, Auffarth GU, Apple DJ. Area of contact between IOL-Optic and Posterior Capsule. Systematic Analysis of Different Hapticparameters. In: Gloor R, et al., eds. *Trans 7th Congress of the German Intraocular Lens Implant Society (DGII).* Zhurich. 1993, pp 222-227.

Wesendahl TA, Auffarth GU, Newland TJ, Brown S, Apple DJ. Einfluss der Kapsulorrhexisgrosse auf der Nachstarentstehung. In: Gloor R, et al, eds., *Trans 7th Congress of the German Intraocular Lens Implant Society (DGII). Zhurich:* 1993:228-236.

Whiteside SB, Apple DJ, Peng Q, Isaacs RT, Guindi A. Fixation elements on plate IOLs. Large positioning holes to improve security of capsular fixation (Part III), *Ophthalmology.* 1998;105:837-842.

Yamada K, Nagamoto T, Yozawa H, et al. Effect of intraocular lens design on posterior capsule opacification after continuous curvilinear capsulorhexis. *J Cataract Refract Surg.* 1995;21:697-700.

Yorston D. Are intraocular lenses the solution to cataract blindness in Africa? *Br J Ophthalmol.* 1998;82:469-471.

Zaczek A, Zetterstrom C. Posterior capsule opacification after phacoemulsification in patients with diabetes mellitus. *J Cataract Refract Surg.* 1999;25:233-237.

Chapter 8

Selected Miscellaneous Complications

SILICONE OIL ADHERENCE TO INTRAOCULAR LENSES

In the mid 1990s we described a rare condition characterized by adherence of silicone oil used in vitreoretinal surgery to an IOL that had been previously implanted in the eye undergoing treatment (Figures 8-1 and 8-2).[1] All lenses examined in our laboratory and almost all cases published to-date have involved IOLs with silicone optics (Figures 8-1 and 8-2). To determine the nature of this phenomenon, we performed in vitro testing by immersing six commonly implanted IOL styles as well as human crystalline lenses in a solution of silicone oil (Figures 8-3 to 8-8).[2] We found that the degree of adherence was multifactorial, but primarily based on the hydrophilic versus hydrophobic nature of the IOL biomaterial. In other words, the greater the contact angle (hydrophobic) (Figures 8-3A and B), the greater the silicone oil adherence. With non-implanted silicone IOLs taken directly out of the manufacturer's package, the amount of coating of silicone oil was virtually 100% (Figures 8-4A and B). It is important to note, however, that with previously implanted IOLs that had existed for a time in the milieu of the aqueous humor, a thin proteinaceous coating derived from the aqueous formed a partial surface film on the IOL optic. This can alter the surface from being hydrophobic with a potential for 100% silicone oil adherence to a more hydrophilic surface with reduced adherence of silicone oil to the lens (Figure 8-4C).

Figures 8-4 through 8-8 document the results obtained after exposure of several IOLs to silicone oil. These results, and results obtained following silicone oil exposure to a human crystalline lens, are tabulated in Figure 8-3. The important point is that although the most adherence occurs with the silicone IOL, other IOLs, with the probable exception very hydrophilic hydrogel designs and the heparin surface modified (HSM) design of Pharmacia-Upjohn, are not immune to this process. We have noted that perfluorocarbon (Figure 8-9), which is another important tool of the retinal surgeon, does not significantly adhere to silicone IOLs.

Figure 8-1A. Clinical photograph of an eye containing a silicone IOL. In Figures 8-1A and B, vitreoretinal procedures requiring silicone oil were performed years after the original IOL had been implanted. Note the obvious deposits and droplets of silicone oil on the IOL optic. The irreversible silicone oil adhesion to the IOL surface that occurred in these figures not only diminished the patient's visual acuity but also the surgeon's ability to view inside each eye.

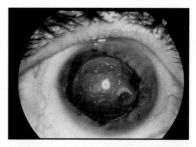

Figure 8-1B. Clinical photograph of an eye containing a silicone IOL. In Figures 8-1A and B, vitreoretinal procedures requiring silicone oil were performed years after the original IOL had been implanted. Note the obvious deposits and droplets of silicone oil on the IOL optic. The irreversible silicone oil adhesion to the IOL surface that occurred in these figures not only diminished the patient's visual acuity but also the surgeon's ability to view inside each eye.

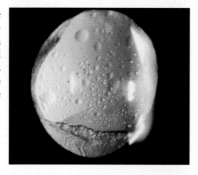

Figure 8-2A. Gross photograph of a silicone IOL explanted because of irreversible silicone oil adhesion to the IOL optics. The deposits and droplets are tenaceous and almost impossible to remove clinically.

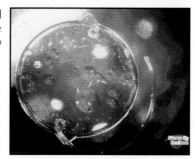

Figure 8-2B. Gross photograph of a silicone IOL explanted because of irreversible silicone oil adhesion to the IOL optics. The deposits and droplets are tenaceous and almost impossible to remove clinically.

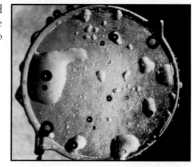

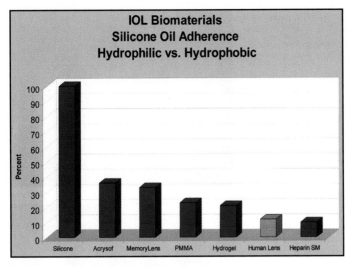

Figure 8-3A. We performed an in vitro study, exposing several IOL styles to silicone oil, then determined the percentages of silicone oil coverage for these IOL styles, finding that the percentage of coating corresponded closely with the wettability of the IOL biomaterial surface (hydrophilic versus hydrophobic). Although the value for silicone was highest in this study, other lenses were not immune to this. According to this exam, a hydrogel or the heparin surface modified (HSM) IOL by Pharmacia-Upjohn would be lenses of choice for patients with severe active or potential vitreo-retinal disease that might be expected to require future treatment with silicone oil. (Bar graph showing relative percentages of silicone oil adherence comparing six IOL designs and the crystalline lens.)

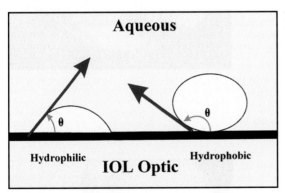

Figure 8-3B. Schematic illustration showing the concept of a small contact angle (hydrophilic) versus a large contact angle (hydrophobic) of a biomaterial.

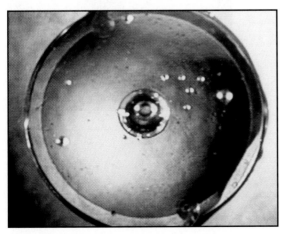

Figure 8-4A. The in vitro silicone oil incubation study noted in Figure 8-3 is presented in Figures 8-4 through 8-9. In each instance, the IOL was incubated with silicone oil and the percentage surface area coated by the oil after removal from the oil solution was noted. With each lens a gross photograph of the incubated IOL was made and a digitized computer analysis of percentage and area cover was determined. The actual percentage is shown graphically in Figure 8-3. In this figure, we demonstrate a gross photograph of a silicone IOL showing virtually 100% coverage by the oil coating.

Figure 8-4B. In each instance in the in vitro study (see Figures 8-3A and B), the IOL was incubated with silicone oil and the percentage surface area coated by the oil after removal from the oil solution was noted. With each lens a gross photograph of the incubated IOL was made and a digitized computer analysis of percentage and area cover was determined. The actual percentage is shown graphically in Figure 8-3A. In this figure, we demonstrate a silicone IOL. Same lens as Figure 8-4A. Computer digital analysis confirms the 100% coating. Yellow = silicone oil.

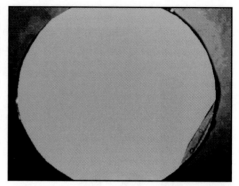

Figure 8-4C. In each instance int he in vitro study (see Figures 8-3A and B), the IOL was incubated with silicone oil and the percentage surface area coated by the oil after removal from the oil solution was noted. With each lens a gross photograph of the incubated IOL was made and a digitized computer analysis of percentage and area cover was determined. The actual percentage is shown graphically in Figure 8-3A. When silicone oil adherence to a previously clinically-implanted silicone IOL (as opposed to a nonimplanted IOL taken directly from the manufacturer's package) was analyzed, the percentage coating was significantly less than the 100% noted in vitro (Figures 8-4A and B). This digitized analysis (yellow = silicone oil) is shown to be in the range of 60 to 70%. This is because IOLs within the aqueous humor of eyes absorb a proteinaceous coating that changes the surface characteristics of the IOL. In this scenario it has transformed the status of the IOL surface from a totally hydrophilic nature to an intermediate value.

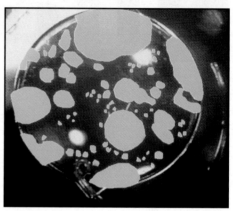

Figure 8-5. The in vitro test (see Figures 8-3A and B) performed on an Alcon AcrySof IOL showed a mean coating of approximately 35%.

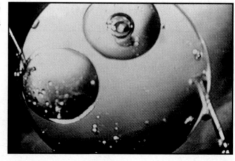

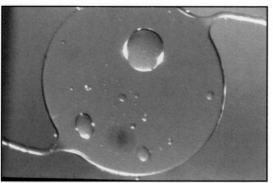

Figure 8-6. The same in vitro study (see Figures 8-3A and B) performed on one-piece all-PMMA designs showed a mean coating of approximately 20%.

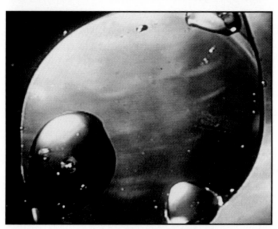

Figure 8-7. The same in vitro study (see Figures 8-3A and B) performed on a Bausch and Lomb Hydroview hydrogel IOL, showing a mean coating of slightly less than 20%.

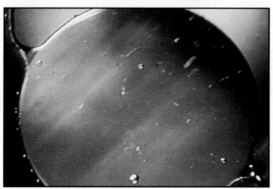

Figure 8-8. The same in vitro analysis (see Figures 8-3A and B) of the Pharmacia-Upjohn HSM IOL, a very hydrophilic design, showed a value of less than 5%. According to this experimental finding, this lens would be an ideal design for implantation in patients with actual or potential vitreoretinal disease.

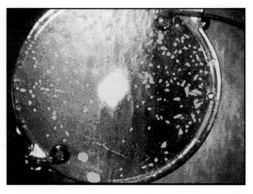

Figure 8-9. Another tool used by the vitreoretinal surgeon in addition to silicone oil is perfluorocarbon. This is a silicone IOL incubated in perfluorocarbon showing minimal adherence of this compound to the lens (yellow flecks= scattered deposits of silicone oil).

A major clinical pearl regarding this condition would be to not implant a relatively hydrophobic implant into a patient with severe present or potential vitreoretinal disease that may require later silicone oil therapy. In such cases, the lens of choice should be based on the results documented in Figure 8-3A; namely, a hydrogel IOL (or hydrophilic acrylic IOL) or a Pharmacia-Upjohn HSM IOL. It must be strongly emphasized, however, that this condition is rare. The factor of silicone oil adherence should not be an important factor in choosing an IOL for routine implantations in healthy patients in the absence of retinal disease. In patients without pre-existing disease, there are numerous other factors that are of much higher priority to the implant surgeon in choosing a foldable design (including both medical factors and factors related to service and costs). The existence of this condition should be known to all cataract-IOL surgeons, but its significance should not be overemphasized or overly exaggerated. This condition should not be construed as a reason for any form of general comdemnation of silicone IOLs.

INTERLENTICULAR OPACIFICATION OF PIGGYBACK INTRAOCULAR LENSES

Opacification between two piggyback IOLs, which we have termed interlenticular opacification (ILO), also known as interpseudophakic opacification of polypseudophakia, was recently presented for the first time in a clinicopathologic report by Gayton, Apple, and associates at the annual meeting of the American Society of Cataract and Refractive Surgery in Seattle, Wash., April 1999[3] (Figures 8-10 to 8-17). The implantation of two IOLs in a single capsular bag (piggyback implantation) has been used successfully for several years as a means to obtain a beneficial refractive result, especially in highly ametropic individuals. The lenses may be implanted primarily (until recently, usually with both lenses placed into the capsular bag), or the second may be implanted secondarily; e.g., to correct for a poor refractive result after performing cataract surgery. The latter of the two lenses is sometimes implanted into the ciliary sulcus, anterior to the primarily implanted lens situated in the capsular bag.

Opacification between these lenses has been a concern, but only recently described, in the above-mentioned clinicopathologic report (Figures 8-10 to 8-15). Most noteworthy,

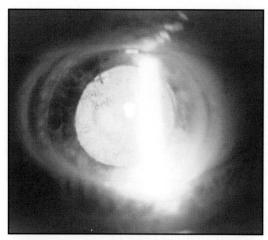

Figure 8-10. Clinical photograph of an eye of a patient with a "piggyback" IOL pair; namely, 2 Alcon AcrySof IOLs, implanted by Dr. Johnny Gayton of Warner Robins, Ga, the inventor of this procedure. These lenses were in the eye for 2 years and the opacification which ensued and is seen here was nonresponsive to Nd:YAG laser treatments and other modalities. The pair of IOLs had to be explanted.

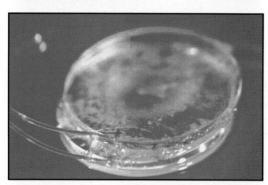

Figure 8-11A. Gross photograph of the pair of piggyback Alcon AcrySof IOLs removed by Dr. Johnny Gayton and referred to the Center for Research on Ocular Therapeutics and Biodevices (same case as shown in Figure 8-10.) This figure shows an oblique view of the gray-white membrane sandwiched between the two lens optics. Some areas appear clear, whereas other areas show dense accumulations of the gray-white material.

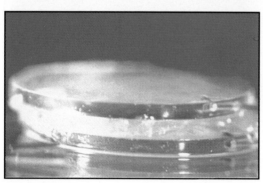

Figure 8-11B. Gross photograph of the pair of piggyback Alcon AcrySof IOLs removed by Dr. Johnny Gayton and referred to the Center for Research on Ocular Therapeutics and Biodevices (same case as shown in Figure 8-10.) This figures shows a sagittal (side view) photograph of the two lenses with the thick gray-white accumulation of the material between the two optics. The accumulation is approximately 0.5 mm in thickness[3]

Figure 8-12A. Photomicrograph of the area between the two IOLs in regions where the accumulation of white material was minimal and in regions where the interpseudophakic opacity was more dense (Figures 8-12A and B). In this area of scanty pearl formation, the anterior acrylic lens is above and remnants of acrylic biomaterial can be seen at the top. The posterior lens is below, and residual acrylic material is also seen at the bottom of this photograph. Most of the space between the two lenses in this region is clear, although a few residual remnants of lens material are seen on each IOL surface. (Hematoxylin and eosin stain, original magnification x200.)

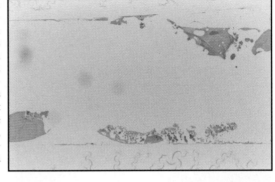

Figure 8-12B. Photomicrograph of the area between the two IOLs in regions where the accumulation of white material was minimal (Figure 8-12A) and in regions where the interpseudophakic opacity was more dense (Figures 8-12A and B). This photomicrograph of the interlenticular space shows total filling of the space by a pink material recognizable as retained lens cortex and cells. (Hematoxylin and eosin stain; original magnification x200.)

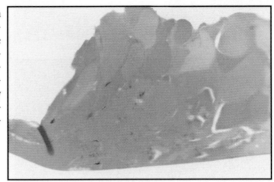

Figure 8-12C. Photomicrograph of the area between the two IOLs in regions where the accumulation of white material was minimal (Figure 8-12A) and in regions where the interpseudophakic opacity was more dense (Figures 8-12A and B). High power photomicrograph through the interlenticular mass, showing details of lens cortical material and retained lens epithelial cells. (Hematoxylin and eosin stain; original magnification x200.)

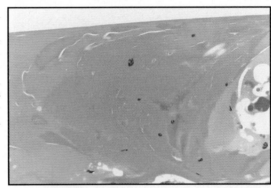

Figure 8-13A. Gross photograph from two piggyback IOLs explanted by Dr. Johnny Gayton, Warner Robins, Ga, and referred to our laboratory. The opacification between these two Alcon AcrySof IOLs was much thinner than that illustrated in the cases shown in Figures 8-10 to 8-12. Note that the central clear area represents the site of central touch of the two IOL optics. In contrast to the first case shown, Figures 8-10 and 8-11, it was possible to separate the two lenses. (Anterior piggyback IOL.)

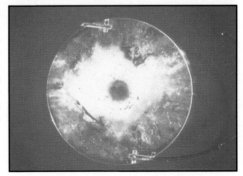

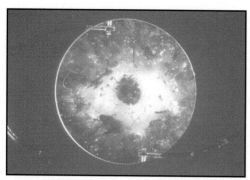

Figure 8-13B. Gross photograph from two piggyback IOLs explanted by Dr. Johnny Gayton, Warner Robins, Ga, and referred to our laboratory. The opacification between these two Alcon AcrySof IOLs was much thinner than that illustrated in the cases shown in Figures 8-10 to 8-12. Note that the central clear area represents the site of central touch of the two IOL optics. In contrast to the first case shown, Figures 8-10 and 8-11, it was possible to separate the two lenses. (Posterior piggyback IOL.)

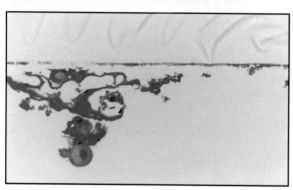

Figure 8-14. High-power photomicrographs through the anterior part of the two lenses shown in Figure 8-13, pointed out the presence of retained lens epithelial cells. The posterior surface of the anterior (front) lens (acrylic material seen above) shows a few clusters of retained lens epithelial cellular elements. (Hematoxylin and eosin stain; original magnification x225.)

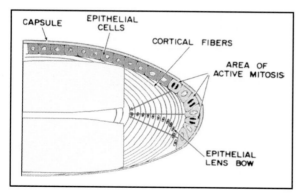

Figure 8-15. Schematic illustration of the equatorial region of a crystalline lens showing location of important cellular elements. The optics of two piggyback IOLs have been sketched in the lens substance. The point of this diagram is to demonstrate how near the edges of the IOL optics (and hence the interlenticular spaces (ILS)) are to the peripheral anterior epithelial cells as well as the equatorial bow. It follows that entrance of retained cells between the lenses into this space does not require an extensive migration. This complication is therefore a potential danger. The best way to prevent this phenomenon is to attain thorough removal of lens material and cells with hydrodissection-enhanced cortical removal.

Figure 8-16A. Schematic illustration of various scenarios of a single and piggyback pair of IOLs. Control: Implantation of a single IOL with a relatively small CCC. The edge of the CCC is in contact with the anterior surface of the IOL optic. This is a common technique used to implant single IOLs and appears to be efficacious in the retained cells and cortex (yellow) remained segregated peripheral to the IOL optic.

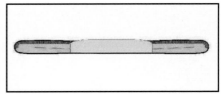

Figure 8-16B. Schematic illustration of various scenarios of a single and piggyback pair of IOLs. Piggyback IOLs: Both IOLs implanted in the capsular bag as with A, the CCC diameter was made relatively small so that the edge of the CCC rests in the front of the IOL optic, placing both lenses totally within the capsular bag compartment. Note, however, that with this scenario the retained/proliferative equatorial lens epithelial cells and cortex (yellow) have direct access to the ILS. [IOL optic= gray; IOL haptic= blue; capsular bag and cells= red; retained/proliferative equatorial lens epithelial cells/cortex= yellow].

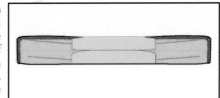

Figure 8-17A. Schematic illustration of a piggyback implantation scenario, which we believe may be useful in helping avoid this complication. This scenario is based on collections of John Gayton, David Apple, Joel Shugar, Paul Ernest and other surgeons. Werner and associates[4] have shown that with the Acrysof IOL there is almost no proliferation of residual anterior epithelial cells, so theanterior capsule around the cut CCC edge between the IOL optics is devoid of cells and hence should not be expected to produce cells within ILS. (Piggyback IOLs, both IOLs implanted in the capsular bag but with a relatively large diameter CCC. In this scenario, there is a possibility that the cut edge of the CCC may fuse with the posterior capsule. This would sequester the retained/proliferating equatorial lens epithelial cells/cortex within the equtorial fornix (yellow material forming Soemmering's ring) and this lessens the liklihood of migration of cells into the ILS. Note that this space (the ILS) remains clear (white) with this scenario.

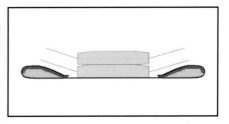

Figure 8-17B. Piggyback IOLs: The posterior (rear) IOL is implanted in the capsular bag with the cut edge of the relatively small diameter CCC resting on its anterior optical surface. The anterior (front) IOL is placed in the ciliary sulcus, anterior to the CCC. Retsined/proliferative lens epithelial cells/cortex (yellow) are confined to the compartment of the capsular bag around the rear IOL and the ILS in front of the CCC is likely to be spared (white). (IOL optic=gray, IOL haptic=blue, capsular bag and cells=red, retained/proliferatice equatorial lens epithelial cells/cortex=yellow)

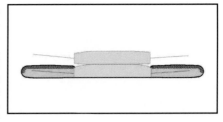

histopathologic analysis in the 2 cases reported by Apple, Gayton, and associates revealed that this membrane was not primarily a fibrosis, but rather an ingrowth of lens epithelial cells from the equatorial lens bow, taking the form of "pearls" (bladder-Wedl cells; Figure 8-12). The opacification in Figures 8-10 or 8-12 consisted of clear-cut, easily identifiable "pearls." The "membrane" in the second case we have examined was less massive (Figures 8-13 and 8-14).

It is not entirely clear whether the process is related to IOL design or material (e.g., PMMA, silicone, acrylic) or other factors. There is no doubt, however, that cells of the equatorial lens bow (E-cells, see Figure 8-15), the source of bladder cells and pearls as seen in routine posterior subcapsular cataracts and also the precursor of the "pearl" form of PCO, are situated in close proximity to the interlenticular space, the potential space between the two IOLs (illustrated schematically in Figure 8-15). With this in mind, a logical conclusion would be that this condition might be closely related to the quality of cortical cleanup. We recommend that extra time and attention be given to removal of lens material with hydrodissection-enhanced cortical cleanup (see Chapter 7). Figures 8-16 and 8-17 reveal several implantation scenarios that in our opinion suggest in addition to thorough cleanup, two additional surgical means that may help minimize ILD, namely, 1) attention to the size of the CCC-in particular creation of a CCC layer than the IOL's optic diameter (Figure 8-17A) and 2) placement of the anterior (front) IOL in the ciliary sulcus with the CCC edge situated between the 2 IOL optics (Figure 8-17B). The rationale for these procedures is described in detail in the legends to Figures 8-1 and 8-17.

We are almost to the point of eradicating the much more common form of intracapsular opacification-namely, secondary cataract or PCO (see Chapter 7). It is important that we recognize, understand, and prevent or treat this new condition of interlenticular opacification early in its course.

COMPLICATIONS OF FOLDABLE PHAKIC INTRAOCULAR LENSES

There are three forms of phakic IOL implantation that are currently being investigated; namely, AC IOLs (Figure 8-18), an iris support design such as the Artisen (Ophthec Corporation, Holland) (Figure 8-19), and phakic posterior chamber lenses (P PC IOLs). The model being implanted in clinical studies at the time of this writing, from Staar Surgical Corporation, is the so-called implantable contact lens (Figure 8-20).

The implantable contact lens is a very thin plate lens manufactured from hydrophilic material that is designed for insertion between the posterior pigment epithelial lining of the iris and the anterior capsule of the crystalline lens. Whereas clinical reports to date have been promising, we have not yet received any explanted or autopsy specimens for pathologic examination.

Among the theoretical and actual complications observed with this phakic posterior PC IOL, there have been rare reports of secondary glaucoma, pigmentary dispersion secondary to touch of the iris epithelium, and, potentially most important, anterior subcapsular anterior lens opacities[4] due to contact of the pseudophakos with the anterior capsule. Reports of this have been relatively unusual and sporadic with the Staar Surgical IOL. However, we

Figure 8-18A. There are three basic types of refractive phakic intraocular lenses. In this figure we show a manufacturer's illustration of the Baikoff style four-point fixation AC IOL design for refractive purposes.

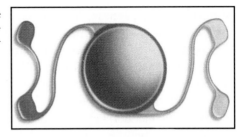

Figure 8-18B. There are three basic types of refractive phakic intraocular lenses. In this figure we show a manufacturer's illustration of the Baikoff style four-point fixation AC IOL the manufacturer's illustration.

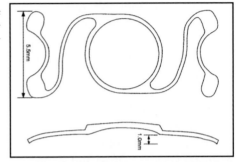

Figure 8-19. The Worst-Fechner iris claw IOL has been modified for use in phakic refractive purposes. It is now marketed as the Artisen IOL. Ophthec in Holland manufactures this lens. This is a manufacturer's illustration of this design.

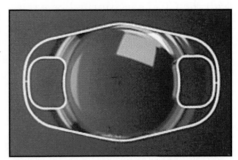

Figure 8-20A. Most experience with phakic PC IOLs has been gained through implantation of the Staar Surgical collamer plate style phakic PC IOL, commonly termed the implantable contact lens. This lens is being implanted widely worldwide and results to date have been favorable. This is a manufacturer's illustration.

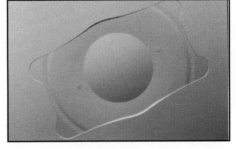

have had the opportunity to examine an earlier model manufactured by another company (Adatomed, Germany), which we have determined to be clearly unsatisfactory.

Adatomed manufactured a silicone plate design for phakic PC IOL implantation. Three lenses of this type were explanted by Drs. Ralf Gerl and Stephanie Schminckler, Ahaus, Germany, and sent to our laboratory. Figure 8-21A illustrates in one of the patients a secondary complicated cataract (a conflict that had actually ensued in all three cases). Figure 8-21B illustrates the removal of the phakic IOL shown in Figure 8-21A.

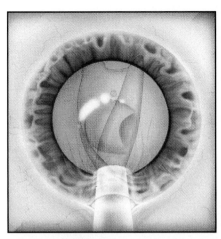

Figure 8-20B. Most experience with phakic PC IOLs has been gained through implantation of the Staar Surgical collamer plate style phakic PC IOL, commonly termed the implantable contact lens. This lens is being implanted widely worldwide and results to date have been favorable. This is a schematic illustration showing the unfolding of the IOL during insertion.

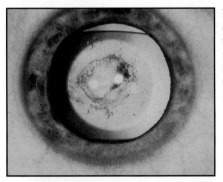

Figure 8-21A. We have had the opportunity to examine explanted phakic PC IOLs fabricated from silicone manufactured by Adatomed Corporation in Germany. This IOL is now off the market. Dr. Ralf Gerl, Ahaus, Germany, removed the lenses. The patient, a young woman, developed complicated cataract as seen here two years post-implantation of the phakic PC IOL.

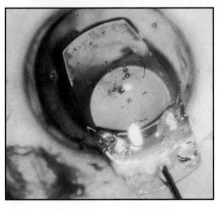

Figure 8-21B. We have had the opportunity to examine explanted phakic PC IOLs fabricated from silicone manufactured by Adatomed Corporation in Germany. This IOL is now off the market. Dr. Ralf Gerl, Ahaus, Germany, removed the lenses. Photograph of the explantation of the IOL shown in Figure 8-21A by Dr. Ralf Gerl.

Gross examination of the explant (Figure 8-22) revealed good polish and surface finish, but measurements determined that this lens was far too thick (maximum anterior-posterior dimension=1.15 mm) to be suitable for implantation in the narrow confines of the posterior chamber. We also implanted this P PC-IOL in cadaver eyes utilizing anterior views (Figures 8-23A and B) and the Miyake-Apple posterior photographic technique (Figure 8-23C). Most noteworthy, in these cadaver eye implantations, it was demonstrated that the fixation did not occur in the ciliary sulcus but rather onto the peripheral zonular fibers

Figure 8-22. Gross photograph of the explanted phakic PC IOL shown in Figure 8-20. This IOL was well polished, but in general was unsuitable because it was too thick in its anterior-posterior dimension, too long, and fabricated from a hydrophobic silicone, which appears not to be the correct material for this particular procedure.

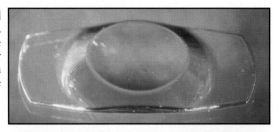

Figure 8-23A. The explanted Adatomed phakic IOL (Figure 8-21) was experimentally implanted into human eyes obtained postmortem. Implantation of the IOL in a human cadaver eye, frontal or surgeon's view.

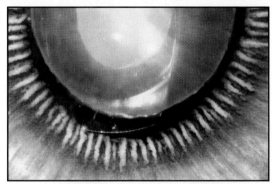

Figure 8-23B. The explanted Adatomed phakic IOL (Figure 8-21) was experimentally implanted into human eyes obtained postmortem. Gross photograph from in front after removal of the cornea and iris showing the lens in place. Note that it appears too long, extending past the lens equator.

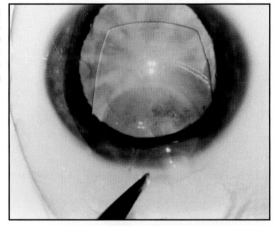

Figure 8-23C. The explanted Adatomed phakic IOL (Figure 8-21) was experimentally implanted into human eyes obtained postmortem. Gross photograph from behind (Miyake-Apple posterior photographic view) showing the phakic PC IOL in place. Note that the lens is very long and extends past the crystalline lens equator (below) with the edge encroaching on the zonules. This, therefore, represents a zonular fixation, as opposed to a ciliary sulcus or capsular bag fixation.

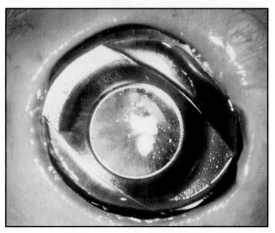

(Figure 8-23C). This illustrates the clinical issue that sizing and fixation are important factors that require further study. It is probable that most phakic PC IOLs now being implanted are actually fixated in the zonules (zonular fixation) rather than the ciliary sulcus as often assumed.

REFERENCES

1. Apple DJ, Federman JL, Krolicki TJ, et al. Irreversible silicone oil adhesion to silicone intraocular lenses. Part I: Clinicopathologic analysis. *Ophthalmology* 1996;103(10):1555-1562.

2. Apple DJ, Isaacs RT, Kent DG, et al. Silicone oil adhesion to intraocular lenses: An experimental comparing various biomaterials. *J Cataract Refract Surg* 1997;23:536-544.

3. Gayton JL, Apple DJ, Peng Q, et al. Interlenticular Opacification: A clinicopathological correlation of a new complication of piggyback posterior chamber intraocular lenses. *J Cataract Refract Surg.* 2000 [In Press].

4. Werner L, Pandey SK, Escobar-Gomez M, Visessook N, Peng Q, Apple DJ. Anterior capsular opacification: A histopathological study comparing different IOL styles. *Ophthalmology.* 1999; 107(3):463-471.

5. Visessook N, Peng Q, Apple DJ, Gerl R, Guindi A. Pathological examination of an explanted phakic posterior chamber intraocular lens. *J Cataract Refract Surg.* 1999;25(2):216-222.

BIBLIOGRAPHY

Silicone Oil Adherence to Intraocular Lenses

Bartz-Schmidt KU, Kirchhof B, Heimann K. Condensation on IOLs during fluid-air exchange. *Ophthalmology.* 1996;103:199.

Bartz-Schmidt KU, Konen W, Esser P, Walter P, Heimann K. Intraocular silicone lenses and silicone oil. *Klinische Monatsblatter fur Augenheilkunde.* 1995;207:162-166.

Cunanan CM, Ghazizadeh M, Buchen SY, Knight PM. Contact-angle analysis of intraocular lenses. *J Cataract Refract Surg* . 1998;24:341-51.

Dick B, Stoffelns B, Pavlovic S, et al. Interaction of silicone oil with various intraocular lenses. A light and scanning electron microscopy study. *Klin Monatsbl Augenheilkd.* 1997;211:192-206.

Eaton AM, Jaffe GJ, McCuen BW, 2nd, Mincey GJ. Condensation on the posterior surface of silicone intraocular lenses during fluid-air exchange. *Ophthalmology.* 1995;102:733-736.

Francese J, Christ FR, Buchen SY, Gwon A, Robertson JE. Moisture droplet formation on the posterior surface of intraocular lenses during fluid/air exchange. *J Cataract Refract Surg.* 1995;21(6):685-689.

Hainsworth D, Chen SN, Cox TA, Jaffe GJ. Condensation on poly(methyl methacrylate), acrylic polymer, and silicone intraocular lenses after fluid-air exchange in rabbits. *Ophthalmology.* 1996;103:1410-1418.

Jaffe GJ. Management of condensation on a foldable acrylic intraocular lens after vitrectomy and fluid-air exchange. *Am J Ophthalmol.* 1997;124:692-693.

Khawly JA, Lambert RJ, Jaffe GJ. Intraocular lens changes after short-and long-term exposure to intraocular silicone oil. An in vivo study. *Ophthalmology* 1998;105:1227-1233

Kusaka S, Kodama T, Ohashi Y. Condensation of silicone oil on the posterior surface of a silicone intraocular lens during vitrectomy. *Am J Ophthalmol.* 1996;121:574-575.

Langefeld JM, Kirchhof B, Meinert H, et al. A new way of removing silicone oil from the surface of silicone intraocular lenses. *Graefes Arch Clin Exp Ophthalmol.* 1999;237:201-206.

Obstbaum SA. Foldable intraocular lenses and vitreoretinal surgery [editorial; comment]. *J Cataract Refract Surg.* 1997;23:457

Slusher MM, Seaton AD. Loss of visibility caused by moisture condensation on the posterior surface of a silicone intraocular lens during fluid/gas exchange after posterior vitrectomy. *Am J Ophthalmol.* 1994;118:667.

Tanner V, Haider A, Rosen P. Phacoemulsification and combined management of intraocular silicone oil. *J Cataract Refract Surg.* 1998;24:585-591.

Interlenticular Opacification of Piggyback Intraocular Lenses

Apple DJ, Solomon KD, Tetz MR, et al. Posterior capsule opacification. *Surv Ophthalmol.* 1992; 37: 73-116.

Behrendt S, Rochels R, Winter M. Sandwich intraocular lens implant: A concept for aphakia correction in children. *Klinische Monatsblatter fur Augenheilkunde.* 1995;207:42-45.

Brint SF. Refractive cataract surgery. *Int Ophthalmol Clin.* 1994;34:1-11.

Fenzl RE, Gills JP, Cherchio M. Refractive and visual outcome of hyperopic cataract cases operated on before and after implementation of the Holladay II formula. *Ophthalmology.* 1998; 105:1759-1764.

Gayton JL, Sanders V, Van der Karr M, Raanan MG. Piggybacking intraocular implants to correct pseudophakic refractive error. *Ophthalmology.* 1999;106:56-59.

Gayton JL, Sanders VN. Implanting two posterior chamber intraocular lenses in a case of microphthalmos. *J Cataract Refract Surg.* 1993; 19:776-777.

Gayton JL. Secondary implantation of a double intraocular lens after penetrating keratoplasty. *J Cataract Refract Surg..* 1998;24:281-282.

Gills JP, Gayton JL, Raanan M. Multiple intraocular lens implantation. In: Gills JP, Fenzl R, Marrin RG, eds., *Cataract Surgery; the State of the Art.* Thorofare, NJ, SLACK Incorporated. 1998, 183-195.

Gills JP. Piggyback minus-power lens implantation in keratoconus. *J Cataract Refract Surg.* 1998; 24:566-568.

Grabow HB. Phakic IOL terminology. *J Cataract Refract Surg..* 1999;25:159-160.

Holladay JT, Gills JP, Leidlein J, Cherchio M. Achieving emmetropia in extremely short eyes with two piggyback posterior chamber intraocular lenses. *Ophthalmology.* 1996; 103:1118-1123.

Kohnen T, Magdowski G, Koch DD. Scanning electron microscopic analysis of foldable acrylic and hydrogel intraocular lenses. *J Cataract Refract Surg.* 1996;22(suppl 2):1342-1350.

Kohnen T. Complications and complication management with foldable intraocular intraocular lenses. *J Cataract Refract Surg.* 1998;24:1167-1168.

Masket S. Piggyback intraocular lens implantation. *J Cataract Refract Surg.* 1998; 24:569-570.

Mittelviefhaus H. Piggyback intraocular lens with exchangeable optic. *J Cataract Refract Surg.* 1996; 22:676-681.

Nishi O. Posterior capsule opacification. Part 1: Experimental investigations. *J Cataract Refract Surg.* 1999; 25:106-117.

Shugar JK, Lewis C, Lee A. Implantation of multiple foldable acrylic posterior chamber lenses in the capsular bag for high hyperopia. *J Cataract Refract Surg.* 1996; 22:1368-1372.

Shugar JK, Schwartz T. Interpseudophakos Elschnig pearls associated with late hyperopic shift: A complication of piggyback posterior chamber intraocular lens implantation. *J Cataract Refract Surg.* 1999; 25:863-867.

Werner L, Shugar JK, Pandey SK, Escobar-Gomez M, Apple DJ. Opacification of piggyback IOLs. Analysis of an amorphous material between the lenses. *J Cataract Refract Surg.* 1999 (submitted).

Complications of Foldable Phakic Intraocular Lenses.

Brown DC, Grabow HB, Martin RG, et al. Staar Collamer intraocular lens: Clinical results from the Phase I FDA core study. *J Cataract & Refract Surg.* 1998;24:1032-1038.

Davison JA. Capsule contraction syndrome. *J Cataract Refract Surg.* 1993; 19:582-589.

Erturk H, Ozcetin H. Phakic posterior chamber intraocular lenses for the correction of high myopia. *Journal of Refractive Surgery.* 1995;11:388-391.

Gills JP, Fenzel RE. Minus power intraocular lenses to correct refractive errors in myopic pseudophakia. *J Cataract Refract Surg.* 1999;25:1205-1208.

Halpern BL, Gallagher SP. Refractive error consequences of reversed-optic AMO SI-40NB intraocular lens. *Ophthalmology.* 1999;106:901-903.

Kent DG, Solomon KD, Peng Q, Apple DJ. Pathology of refractive surgery. In: Ocular pathology. *Clinical Applications and Self Assessment.* 5th ed. St. Louis, Mo: Mosby-Year Book, Inc.; 1998:205-260.

Trindade F, Pereira F. Cataract formation after posterior chamber phakic intraocular lens implantation. *J Cataract Refract Surg.* 1998;24:1661-1663.

Recapitulation

Section

5

Recapitulation

Chapter
9

Recapitulation

SECTION 1

A familiarity with the history of cataract surgery-IOL implantation (Chapter 2) helps one understand the mechanisms and rationale for today's surgery, and helps avoid repeating the missteps and mistakes of the past. All of the currently implanted foldable IOLs studied in our database have provided exemplary clinical results, especially after implantation with good surgical technique. However, they are not perfect, and there are subtle differences among the various modern foldable designs. One example relates to an IOL's suitability in helping control postoperative reactivity/proliferation of retained lens epithelial cells within the capsular bag. This helps avoid the common complication of PCO and other various complications such as post-fibrotic IOL decentration. Today's research on foldable IOLs is focused on fine-tuning the technology. A careful perusal of the text, tables, and illustrations with their legends in this book should help surgeons discern and evaluate some of the subtle differences and then ascertain in his or her mind which IOL(s) may be the best for his or her practice.

SECTION 2

Recall that we can only provide direct clinicopathologic analysis and conclusions based on the database of specimens available to us in the United States (Chapters 3 to 5). A recapitulation of findings on the major foldable IOL designs in this group is as follows.

SILICONE PLATE INTRAOCULAR LENSES

Because of their relatively narrow and rectangular geometric profile, plate IOLs are easy to fold and insert with an injector through a small incision. The small hole plate lenses have

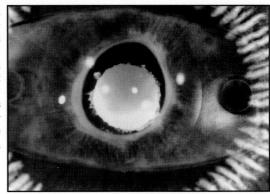

Figure 9-1. Gross photograph from behind of a human eye obtained postmortem (Miyake-Apple posterior photographic technique) showing a Staar Surgical-Bausch and Lomb Surgical large-hole silicone plate lens (Chapter 3). Although this design often shows evidence of significant lens anterior epithelial cell proliferation (ACO) and Soemmering's ring formation, overall results have been impressive. The PCO rate is relatively low (8.2%) (see Figures 7-79 and 7-80). Note perfect centration and clear media. A toric design is now available for astigmatism correction.

largely been removed from the market because these occasionally decentered in the capsule bag or actually dislocated after Nd:YAG laser posterior capsulotomy. They had a Nd:YAG laser posterior capsule rate of 20.7% as determined in our autopsy globes (see Figures 7-79, and 7-80).

The small hole silicone plate IOLs have been superseded by the large hole plate designs (Figure 9-1). In general, the latter fixate more securely in the capsular bag as soon as the postoperative fibrotic process occurs, usually after 4 to 6 weeks postoperatively. This has lowered the incidence of long-term IOL rotation (very important with the toric IOL), decentration, and dislocation. The explantation rate is now very low. Although ACO is a common occurrence (see Figure 3-12), the rate of central visually significant PCO as measured by the Nd:YAG laser posterior capsulotomy rate is relatively low (8.2%, see Figures 7-79, 7-80). When implanted precisely in the capsular bag after sufficient cortical cleanup, these IOLs provide reliable results. At present, this is the only IOL model that offers a toric design.

THREE-PIECE SILICONE INTRAOCULAR LENSES

The elastimide-polyimide design of Staar Surgical-Bausch and Lomb Surgical (Chapter 4, Figure 9-2) has provided consistently good results with a low complication rate. The relatively rigid high memory yellow polyimide haptics appear to be efficacious in helping stabilize the IOL in the bag and in enhancing the barrier effect created by the IOLs' truncated optic edge. It centers well and to date has shown a relatively low rate of PCO (11.1%, see Figures 7-79 and 7-80). Explantations necessitated by IOL-induced complications have been rare.

The SI series of Allergan silicone optic IOLs (Chapter 4, Figure 9-3) has a long history of providing admirable results. Over 4 million have been implanted, far more than any other foldable IOL. There have been steady improvements throughout the last decade. The current SI-40 lens and the SA-40 ("Array") multifocal design, both with PMMA haptics, are popular with many surgeons. These lenses, in association with the improved surgical techniques evolving during the past decade, have produced results that have improved from very good with the SI-30 to excellent with the SI-40 (Figure 9-3). In our database, the PCO rate is low by historic comparison with earlier published rates of 30% to 50 50% over the past two decades. Very few explanted SI-40 lenses have been submitted to our laboratory. Those that have had usually been removed for surgical issues unrelated to IOL safety

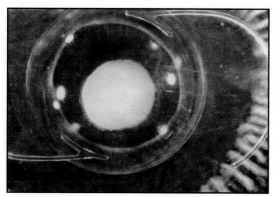

Figure 9-2. Gross photograph from behind of a human eye obtained postmortem (Miyake-Apple posterior photographic technique), showing the Staar Surgical-Bausch and Lomb Surgical elastimide-polyimide IOL (Chapter 4). The IOL is well-centered, with total clarity of the media. The PCO rate of this IOL is 11.1% (see Figures 7-79 and 7-80).

issues. The SI series of Allergan IOLs has had a tried-and-true history and the SI-40 design and its cousin the SA-40 "Array" multifocal continue this tradition. The number of accessions is still low, so further study and evaluation are necessary. The SA-40 is the only currently approved multifocal design on the market and results with this lens have been excellent with good patient satisfaction.

HYDROPHOBIC ACRYLIC INTRAOCULAR LENS

One of the most notable and advantageous characteristics of the Alcon AcrySof IOL (Figure 9-4) is the apparent lack of postoperative lens epithelial cellular reactivity that occurs within the capsule around the IOL. Cellular proliferation of both anterior and posterior lens epithelial cells is the lowest that we have noted with any biomaterial (see Figure 5-13). Decreased reactivity of the anterior capsule is important in improving the view of the peripheral retina by the vitreoretinal surgeon, as well as preventing such sequelae as fibrosis-induced decentration and capsular contraction syndrome (capsular phimosis-see Chapter 7). The lack of proliferation of cells across the posterior capsule is of course of paramount importance in helping reduce the incidence of PCO (see Chapter 7).

The apparently good biocompatibility of this IOL is perhaps at least partially related to its optic's close adherence to both the anterior and posterior capsules. This material has an adhesive, "sticky" characteristic (termed a bio-adhesion). This helps explain the fact that, following good removal of cells by hydrodissection-enhanced cortical cleanup, the vast majority of capsular bags associated with this design remain clear. The second line of defense against PCO, the square-truncated optic edge, apparently further enhances the ability of this design in lowering the incidence of PCO. The 1.3% Nd:YAG laser rate we have noted with this IOL as of August 1, 1999 (see Figures 7-78,7-79, 7-80, and 7-85) represents the lowest Nd:YAG rate observed with any current or former IOL.

Characteristics purported to cause visual disturbances (eg, "glistenings", folding creases, problems related to the square optic edge) have been reported. However, these have been rare and significant clinical sequelae are unusual.

Figure 9-3. Gross photomicrograph from behind of a human eye obtained postmortem (Miyake-Apple posterior photographic technique) showing an Allergan SI-40 three-piece PMMA-haptic silicone-optic IOL (see Chapter 4). Note perfect centration and clear media. The SA-40 multifocal equivalent of this design is the only approved multifocal IOL on the market and this lens plays a special role in refractive management of selected patients.

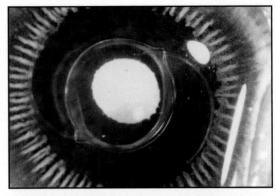

Figure 9-4. Gross photograph from behind of a human eye obtained postmortem (Miyake-Apple posterior photographic technique), showing the Alcon AcrySof acrylic foldable IOL (see Chapter 5). Note the perfect centration and clarity of the media. This IOL has the lowest anterior capsular and posterior capsular opacification rates of all IOLs available to us for study in our United States autopsy database (see Figure 5-13). It appears to be suitable for pediatric implantation and for use as a "piggyback" IOL.

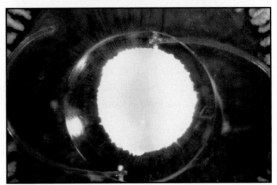

SECTION 3

A clinicopathologic evaluation of foldable IOLs not yet available to us in significant numbers in our United States database will naturally have to wait until a later date. In this text we have cataloged them and established a baseline for a future database. At the time of publication, there has been some concern with calcification of some new hydrgel designs, so careful follow-up is warranted.

SECTION 4

As we enter the 21st century, efficient surgical tools and appropriate IOLs are available to allow a new standard in the prevention of PCO (see Chapter 7). Nd:YAG laser posterior capsulotomy rates reaching down into single digits (e.g. 1.3%) (see Figures 7-79 and 7-80) are now within reach.

The complication of silicone adherence to a previously implanted IOL (see Chapter 8) has been well described in the literature. Simple awareness of this complication should enable one to avoid it. The main factor is clinical judgment in selecting the appropriate IOL for patients with current or potential severe vitreoretinal disease that may require silicone oil in the future. In the overwhelming majority of cases, this entity is not a significant factor in choosing an IOL.

The use of "piggyback" IOLs and foldable phakic IOLs (Chapter 8) are exciting opportunities for future pseudophakic refractive procedures. Hard data on outcome studies for these modalities should become available in the near future.

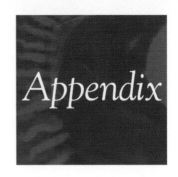

Cataract and Intraocular Lens-Related Publications

Selected cataract IOL-related publications from the Center for Research on Ocular Therapeutics and Biodevices, 1984 to 2000 (arranged by type and date).

BOOKS

1. Apple DJ, Gieser SC, Isenberg RA. *Evolution of Intraocular Lenses.* Salt Lake City, Ut: University of Utah Printing Services; 1985.

2. Apple DJ, Kincaid MC, Mamalis N, Olson RJ. *Intraocular Lenses. Evolution, Designs, Complications, and Pathology.* Baltimore, MD: Williams & Wilkins; 1989.

3. Apple DJ, Rabb MF. *Ocular Pathology, Clinical Applications, and Self-Assessment.* 4th ed. (Formerly *Clinico-Pathologic Correlation of Ocular Disease: A Text and Stereo Atlas.* 4th ed.) St. Louis, Mo: CV Mosby; 1991.

4. Apple DJ, Rabb MF. *Ocular Pathology, Clinical Applications, and Self-Assessment.* 5th ed. St. Louis, Mo: Mosby-Year Book, Inc.; 1998.

5. Apple DJ, Ram J, Foster A, et al. *Elimination of Cataract Blindness: A Global Perspective Entering the New Century.* MONOGRAPH (SPECIAL issue). Surv Ophthalmol. 2000.

BOOK CHAPTERS

6. Crandall AS, Richards SC, Apple DJ. Extracapsular cataract extraction: In-the-bag versus ciliary sulcus fixation. In: *Transactions of the Pacific Coast Oto-Ophthalmological Society.* 1985;66:73-79.

7. Apple DJ. Pathology of intraocular lenses. Polypropylene vs PMMA. In: Jeffe MS, ed. *Intraocular Lens Complications; Self-Study Program. Module II: Proceedings of Symposium on IOL Complications.* Stockholm, Sweden: Pharmacia monograph; Aug 17-24, 1985.

8. Popham JK, Apple DJ, Newman DA, Isenberg RA, Deacon J. Advantages and limitations of soft intraocular lenses: A scientific perspective (Chapter 2). In: Mazzocco TR, Rajacich GM, Epstein E, eds. *Soft Implant Lenses In Cataract Surgery.* Thorofare, NJ: SLACK Incorporated; 1986:11-30.

9. Apple DJ, Tetz M, Hunold W. Lokalisierte endophthalmitis: Eine bisher nicht beschriebene komplikation der extrakapsularen kataraktextraktion. In: Jacobi KW, Schott K, Gloor B, eds. *Proceedings of the First Congress of the Deutsche Gesselschaft für Intraokularlinsen Implantation.* Berlin, Germany: Springer-Verlag; 1987:6-14.

10. Apple DJ, Tetz MR, Hansen SO. Use of viscoelastics intraocular lens removal. In: Rosen E, ed. *Viscoelastic Materials.* Oxford, England: Pergamon Press; 1988.

11. Apple D, Hansen S, Richard S, Tetz M. Histopathological and experimental aspects of modern lens implant surgery. In: Rosen E, Kalb I, eds. *Intercapsular Cataract Extraction.* Oxford, England: Pergamon Press; 1988:1-11.

12. Apple DJ, Brems RN, Ellis GW, et al. Posterior chamber intraocular lens fixation. In: Buratto L, ed. *Extracapsular Cataract Microsurgery and Posterior Chamber Intraocular Lenses (vol 2).* Milano, Italy: Centro Ambrosiano Microchirurgia Oculare; 1989:Chapter 12, 473-478.

13. Carlson AN, Tetz MR, Apple DJ. Infectious complications of modern cataract surgery and intraocular lens implantation. In: Moellering RC Jr, Westenfelder GO eds. *Infectious Disease Clinics of North America. Infections of Prosthetic Devices.* Philadelphia, Pa: W. B. Saunders; 1989; Vol 3(2):339-355.

14. Apple DJ. Histopathological findings. In: Hoffmann K, Hockwin O, eds. *Viscoelastic Substances.* Berlin, Germany: Springer-Verlag; 1990:69-77.

15. Apple DJ, Morgan RC, Tsai JC. Histology of posterior chamber fixation. In: Percival SPB, ed. *A Colour Atlas of Lens Implantation.* London, England: Mosby Year Book; 1991: Chapter 36.

16. Apple DJ, Assia EI, Wasserman D, et al. Evidence in support of the continuous tear anterior capsulectomy (capsulorhexis technique). In: Cangelosi GC, ed. *Advances In Cataract Surgery. New Orleans Academy of Ophthalmology.* Thorofare, NJ: SLACK Incorporated; 1991:Chapter 3, 21-47.

17. Apple DJ, Tsai JC, Castaneda VE, et al. Posterior chamber intraocular lens (PC IOL): A clinical goal with bifocal and multifocal IOLs. In: Maxwell WA, Nordan LT, eds. *Current Concepts of Multifocal Intraocular Lenses.* Thorofare, NJ: LACK Incorporated; 1991: Chapter 19, 219-231.

18. Legler UFC, Apple DJ, Assia EI, Tetz MR. Linsendislokation und-explantation. Komplikationen bei Intraokularlinsen eine Analyse an explantierten Kunstlinsen. In: Transactions of the German Ophthalmol Soc March 8 and 9, 1991; Aachen, Germany. Wenzel HVM, Reim M, Freyler H, Hartman C, eds. *Kongress der Deutschsprachigen Gesellschaft für Intraokularlinsen Implantation.* Berlin, Germany: Springer-Verlag; 1991:743-753.

19. Apple DJ, Assia EI, Blumenthal M, Legler UFC: Verformbare Linsen. Das konzept der ausdehnbaren Hydrogellinse und die Wiederherstellung der natürlichen Kapselsackanatomie. In *Transactions of the German Ophthalmol Soc*, March 8 and 9, 1991; Aachen, Germany. In: Wenzel HVM, Reim M, Freyler H, Hartmann C, eds. Kongress der Deutschsprachigen Gesellschaft fhr Intraokularlinsen Implantation. Berlin, Germany: Springer-Verlag; 1991; 375-380.

20. Assia EI, Castaneda VE, Legler UFC, et al. Studies on cataract surgery and intraocular lenses at the center for intraocular lens research. In: Obstbaum SA, ed. *Cataract and Intraocular Lens Surgery; Ophthalmology Clinics of North America.* Vol. 4, Num. 2. Philadelphia, Pa: WB Saunders; 1991:251-266.

21. Apple D, Davison JA, Nordan LT, Maxwell WA. Capsulorhexis, PC IOL centration, and transscleral PC IOL fixation. In: Nordan LT, Maxwell WA, Davison JA, eds. *The Surgical Rehabilitation of Vision: An Integrated Approach to Anterior Segment Surgery.* London, New York: Gower Medical Publishing; 1992:Chapter 9, 1-12.

22. Apple DJ, Morgan RC, Tsai JC, Lim ES. Update on implantation of posterior chamber intraocular lenses. In: Weinstock FJ, ed. *Management and Care of the Cataract Patient.* Boston, MA: Blackwell Scientific Publications; 1992:Chapter 12, 128-134.

23. Wesendahl TA, Auffarth GU, Newland TJ, Brown S, Apple DJ. Einfluss der kapsulorrhexisgrösse auf der nachstarentstehung. In: Gloor R, et al., eds. *Trans 7th Congress of the German Intraocular Lens Implant Society (DGII).* Zhürich, Switzerland; 1993:228-236.

24. Auffarth GU, Schmidt JA, Wesendahl TA, Recum AV, Apple DJ. Untersuchungen an IOL-oberflächenstruckturen mit rasterelektronenmikroskopie und quantitativer dreidimensionaler non-contact profilometrie (TOPO). In: Gloor R, et al., eds. *Trans 7th Congress of the German Intraocular Lens Implant Society (DGII).* Zhürich, Switzerland; 1993:243-248.

25. Newland TJ, Auffarth GU, Wesendahl TA, Blotnik CA, Apple DJ. Oberflächenschäden an silikon IOL-Optiken durch Nd:YAG-Laser: Befunde bei explantierten intraocularlinsen. In: Gloor R, et al., eds. *Trans 7th Congress of the German Intraocular Lens Implant Society (DGII).* Zhürich, Switzerland; 1993:391-396.

26. Wesendahl TA, Hunold W, Auffarth GU, Newland T, Blotnick C, Apple DJ. Einfluss von optikgeometrie und haptikabwiklung auf die lagebeziehungen, on IOL und hiterem kapselblatt. In: Gloor R, et al., eds. *Trans 7th Congress of the German Intraocular Lens Implant Society (DGII).* Zhürich, Switzerland; 1993:222-227.

27. Wesendahl TA, Auffarth GU, Apple DJ. Area of contact between IOL-optic and posterior capsule. Systematic analysis of different haptic parameters. In: Gloor R, et al., eds. *Trans 7th Congress of the German Intraocular Lens Implant Society (DGII).* Zhürich, Switzerland; 1993:222-227.

28. Apple DJ. Foreword. In: Wenzel M. *Specular Microscopy of Intraocular Lenses. Atlas and Textbook for Slit-Lamp and Specular Microscopic Examinations.* New York, NY; Thieme Medical Publishers Inc.:1993.

29. Apple DJ, Auffarth GU, Wesendahl TA. Pathophysiology of modern capsular surgery. In: Steinert, Auffarth GU, Wesendahl TA, Assia EI, Apple DJ, eds. *Textbook of Modern Cataract Surgery: Technique, Complications, & Management.* Philadelphia, PA: W. B. Saunders Company; 1995: Chapter 26, 314-324.

30. Auffarth GU, Apple DJ. Einflub von intraokularlinsendesign und operativen techniken auf die nachstarentwicklung. In: Ohrloff Ch, Hartmann C, eds. *Kongressband: 11. Kongress der Deutschsprachigen Gesellschaft für Intraokularlinsen Implantation unde refraktive Chirurgie.* Frankfurt, Germany (1997). Berlin, Heidelberg, New York: Springer (Publ.); 1997.

31. Apple DJ. Lens replacement. In: Yanoff M, Duker J. *Ophthalmology.* Philadelphia, Pa: Mosby-Year Book, Inc.; 1998.

32. Auffarth GU, Wesendahl TA, Brown SJ, Apple DJ. häufigkeit und art von explantationsgründen von einstückigen und dreistückigen hinterkammerlinsen. In: Wollensak J, et al., eds. *Transactions of the 8th Congress of the German Intraocular Lens Implant Society (DGII) in Berlin (1994).* Berlin, Heidelberg, New York: Springer Verlag Publishing; 1994:501-507.

33. Auffarth GU, Tsao K, Wesendahl TA, Apple DJ. Zentrierung von hinterkammerlinsen bei patienten mit pseudoexfoliationssyndrom: Befunde in explantierten autopsieaugen, In: Wollensak J, et al., eds. *Transactions of the 8th Congress of the German Intraocular Lens Implant Society (DGII) in Berlin (1994).* Berlin, Heidelberg, New York: Springer Verlag Publishing; 1994;530-537.

34. Auffarth GU, Beischel CJ, Wesendahl TA, Apple DJ. Soemmerring's Ring bildung nach kataraktoperation und HKL implantation: Eine studie von 827 autopsieaugen. In: Rochels R, Dunker G, Hartmann Ch., eds. *Transactions of the 9th Congress of the German Intraocular Lens Implant Society, Kiel, 1995.* Heidelberg, Berlin, New York: Springer Verlag Publishing; 1995.

35. Auffarth GU, Wilcox CM, Sims JC, et al. Komplikationen von 100 explantierten silikonhinterkammerlinsen. In: Rochels R, Dunker G, Hartmann Ch, eds. *Transactions of the 9th Congress of the German Intraocular Lens Implant Society, Kiel, 1995.* Heidelberg, Berlin, New York: Springer Verlag Publishing; 1995.

36. Auffarth GU, McCabe C, Tetz MR, Apple DJ. Die modifizierte disk-linse nach anis: Befunde bei 15 menschlichen autopsieaugen. In: Rochels R, Dunker G, Hartmann Ch, eds. *Transactions of the 9th Congress of the German Intraocular Lens Implant Society, Kiel, 1995.* Heidelberg, Berlin, New York: Springer Verlag Publishing; 1995.

37. Apple DJ, Kent DG, Peng Q, Isaacs RT, Auffarth GU. Verbesserung der befestigung von silikonschiffchenlinsen durch den gebrauch von positionierungslöchern. In: *der Linsenhaptik. Proceedings of the 10th Annual Deutche Gesellschaft fuer Intraokularlinsen Implantation Meeting.* Budapest, Hungary: March 1996.

38. Auffarth GU, Apple DJ. Einfluss von intraokularlinsendesign und operativen techniken auf die nachstarentwicklung. In: Ohroloff C, et al., eds. *Transactions of the 11th Congress of the German Intraocular Lens Implant Society (DGII).* Berlin, (1997). Berlin, Heidelberg, New York: Springer-Verlag Publishing; 1998;241-249.

39. Auffarth GU, Ram J, Apple DJ, Peng Q, Visessook N. *EinfluB der Kapselsackfixation von Intraokularlinsen auf die Ausbildung der Cataracta Secundaria.* Paper presented at the DGII 1998 Meeting. Germany: 1998.

40. Kent DG, Solomon KD, Peng Q, Apple DJ. Pathology of refractive surgery (Chapter 5). In: *Ocular Pathology. Clinical Applications and Self Assessment.* 5th ed. St. Louis, Mo: Mosby-Year Book, Inc; 1998:205-260.

41. Werner L, Apple DJ, Pandey SK, Esocobar-Gomez M, Peng Q, Visessook N. Postoperative proliferation of anterior and equatorial lens epithelial cells: A comparison between various foldable IOL designs. In: Buratto L, ed. *Cataract Surgery in Complicated Cases.* Thorofare, NJ: SLACK Incorporated; 2000: Chapter 18. (In Press)

42. Wilson ME, Pandey SK, Werner L, Ram J, Apple DJ. Pediatric Cataract Surgery: Current techniques, complications and management. In: Agarwal S, Agarwal A, Apple DJ, Buratto L, Agarwal A, eds. *Textbook of Ophthalmology.* Thorofare, NJ: SLACK Incorporated; 2000 (in press).

JOURNAL ARTICLES

43. Apple DJ, Mamalis N, Brady SE, et al. Biocompatability of implant materials: A review and scanning electron microscopic study. *J Am Intraocul Implant Soc.* 1984;10:53-66.

44. Mamalis N, Apple DJ, Brady SE, Notz RG, Olson RJ. Pathological and scanning electron microscopic evaluation of the 91Z intraocular lens. *J Am Intraocul Implant Soc.* 1984;10:191-199.

45. Googe JM, Mamalis N, Apple DJ, Olson RJ. BSS warning (letter to the editor). *J Am Intraocul Implant Soc.* 1984;10:202.

46. Apple DJ, Craythorn JM, Olson RJ, et al. Anterior segment complications and neovascular glaucoma following implantation of posterior chamber intraocular lens. *Ophthalmology.* 1984;91:403-419.

47. Apple DJ, Mamalis N, Loftfield K, et al. Complications of intraocular lenses. A historical and histopathological review. *Surv Ophthalmol.* 1984;29:1-54.

48. Apple DJ, Mamalis N, Steinmetz RL, et al. Phacoanaphylactic endophthalmitis associated with extracapsular cataract extraction and a posterior chamber intraocular lens. *Arch Ophthalmol.* 1984;102(10):1528-1532.

49. Ohrloff C, Duffin RM, Apple DJ, Olson RJ. Opacification, vascularization, and chronic inflammation produced by hydrogel corneal lamellar implants. *Am J Ophthalmol.* 1984; 98:422-425.

50. Apple DJ, Mamalis N, Steinmetz RL, et al. Phacoanaphylactic endophthalmitis following ECCE and IOL implantation (guest editorial). *J Am Intraocul Implant Soc.* 1984;10:423-424.

51.   Apple DJ, Cameron JD, Lindstrom RL. Loop fixation of posterior chamber intraocular lenses. *Cataract.* 1984;2(1):7-10.

52.   Apple DJ. *Utah Center for Intraocular Lens Research.* Proceedings of the Research to Prevent Blindness Science Writer's Seminar. 1984;35-36.

53.   Apple DJ, Reidy JJ, Googe JM, et al. A comparison of ciliary sulcus and capsular bag fixation of posterior chamber intraocular lenses. *J Am Intraocul Implant Soc.* 1985;11:44-63.

54.   Kincaid MC, Apple DJ, Mamalis N, Brady SE, Rashid ER. Histopathologic correlative study of Kelman-Style flexible anterior chamber intraocular lenses. *Am J Ophthalmol.* 1985;99:159-169.

55.   Reidy JJ, Apple DJ, Googe JM. An analysis of semiflexible, closed-Loop anterior chamber intraocular lenses. *J Am Intraocul Implant Soc.* 1985;11:344-352.

56.   Gieser SC, Apple DJ, Loftfield K. Richey MA, Rivera RP. Phthisis bulbi after intraocular lens implantation in a child. *Can J Ophthalmol.* 1985;20(5):184-185.

57.   Isenberg RA, Weiss RL, Apple DJ, Lowrey DB. Fungal contamination of balanced salt solution. *J Am Intraocul Implant Soc.* 1985;11:485-486.

58.   Apple DJ, Kincaid MC. Histopathology of intraocular lens explantation. *Cataract.* 1985;2(7):7-11.

59.   Welch DB, Apple DJ, Mendelsohn AD, et al. Lens injury following iridotomy with a Q-switched Neodymium-YAG laser. *Arch Ophthalmol.* 1986,104:123-125.

60.   Isenberg RA, Apple DJ, Reidy JJ. Histopathologic and scanning electron microscopic study of one type of intraocular lens. *Arch Ophthalmol.* 104:683-686, 1986.

61.   Richburg FA, Reidy JJ, Apple DJ, Olson RJ. Sterile hypopyon secondary to ultrasonic cleaning solution. *J Cataract Refract Surg.* 1986;12:248-251.

62.   Newman DA, McIntyre DJ, Apple DJ. Pathologic findings of an explanted silicone intraocular lens. *J Cataract Refract Surg.* 1986;12:292-297.

63.   Apple DJ, Park SB, Merkley KH, et al. Posterior chamber intraocular lenses in a series of 75 autopsy eyes. Part I: Loop Location. *J Cataract Refract Surg.* 1986;12:358-362.

64.   Park SB, Brems RN, Parsons MR, et al. Posterior chamber intraocular lenses in a series of 75 autopsy eyes. Part II: Post-implantation loop configuration. *J Cataract Refract Surg.* 1986;12:363-366.

65.   Brems RN, Apple DJ, Pfeffer BR, et al. Posterior chamber intraocular lenses in a series of of 75 autopsy eyes. Part III: Correlation of positioning holes and optic edges with the pupillary aperture and visual axis. *J Cataract Refract Surg.* 1986;12:367-371.

66.   Apple DJ, Osher RH, Lichtenstein SB, Koch DD. IOL *Materials and Complications.* Proceedings of symposium on IOL materials and complications. Orlando, Fla:, Coburn monograph; January 31-February 2, 1986.

67.   Apple DJ, Brems RN, Ellis GW, Spencer DA. A review of the histopathology of intraocular lens fixation. *Curr Can Ophthalmic Prac.* 1986;4:54-56, 78-79.

68.   Apple DJ. Intraocular lenses: Notes from an interested observer. *Arch Ophthalmol.* 1986;104:1150-1152.

69.   Deacon J, Apple DJ. Integrity of polydiaxonone sutures: A case report. *J Cataract Refract Surg.* 1986;12:540-542.

70.   Apple DJ, Olson RJ. Closed-loop anterior chamber lenses (Letter to the Editor). *Arch Ophthalmol.* 1987;105:19-20.

71.   Park SB, Kratz RP, Olson PF, Pfeffer BR, Apple DJ. In vivo fracture of an extruded oolymethylmethacrylate intraocular lens loop. *J Cataract Refract Surg.* 1987;13:194-197.

72.   Apple DJ, Brems RN, Park RB, et al. Anterior chamber lenses: Part I: Complications and pathology and a review of designs. *J Cataract Refract Surg.* 1987;13:157-174.

73.   Apple DJ, Hansen SO, Richards SC, et al. Anterior chamber lenses. Part II: A laboratory study. *J Cataract Refract Surg.* 1987;13:175-189.

74. Pfeffer BR, Richards SC, Kersten RC, Olson RJ, Apple DJ. Histopathological examination of a cornea with an uncomplicated radial keratotomy. *Int Intraocular Implant Refract Surg.* 1987;1:8-10.

75. Apple DJ. *Different Aspects of Extracapsular Intraocular Lens Surgery: Pros and Cons.* Panama City, Republic of Panama: Highlights of Ophthalmology; 1987.

76. Apple DJ. *"Injectable" Intraocular Lenses. Research to Prevent Blindness, Inc., Science Writers Seminar.* Washington, D.C. 1987;19-20.

77. Apple DJ, Lichtenstein SB, Heerlein K, et al. Visual aberrations caused by optic components of posterior chamber intraocular lenses. *J Cataract Refract Surg.* 1987;13:431-435.

78. Apple DJ, Hansen SO, Tetz MR, Olson RJ, Richards SC. Complications of closed-loop lens removal (Reply to letter to the editor). *Arch Ophthalmol.* 1987;105:887-889.

79. Gobel RJ, Janatova J, Googe JM, Apple DJ. Activation of complement in human serum by some synthetic polymers used for intraocular lenses. *Biomaterials.* 1987;8:285-288.

80. Cameron JD, Apple DJ, Sumsion MA, et al. Pathology of iris support intraocular lenses. implant. *Eur J Implant Refrac Surg.* 1987;5(1):15-24.

81. Piest KL, Kincaid MC, Tetz MR, et al. Localized endophthalmitis: A newly documented cause of toxic lens syndrome. *J Cataract Refract Surg.* 1987;13:498-510.

82. Apple DJ. Stableflex lens report (Reply to letter to editor by ML Furillo). *J Cataract Refract Surg.* 1987;13:455-458.

83. Apple DJ, Tetz MR, Hansen SO, et al. Intercapsular implantation of various posterior chamber IOLs: Animal test results. *Ophthalmic Prac.* 1987;5(3):100-104, 132-134.

84. Apple DJ, Tetz M, Hunold W. *Lokalisierte Endophthalmitis: Eine bisher nicht Beschriebene Komplikation der Extrakapsulären Kataraktextraktion.* Proceedings of the Deutsche Gesellschaft für Intraokularlinsen Implantation Meeting, Giessen, West Germany, March 7, 1987.

85. Tetz MR, Apple DJ, Hansen SO, et al. "Localized endophthalmitis": A complication of extracapsular cataract extraction. *Implants In Ophthalmol.* (Singapore) 1987;1(3):93-97.

86. Tetz MR, Apple DJ, Price FW Jr, et al. A newly described complication of Neodymium:YAG laser capsulotomy: Exacerbation of an intraocular infection. *Arch Ophthalmol.* 1987;105:1324-1325.

87. Bath PE, Mueller G, Apple DJ, Brems RN. Excimer laser lens ablation. *Arch Ophthalmol.* 1987;105:1164-1165.

88. Reidy OJJ, Bode D, Kincaid MC, Notz RG, Apple DJ. Fulminant band keratopathy associated with preexisting corneal anesthesia. *Ophthalmic Surg.* 1987;18.

89. McKnight GT, Richards SC, Apple DJ, et al. Transcorneal extrusion of anterior chamber intraocular lenses: A report of three cases. *Arch Ophthalmol.* 1987;105:1656-1659.

90. Hansen SO, Apple DJ, Tetz MR, et al. Comparative histopathologic study of various lens biomaterials in primates after Nd:YAG laser treatment. *J Cataract Refract Surg.* 1987;13:657-661.

91. Bath PE, Kar H, Apple DJ, Hansen SO, et al. Endocapsular excimer laser phakoablation through a 1-mm incision. *Ophthalmic Laser Therapy* 1987;2(4):245-248.

92. Olson RJ, Apple DJ. Unexplained intraocular toxicity after cataract-intraocular lens surgery (Letter to the Editor). *J Cataract Refract Surg.* 1987;13:688-689.

93. 'Localized' endophthalmitis: New risk in ECCE. *Ocular Surgery News.* 1987;5(15):1,18, 19.

94. Bath PE, Apple DJ, Muller-Stolzenburg N. Excimer laser application for cataract surgery. Laser interaction with tissue. *Proceedings of SPIE-The International Society for Optical Engineering.* 1988;908:72-74.

95. Hansen SO, Tetz MR, Solomon KD, et al. Decentration of flexible loop posterior chamber intraocular lenses in a series of 222 postmortem eyes. *Ophthalmology.* 1988;95:344-349.

96. Hansen SO, Tetz MR, Mamalis N, Apple DJ. A new surgical technique for managing sunset syndrome (Letter to the Editor). *Ophthalmic Surg.* 1988;19:295.

97. Solomon KD, Gwin TD, Hansen SO, et al. Preliminary report of ultrasound and laser energy applications to small incision cataract surgery: SEM and histopathologic study. *Ophthalmic Prac.* 1988;6(2):52-91.

98. Apple DJ, Tetz MR, Hansen SO, et al. Intercapsular (endocapsular) intraocular lens implantation: Results of animal studies. Proceedings of the endocapsular symposium, IOIS Meeting, Fukuoka, Japan, June 17-21, 1987. *Jpn IOL Soc J.* 1988; 2(1):45-61.

99. Hansen SO, Solomon KD, McKnight GT, et al. Posterior capsular opacification and intraocular lens decentration. Part I: Comparison of various posterior chamber lens designs implanted in the rabbit model. *J Cataract Refract Surg.* 1988;14:605-614.

100. Tetz MR, O'Morchoe DJC, Gwin TD, et al. Posterior capsular opacification and intraocular lens decentration. Part II: Experimental findings on a prototype circular IOL design. *J Cataract Refract Surg.* 1988;14:614-623.

101. Deacon J, Buchen SY, Apple DJ. *Evaluation of Silicone Intraocular Lenses in a Feline Model and Clinical Trials. Proceedings of the Society for Biomaterials Symposium on Retrieval and Analysis of Surgical Implants and Biomaterials.* Snowbird, Utah; 1988.

102. Apple DJ. Center for Intraocular Lens Research transfers to Medical University of South Carolina (Editorial). *J Cataract Refract Surg.* 1988;14:481.

103. Nishi K, Apple DJ, Tetz MR. A case of localized endophthalmitis due to Propionibacterium acnes and Staphylococcus epidermidis following extracapsular cataract extraction. *Jpn J Clin Ophthalmol.* 1988;42(8):931-935.

104. Tetz M, Imkamp E, Hansen SO, Solomon KD, Apple DJ. Experimentelle studie zur hinterkapseltrübung und optischen dezentrierung verschiedener hinterkammerlinsen nach interkapsulärer implantation. *Fortschr Ophthalmol.* 1988;85:682-688.

105. Solomon KD, Gwin TD, O'Morchoe DJC, et al. Protective effect of the anterior lens capsule during extracapsular cataract extraction. Part I: Experimental animal study. *Ophthalmology.* 1989;96(5):591-597.

106. Patel J, Apple DJ, Hansen SO, et al. Protective effect of the anterior lens capsule during extracapsular cataract extraction. Part II: Preliminary results of clinical study. *Ophthalmology.* 1989;96(5):598-602.

107. Hunold W, Tetz MR, Kleine E, et al. A method to study the interaction between intraocular lens loops and anterior segment vasculature. *J Cataract Refract Surg.* 1989;15(3):289-296.

108. Apple DJ. *Capsulorhexis. Proceedings of The Third International, Implant, Microsurgical & Refractive Keratoplasty Meeting.* Fukuoka, Japan. May 26-28, 1989.

109. Apple DJ. *Pea-podding. Proceedings of The Third International, Implant, Microsurgical & Refractive Keratoplasty Meeting.* Fukuoka, Japan. May 26-28, 1989.

110. Apple DJ, Price FW, Gwin T, et al. Sutured retropupillary posterior chamber IOLs for exchange or secondary implantation. *Ophthalmology.* 1989;96(8):1241-1247.

111. Madsen K, Stenevi U, Apple DJ, Härfstrand A. Histochemical and receptor binding studies of hyaluronic acid and hyaluronic acid binding sites on corneal endothelium. *Ophthalmic Prac.* 1989;7(3):1-8.

112. Imkamp E, Apple DJ, Tetz M, Solomon KD, Gwin TD. Protektiver effekt der vorderen linsenkapsel: Corneaendothelzellverluste nach interkapsulärer phakoemulsifikation verglichen mit phakoemulsifikation mit grosser offener kapsulotomie. *Fortschritte der Ophthalmologie.* 1989;86(1):15-18.

113. Buchen SY, Richards SC, Solomon KD, et al. Evaluation of the biocompatibility and fixation of a new silicone intraocular lens in the feline model. *J Cataract Refract Surg.* 1989;15:545-553.

114. Apple DJ, Lim ES, Morgan RC, et al. Preparation and study of human eyes obtained postmortem with the Miyake posterior photographic technique. *Ophthalmology.* 1990;97:810-816.

115. Harfstrand A, Stenevi U, Schenholm M, et al. Sodium hyaluronate is naturally occurring on corneal endothelial cells of various species including man. *3rd Int Symp Ocular Microsurgery.* 1990;41-46.

116. Legler UFC, Apple DJ, Hund P, Kirkconnell WS. Chronic ciliary pain secondary to posterior chamber Intraocular lens loop incarceration (Letter to the Editor). *Am J Ophthalmol.* 1991;111(4):513-515.

117. Lim ES, Apple DJ, Tsai JC, et al. An analysis of flexible anterior chamber lenses with special reference to the normalized rate of lens explantation. *Ophthalmology.* 98:243-246, 1991.

118. Wasserman D, Apple DJ, Castaneda VE, et al. Anterior capsular tears and loop fixation of posterior chamber intraocular lenses. *Ophthalmology.* 1991;98:425-431.

119. Assia EI, Apple DJ, Tsai JC, Morgan RC. Mechanism of radial tear formation and extension after anterior capsulotomy. *Ophthalmology.* 1991;98:432-437.

120. Assia EI, Apple DJ, Barden A, et al. An experimental study comparing various anterior capsulectomy techniques. *Arch Ophthalmol.* 1991;109:642-647.

121. Assia EI, Apple DJ, Barden A, et al. An experimental study comparing various anterior capsulectomy techniques. *Arch Ophthalmol* (Chinese Edition). 1991;109:642-647.

122. Assia EI, Apple DJ, Barden A, et al. Estudio experimental comparando diversas tecnicas de capsulectomia anterior. *Arch Ophthalmol* (Spanish Edition). 2:280-285, 1991.

123. Assia EI, Apple DJ, Tsai JC, Lim ES. The elastic properties of the lens capsule in capsulorhexis. *Am J Ophthalmol.* 1991;111:628-632.

124. Assia EI, Hoggatt J, Apple DJ. Experimental nucleus extraction through a capsulorhexis in an eye with pseudoexfoliation syndrome. *Am J Ophthalmol.* 1991;111:645-647.

125. Solomon KD, Apple DJ, Mamalis N, et al. Complications of intraocular lenses with special reference to an analysis of 2500 explanted intraocular lenses (IOLs). *Eur J Implant Refract Surg.* 1991;3:195-200.

126. Hennis HL, Assia EI, Stewart WC, Legler UFC, Apple DJ. A transscleral cyclophotocoagulation using a semiconductor diode laser in cadaver eyes. *Ocular Surgery.* 1991;22(5):274-278.

127. Assia EI, Castaneda VE, Legler UFC, et al. Studies on cataract surgery and intraocular lenses at the Center for Intraocular Lens Research. *Ophthalmology Clinics of North America.* 1991;4:251-266.

128. Assia EI, Apple DJ, Tsai JC, Lim ES. The elastic properties of the lens capsule in capsulorhexis (Reply to Letter to the Editor). *Am J Ophthalmol.* 1991;112:355.

129. Legler UFC, Apple DJ. Comments on silicone intraocular lens discoloration (Letter to the Editor). *Arch Ophthalmol.* 1991;109:1495.

130. Assia EI, Hennis HL, Stewart WC, et al. A comparison of neodymium:yttrium aluminum garnet and diode laser transscleral cyclophotocoagulation and cyclocryotherapy. *Invest Ophthalmol Vis Sci.* 1991;32:2774-2778.

131. Assia EI, Apple DJ, Morgan RC, Legler UFC, Brown SJ. The relationship between the stretching capability of the anterior capsule and zonules. *Invest Ophthalmol Vis Sci.* 1991;32:2835-2839.

132. Assia EI, Apple EJ, Tsai JC, Lim ES. The elastic properties of the lens capsule in capsulorhexis (Reply to Letter to the Editor). *Am J Ophthalmol.* 1991;112(4):474-475.

133. Assia EI, Apple DJ, Lim ES, Morgan RC, Tsai JC. Removal of viscoelastic material after experimental cataract surgery in vitro. *J Cataract Refract Surg.* 1992;18:3-6.

134. Wenzel MR, Imkamp EM, Apple DJ. Variations in manufacturing quality of diffractive multifocal lenses. *J Cataract Refract Surg.* 1992;18(2):153-156.

135. Assia EI, Apple DJ. Side-view analysis of the lens. Part I: The crystalline lens and the evacuated capsular bag. *Arch Ophthalmol.* 1992;110:89-93.

136. Assia EI, Apple DJ. Side-view analysis of the lens. Part I: The crystalline lens and the evacuated capsular bag. *Arch Ophthalmol* (Spanish Edition). 1992;3:152-156.

137. Assia EI, Apple DJ. Side-view analysis of the lens. Part II: Positioning of intraocular lenses. *Arch Ophthalmol.* 1992;110:94-97.

138. Assia EI, Apple DJ. Side-view analysis of the lens. Part II: Positioning of intraocular lenses. *Arch Ophthalmol* (Spanish Edition). 1992;3:157-161.

139. Castaneda VE, Legler UFC, Tsai JC, et al. Posterior continuous curvilinear capsulorhexis: An experimental study with clinical applications. *Ophthalmology.* 1992;99:45-50.

140. Assia EI, Apple DJ. Capsulorhexis and corneal magnification. (Reply to Letter to the Editor). *Arch Ophthalmol.* 1992;110(2):170.

141. Assia EI, Blumenthal M, Apple DJ. Hydrodissection and visco extraction of the nucleus in planned extracapsular cataract extraction. *Eur J Implant Refract Surg.* 1992;4:3-8.

142. Apple DJ. Intraocular lens biocompatibility (Guest Editorial). *J Cataract Refract Surg.* 1992;18(5):217-218.

143. Tsai JC, Castaneda VE, Apple DJ, et al. Scanning electron microscopic study of modern silicone intraocular lenses. *J Cataract Refract Surg.* 1992;18(5):232-235.

144. Solomon KD, Legler UFC, Kostick MP. Capsular opacification after cataract surgery. *Curr Opin in Ophthalmol.* 1992;3:46-51.

145. Christ FR, Buchen SY, Fencil DA, et al. A comparative evaluation of the biostability of a poly (ether urethane) in the Intraocular, Intramuscular, and subcutaneous environments. *J Biomed Materials Res.* 1992;26:607-629.

146. Harfstrand A, Molander N, Stenevi U, et al. Evidence of hyaluronic acid and hyaluronic acid binding sites on human corneal endothelium. *J Cataract Refract Surg.* 1992;18(5):232-235.

147. Legler UFC, Assia EI, Castaneda VE, Hoggatt JP, Apple DJ. A prospective experimental study on factors related to posterior chamber intraocular lens decentration. *J Cataract Refract Surg.* 1992;18:449-455.

148. Apple DJ, Solomon KD, Tetz MR, et al. Posterior capsular opacification. A review. *Surv Ophthalmol.* 1992;37(2): 73-116.

149. Apple DJ, Legler UFC, Assia EI. Vergleich verschiedener kapsulektomietechniken in der kataraktchirurgie. *Der Ophthalmologe.* 1992;89:301-304.

150. Assia EI, Apple DJ. Update on IOLs, Personal Interview on IOLs. *Highlights of Ophthalmology.* 1992.

151. Apple DJ, Carlson AN. Localized endophthalmitis. Answer. In: Masket S, ed. Consultation Section. *J Cataract Refract Surg.* 1992;18:413-419.

152. Assia EI, Legler UFC, Castaneda VE, Apple DJ. Loop memory of posterior chamber intraocular lenses of various sizes, designs and loop materials. *J Cataract Refract Surg.* 1992;18:541-546.

153. Ohmi S, Uenoyama K, Apple DJ. Implantation of IOLs with different diameters. *Acta Soc Ophthalmol Jpn.* 1992;96(9):1093-1098.

154. McMillan TA, Stewart WC, Nutaitis MJ, Powers TP, Apple DJ. The effect of varying wavelength on subconjunctival scleral laser suture lysis in rabbits. *Ophthalmololgica.* 1992;70:758-761.

155. Kostick AMP, Legler UFC, Bluestein EC, Carlson AN, Apple DJ. *Analysis of Intraocular Lens Haptic Fixation in Human Cadaver Eyes.* Sarasota, Fla: ARVO; 1992:1307.

156. Tetz M, Apple DJ, Price FJ, et al. *Localized endophthalmitis. Proceedings in International Symposium of the German Ophthalmological Society.* Münster, Germany; 1992.

157. Assia EI, Legler UFC, Castaneda VE, et al. Clinicopathologic study on the effect of radial tears and loop fixation on intraocular lens decentration. *Ophthalmology.* 1993;100:153-158.

158. Assia EI, Blumenthal M, Legler UFC, Apple DJ. Photoanalysis of fixation of posterior chamber intraocular lenses. *Eur J Implant Refract Surg.* 1993.

159. Wesendahl TA, Auffarth GU, Brown S, Apple DJ. Textur von IOL-Oberflechen: Ein neues Konzept zur Nachstarprevention. *Der Ophthalmologe.* 1993;90(Suppl I):S140.

160. Apple DJ, Auffarth G, Wesendahl T, Brown S. Komplikationen bei vorderkammerlinsen: Eine analyse von 4000 explantierten IOLs. *Der Ophthalmologe.* 1993;90(Suppl I):S113.

161. Auffarth G, Wesendahl T, Brown S, Apple DJ. Eine analyse von komplikationen bei explantierten hinterkammerlinsen. *Der Ophthalmologe.* 1993;90(Suppl I):S140.

162. Auffarth G, Wesendahl T, Newland T, Apple DJ. Eine kapsulorhexistechnik bei kindlicher katarakt. *Der Ophthalmologe.* 1993;90(Suppl I):S13.

163. Wesendahl TA, Hunold W, Auffarth GU, Apple DJ. Kontaktbereich von IOL-optik und hinterkapsel: Systematische untersuchung unterschiedlicher haptikparameter. *Der Ophthalmologe.* 1993;90(Suppl I):S19.

164. Anonymous. Ehud Assia e os estudos Israelitas (Interview). *Oftalmologia Abr/Mai.* 1993;33:39.

165. Wright M, Apple DJ. How should we approach Third World cataract surgery? Anterior chamber IOLs after ICCE may decrease the extensive backlog of cases. *Ophthalmol Times.* 1993;18(13):28.

166. Apple DJ, Blotnik C. Postoperative lens deposits (Letter to the Editor). *J Cataract Refract Surg.* 1993;19:441.

167. Legler UFC, Apple DJ, Assia EI, et al. Inhibition of posterior capsular opacification: The effect of colchicine in a sustained drug delivery system. *J Cataract Refract Surg.* 1993;19:462-470.

168. Apple DJ, Auffarth GU, Wesendahl TA. Komplikationen bei vorderkammerlinsen: Eine analyse von 4000 explantierten IOLs. In Med-Report 1993;15/17:8.

169. Reidy JJ, Kemp JR, Anthone KD, et al. Histopathology of an excimer laser phototherapeutic keratectomy for HSV stromal keratitis two years post-laser. *Invest Ophthalmol Vis Sci.* 1993;34(4):1245.

170. Auffarth G, Wesendahl T, Apple DJ. Surface characteristics of intraocular lens implants: An evaluation using scanning electron microscopy and quantitative three-dimensional noncontacting profilometry (TOPO). *J Long-term Effect of Med Implants.* 1993;3(4): 321-331.

171. Apple DJ, Williamson. Modern ACLs make ICCE viable in Third World surgery. *Ocular Surg News.* 1993.

172. Stenevi ULF, Gwin T, Anders H, Apple DJ. Demonstration of hyaluronic acid binding to corneal endothelial cells in human eye-bank eyes. *Eur J Implant Ref Surg.* 1993;5:228-232.

173. Auffarth G, Wesendahl T, Brown S, Apple D. Analysis of complications in explanted posterior chamber intraocular lenses. *Ger J Ophthalmol.* 1993;2(4/5):366.

174. Wesendahl T, Hunold W, Auffarth G, Apple DJ. Area of contact between IOL-optic and posterior capsule systematic analysis of different haptic parameters. *Ger J Ophthalmol.* 1993;2(4/5):265.

175. Auffarth GU, Wesendahl T, Newland T, Apple DJ. A capsulorhexis technic in pediatric cataracts. *Ger J Ophthalmol.* 1993;2(4/5):259.

176. Apple DJ, Auffarth G, Wesendahl T, Brown S. Complications in anterior chamber lenses: An analysis of 4000 explanted IOLs. *Ger J Ophthalmol.* 1993;2(4/5):338.

177. Wesendahl T, Auffarth G, Brown S, Apple D. IOL surface texturing a new concept for PCO Prevention. *Ger J Ophthalmol.* 1993;2(4/5):365.

178. Auffarth G, Wesendahl T, Brown S, Apple DJ. Analysis of complications in explanted posterior chamber intraocular lenses. *Ger J Ophthalmol.* 1993; 2(4/5):366.

179. Wesendahl T, Hunold W, Auffarth G, Apple DJ. Area of contact between IOL-optic and posterior capsule systematic analysis of different haptic parameters. *Ger J Ophthalmol.* 1993;2(4/5):265.

180. Auffarth GU, Wesendahl T, Newland T, Apple DJ. A capsulorhexis technic in pediatric cataracts. *Ger J Ophthalmol.* 1993;2(4/5):259.

181. Apple DJ, Auffarth G, Wesendahl T, Brown S. Complications in anterior chamber lenses: An analysis of 4000 explanted IOLs. *Ger J Ophthalmol.* 1993;2(4/5):338.

182. Wesendahl T, Auffarth G, Brown S, Apple DJ. IOL surface texturing a new concept for PCO prevention. *Ger J Ophthalmol.* 1993;2(4/5):365.

183. Auffarth G, Wesendahl T, Brown S, Apple DJ. Analysis of complications in explanted posterior chamber intraocular lenses. *Ger J Ophthalmol.* 1993;2(4/5):366.

184. Wesendahl T, Hunold W, Auffarth G, Apple DJ. Area of contact between IOL-optic and posterior capsule systematic analysis of different haptic parameters. *Ger J Ophthalmol.* 1993;2(4/5):265.

185. Auffarth GU, Wesendahl T, Newland T, Apple DJ. A capsulorhexis technic in pediatric cataracts. *Ger J Ophthalmol.* 1993;2(4/5):259.

186. Apple DJ, Auffarth G, Wesendahl T, Brown S. Complications in anterior chamber lenses: An analysis of 4000 explanted IOLs. *Ger J Ophthalmol.* 1993;2(4/5):338.

187. Wesendahl T, Auffarth G, Brown S, Apple DJ. IOL surface texturing a new concept for PCO prevention. *Ger J Ophthalmol.* 1993;2(4/5):365.

188. Auffarth GU, Newland TJ, Wesendahl TA, Apple DJ. Nd:Yag laser damage on silicone Intraocular lenses confused with pigment deposits on clinical examination. Letter to the Journal. *Am J Ophthalmol.* 1994;118(4):526-528.

189. Newland T, Auffarth G, Wesendahl T, Blotnick C, Apple DJ. Pathology of Nd:YAG laser damage on explanted lenses with experimentally-produced lesions. *J Cataract Refract Surg.* 1994;20:527-533.

190. Koenig SB, Apple DJ, Hyndiuk RA. Penetrating keratoplasty and intraocular lens exchange: Open-loop anterior chamber lenses vs. sutured posterior chamber lenses. *Cornea.* 1994;13(5):418-421.

191. Assia EI, Blotnick CA, Powers TP, Legler UFC, Apple DJ. Clinico-pathologic study on ocular trauma in eyes with intraocular lenses. *Am J Ophthalmol.* 1994;117(11): 30-36.

192. Apple DJ, John T, Powers T, Dado R, Jr. In vivo interaction of extruded intraocular lens (IOL) haptic with human ocular surface environment. *ARVO.* 1994.

193. Auffarth GU, Wesendahl TA, Newland TJ, Apple DJ. Capsulorhexis in the rabbit eye as a model for pediatric capsulectomy. *J Cataract Refract Surg.* 1994;20:188-191.

194. Apple DJ, Auffarth GU, Wesendahl TA. A randomized trial of intraocular lens fixation techniques with penetrating keratoplasty (Letter to the Editor). *Ophthalmology.* 1994;101(5):798-799.

195. Auffarth GU, Wesendahl TA, Apple DJ. Are there indications for open loop anterior chamber IOLs in the 1990s? (Editorial). *Ophthalmic Prac.* 1994.

196. Auffarth G, Wesendahl TA, Apple DJ. Are there acceptable anterior chamber intraocular lenses (AC IOLs) for clinical use in the 1990s? An analysis of 4104 explanted AC IOLs. *Ophthalmology.* 1994;101(12):1913-1922.

197. Ram J, Auffarth GU, Wesendahl TA, Apple DJ. Miyake posterior view video technique; a means to reduce the learning curve in phacoemulsification. *Ophthalmic Practice.* 1994;12(5):206-210.

198. Wang XH, Wilson ME, Bluestein EC, Auffarth G, Apple DJ. Pediatric cataract surgery and IOL implantation techniques in the pediatric age group: A laboratory study. *J Cataract Refract Surg.* 1994;20:607-609.

199. Wilson ME, Wang XH, Bluestein EC, Apple DJ. Comparison of mechanized anterior capsulectomy and manual continuous capsulorhexis (CCC) in pediatric eyes. *J Cataract Refract Surg.* 1994;20:602-606.

200. Wilson ME, Apple DJ, Bluestein EC, Wang XH. Intraocular lenses for pediatric implantation biomaterials, designs, and sizing. *J Cataract Refract Surg.* 1994;20:584-591.

201. Apple DJ, Auffarth GU, Wesendahl TA. Letter to editor. *Ophthalmology.* 1994;101(5):798-799.

202. Auffarth GU, Wesendahl TA, Assia EI, Apple DJ. *The Concept of Modern Capsular Surgery.* Proceedings. Illinois Society of Ophthalmology and Otolaryngology. 1994.

203. Apple DJ. Pathological Aspects of Capsular Surgery. *Eur J Implant Ref Surg.* 1994;6.

204. Auffarth GU, Wesendahl TA, Brown SJ, Apple DJ. Komplikationen nach Vorderkammerlinsenimplantation: Eine Analyse von 4100 explantierten Intraokularlinsen, *Ophthalmologe.* 1994;91:512-517.

205. Auffarth GU, Wesendahl TA, Brown SJ, Apple DJ. Gründe fuer die Explantation von Hinterkammerlinsen. *Ophthalmologe.* 1994;91:507-511.

206. Auffarth GU, Wesendahl TA, Newland TJ, Apple DJ. Eine kapsulorhexistechnik bei kindlicher katarakt: Dargestellt am kaninchenmodell. *Ophthalmologe.* 1994,91:518-520.

207. Auffarth GU, Taso K, Wesendahl TA, Apple DJ. Pathologische befunde in autopsie augen mit pseudoexfoliationssyndrom und implantierten hinterkammerlinsen. *Ophthalmologe.* 1994;91(Suppl.1):35.

208. Wesendahl TA, Shallaby WS, Auffarth GU, Corson DW, Apple DJ. Entwicklung von neuartigen hydrogelintraokularlinsen aus polyvinylpyrrolidone (PVP) polymeren. *Ophthalmologe.* 1994;91(Suppl.1):139.

209. Auffarth GU, Tsao K, Wesendahl TA, Apple DJ. Pathology of autopsy eyes with pseudoexfoliation syndrome: A study of cases with implanted posterior chamber lenses. *Ger J Ophthalmol.* 1994;3:284.

210. Wesendahl TA, Shallaby WS, Auffarth GU, Corson DW, Apple DJ. Suitability of polyvinylpyrrolidone (PVP) as a material for hydrogel intraocular lenses. *Ger J Ophthalmol.* 1994;3:383.

211. Auffarth GU, Hunhold G, Hhrtgen, Wesendahl TA, Mehdorn E. Nachtfahrtauglichkeit pseudophaker patienten. *Der Ophthalmologe.* 1994;91(4):454-459.

212. Newland TJ, Auffarth GU, Wesendahl TA, Apple DJ. Neodymium: YAG laser damage on silicone intraocular lenses. A comparison of lesions on explanted lenses and experimentally produced lesions. *J Cataract Refract Surg.* 1994;20:527-533.

213. Auffarth GU, Newland TJ, Wesendahl TA, Apple DJ. Nd:YAG laser damage to silicone intraocular lenses confused with pigment deposits on clinical examination. *Am J Ophthalmol.* 1994;118(4):526-530.

214. Apple DJ, Auffarth GU, Wesendahl TA, Sakabe I. Modified removal technique best for aspirating Healon GV: Greater viscosity material has unique personality. *Ocular Surgery News* (International Edition). 1994;5(8):29-30.

215. Auffarth GU, Wesendahl TA, Solomon KD, Brown SJ, Apple DJ. A preparation technique of human postmortem eyes for closed system ocular surgery: A new research and teaching tool. *Ophthalmology.* 1994;101:152.

216. Solomon KD, Auffarth GU, Wesendahl TA, Brown SJ, Apple DJ. Sutured posterior chamber lenses in the absence of capsular support: An anatomic study using postmortem human eyes. *Ophthalmology.* 1994;101:149.

217. Wesendahl TA, Auffarth GU, Sakabe I, Apple DJ. Entfernung viskoelastischer substanzen nach linsenimplantation: Eine experimentelle studie an menschlichen autopsieaugen. *Klinische Monatsblätter fhr Augenheilkunde.* 1994;205:397.

218. Wilson ME, Bluestein EC, Wang XH, Apple DJ. Comparison of mechanized anterior capsulectomy and manual continuous capsulorhexis in pediatric eyes. *J Cataract Refract Surg.* 1994;20:602-606.

219. Wesendahl TA, Shalaby WS, Auffarth GU, Corson DW, Apple DJ. Eignung von polyvinylpyrrolidone (PVP) als material fur hydrogel intraocularlinsen. Deutsche Ophthalmologische Gesellschaft Heidelberg 93rd Annual Meeting; Mannheim/Heidelberg, 1994. *Der Ophthalmologe.* 1994;91(Suppl.1):35.

220. Auffarth, Wesendahl TA, Solomon KD, Brown SJ, Apple DJ. Evaluation of different removal techniques of a high-viscosity viscoelastic. (Healon GV). *J Cataract Refract Surg.* 1994:[Special Issue: Best Paper of 1994 ASCRS Meeting];30-32.

221. Auffarth GU, Wesendahl TA, Brown SJ, Apple DJ. Update on complications of anterior chamber intraocular lenses. *J Cataract Refract Surg.* 1994;[Special Issue: Best Paper of 1994 ASCRS Meeting]:70-76.

222. Wesendahl TA, Shalaby WS, Auffarth GU, Corson DW, Apple DJ. Suitability of polyvinylpyrrolidone (PVP) as a material for hydrogel intraocular lenses. *Ger J Ophthalmol.* 1994;3(4/5):383.

223. Auffarth GU, Taso K, Wesendahl TA, Apple DJ. Pathology of autopsy eyes with implanted posterior chamber lenses. *Ger J Ophthalmol.* 1994;3(4/5):284.

224. Golnik KC, Hund PW III, Apple DJ. The atonic pupil following cataract surgery. *J Cataract Refract Surg.* 1995;21:170-175.

225. Apple DJ, Ram J, Wang XH, Brown S. Cataract surgery in the developing world. *Saudi J Ophthalmol.* 1995;(9)1:2-15.

226. Apple DJ, Sims JC. Harold Ridley and the invention of the intraocular lens. *Surv of Ophthalmol.* 1995;40(4):279-292.

227. Auffarth GU, Wesendahl TA, Brown SJ, Apple DJ. Update on complications of anterior chamber intraocular lenses. J *Cataract Refract Surg.* 1995;22:1-7.

228. Auffarth GU, Wilcox M, Sims JCR, et al. Analysis of 100 Explanted one-piece and three-piece silicone intraocular lenses. *Ophthamology.* 1995;102(8):1144-1150.

229. Auffarth GU, Brown SJ, Wesendahl TA, Apple DJ. Letter (Authors' reply to Dr. Drews' letter); Are there acceptable anterior chamber intraocular lenses for clinical use in the 1990s? An analysis of 4104 explanted anterior chamber intraocular lenses. *Ophthalmology.* 1995;102(6): 857-859.

230. Auffarth GU, Brown SJ, Wesendahl TA, Apple DJ. Letter (Authors' reply to Dr. Spencer's letter); Are there acceptable anterior chamber intraocular lenses for clinical use in the 1990s? An analysis of 4104 explanted anterior chamber intraocular lenses. *Ophthalmology.* 1995;102(7):1001-1002.

231. Blotnick CA, Powers TP, Newland T, et al. Case report: Pathology of silicone intraocular lenses in human eyes obtained postmortem. *J Cataract Refract Surg.* 1995;21(4):447-452.

232. Turkalj JW, Carlson AN, Manos JP, Apple DJ. Is the sutureless cataract incision a valve for bacterial inoculation? *J Cataract Refract Surg.* 1995;21(4):472-476.

233. Kent DG, Sims JCR, Apple DJ. Letter. Pediatric capsulorhexis technique. *J Cataract Refract Surg.* 1995;21(5):236.

234. Auffarth GU, Beischel CJ, Wesendahl TA, Apple DJ. Soemmering's Ring Bildung nach kataraktoperation und HKL implantation: Eine studie von 827 autopsieaugen. *Klinische Monatsblätter für Augenheilkunde.* 1995;206(Suppl.1):1-12.

235. Auffarth GU, Wilcox CM, Sims JC, et al. Komplikationen von 100 explantierten silikonhinterkammerlinsen. *Klinische Monatsblätter für Augenheilkunde.* 1995;206(Suppl.1):22-23.

236. Auffarth GU, McCabe C, Tetz MR, Apple DJ. Die modifizierte disk-linse nach anis: befunde bei 15 menschlichen autopsieaugen. *Klinische Monatsblätter für Augenheilkunde.* 1995;206(Suppl.1):13-14.

237. Auffarth GU, Recum AV, Wesendahl TA, Apple DJ. Ultrastrukturoberflächenanalyse von silikon und PMMA intraokularlinsen mittels 3-D profilometrie. *Der Ophthalmologe.* 1995;92(Suppl.1):189.

238. Auffarth GU, McCabe C, Sims JCR, et al. Zentrierverhalten und fixation von eiustüeinsthckigen und dreistückigen silikon hinterkammerlinsen: Eine analyse von 29 menschlichen autopsieaugen. *Der Ophthalmologe.* 1995;92(Suppl.1):191.

239. Wesendahl TA, Ram J, Auffarth GU, Brown SJ, Apple DJ. Verringerung der nachstarrate durch stärkere hapikabwinklung von einstückigen PMMA hinterkammerlinsen. *Der Ophthalmologe.* 1995;92(Suppl.1):108.

240. Auffarth GU, Recum AV, Wesendahl TA, Apple DJ. Ultrastructural analysis of intraocular lens surfaces made of silicone and PMMA using 3-D profilometry. *Ger J Ophthalmol.* 1995;4(Suppl.1):152.

241. Auffarth GU, McCabe C, Sims JCR, et al. Centration and fixation of silicone plate lenses and three piece silicone IOLs: Analysis of 29 human autopsy eyes. *Ger J Ophthalmol.* 1995; 4(Suppl.1):153.

242. Wesendahl TA, Ram J, Auffarth GU, Brown SJ, Apple DJ. Reduction of posterior capsule opacification by increased haptic angulation of one-piece PMMA intraocular lenses. *Ger J Ophthalmol.* 1995;4(Suppl.1):74.

243. Assia EI, Legler UFC, Apple DJ. The capsular bag after short- and long-term fixation of intraocular lenses. *Ophthalmology.* 1995;102(8):1151-1157.

244. Auffarth GU, Tsao K, Wesendahl TA, Apple DJ. Hinterkammerlinsenzentrierung in autopsieaugen mit und ohne pseudoexfoliationssyndrom. *Ophthalmologe.* 1995;92:750-755.

245. Auffarth GU, Mcabe C, Sims JCR, et al. *Zentrierverhalten und Fixation von Einstückigen und Dreistückigen Silikon Hinterkammerlinsen: Eine Analyse von 29 Menschilchen Autopsieaugen.* Deutsche Ophthalmologische Gesellschaft Heidelberg 93rd Annual Meeting. Mannheim/Heidelberg; 1995.

246. Auffarth GU, Beischel CJ, Wesendahl TA, Apple DJ. Soemmerring's Ring-Bildung nach kataraktoperation und HKL-implantation: Eine studie von 827 autopsieaugen. *Klinische Monatsblätter fhr Augenheilkunde.* 1995;206:11-12.

247. Auffarth GU, Wilcox M, Sims JCR, et al. Complications of silicone intraocular lenses. *J Cataract Refract Surg.* 1995;[Special Issue: Best Paper of 1995 ASCRS Meeting]:38-41.

248. Snellingen T, Apple DJ, et.al. The south Asian cataract management study. Part I. The first 662 cataract surgeries: a preliminary report. *Br J Ophthalmol.* 1995;79(11):1029-1035.

249. Ram J, Auffarth GU, Wesendahl TA, Apple DJ. Miyake posterior video technique: A means to reduce the learning curve for phacoemulsification. *Ophthalmic Practice* [Asian Edition, Inaugural Issue]. 1995;1(1):6-10.

250. Auffarth GU, Wesendahl TA, Solomon KD, Brown SJ, Apple DJ. Modified preparation technique for closed system ocular surgery of human eyes obtained post-mortem: An improved research and teaching tool. *Ophthalmology.* 1996;103:977-982.

251. Apple DJ, Federman JL, Krolicki TJ, et al. Irreversible silicone oil adhesion to silicone intraocular lenses. Part I: Clinicopathologic analysis. *Ophthalmology.* 1996;103(10):1555-1562.

252. Auffarth GU, McCabe C, Tetz MR, Apple DJ. Clinicopathological findings in autopsy eyes with the Anis modified disc IOL. *J Cataract Refract Surg.* 1996;22(2):1471-1475.

253. Auffarth GU, McCabe C, Wilcox M, et al. Centration and fixation of silicone intraocular lenses: An analysis of clinicopathological findings in human autopsy eyes. *J Cataract Refract Surg.* 1996;22(2):1281-1285.

254. Wesendahl TA, Shalaby WS, Auffarth GU, Corson DW, Apple DJ. Eignung von polyvinylpyrrolidone (PVP) als material fur hydroge intraocularlinsen. *Ophthalmologe.* 1996;93:22-28.

255. Auffarth GU, Tsoa K, Wesendahl TA, Sugita A, Apple DJ. Centration and fixation of posterior chamber intraocular lenses in eyes with pseudoexfoliation syndrome: An analysis of explanted autopsy eyes. *Acta Ophthalmol Scand.* 1996;74:167-171.

256. Auffarth GU, Wesendahl TA, Apple DJ. Are there indications for open-loop AC IOLs in the 1990s? Editorial. *Ophthalmic Practice* [Asian Edition]. 1996;2(1):2.

257. Bluestein EC, Kent DG, Greene WB, Apple DJ, Solomon KD. Wound healing in infant corneas after photorefractive keratectomy. *Invest Ophthalmol Vis Sci.* 1996;37(3):273,S60.

258. Peng Q, Solomon DK, Kent DG, Ahmad OF, Apple DJ. Comparison of keratocyte activation in laser in situ keratomileusis and photorefractive keratectomy. *Invest Ophthalmol Vis Sci.* 1996;37(3):290,S63.

259. Kent DG, Solomon KD, Peng Q, Apple DJ. Human corneal wound healing after laser in situ keratomileusis. *Invest Ophthalmol Vis Sci.* 1996;37(3):292,S63.

260. James ER, McLean DC, Jr., Kent DG, et al. Cytokine mRNA expression in rabbit lens epithelium following lens extraction and IOL implantation. *Invest Ophthalmol Vis Sci.* 1996;37(3):4536,S988.

261. Wilson ME, Saunders RA, Roberts EL, Apple DJ. Mechanized anterior capsulectomy as an alternative to manual capsulorhexis in children undergoing intraocular lens implantation. *J Pediatric Ophthalmol Strabismus.* 1996;33(7/8):237-240.

262. Apple DJ. Enhancement of silicone plate IOL fixation by the use of positioning holes in the lens haptic. *J Cataract Refract Surg.* 1996;6[Special Issue: Best Paper of 1996 ASCRS Meeting]:21-25.

263. Ram J, Wesendahl T, Auffarth G, Apple DJ. Evaluation of phacoemulsification technique: Divide and conquer versus phaco technique. Indian Ophthalmology. In: Pasricha JK, ed. *Proceedings of AIOS conference, Chandigarh, 1996.* Karnal Eye Institute: Karnal, India; 1996:147-149.

264. Isaacs R, Ram J, Apple DJ. Cataract blindness in the developing world: Is there a solution? *J Agromedicine.* 1996;3(4):7-21.

265. Apple DJ, Isaacs RT, Kent DG, et al. Silicone oil adhesion to intraocular lenses: An experimental comparing various biomaterials. *J Cataract Refract Surg.* 1997;23:536-544.

266. Kent DG, Solomon KD, Peng Q, Brown SR, Apple DJ. The effect of photorefractive keratectomy and laser in situ keratomileusis on the corneal endothelium. *J Cataract Refract Surg.* 1997;23(4):386-397.

267. Kent DG, Peng Q, Isaacs RT, et al. Security of capsular fixation: Small- versus large-hole plate-haptic lenses. *J Cataract Refract Surg.* 1997;23(11):1371-1375.

268. Solomon KD, Turhalj JW, Whiteside SB, Stewart JC, Apple DJ. Topical 0.5% Ketorolac vs 0.03% Flurbiprofen for inhibition of miosis during cataract surgery. *Arch Ophthalmol.* 1997;115(9):1119-1122.

269. Apple DJ. Irreversible silicone oil [Reply to a letter to the editor]. *Ophthalmology.* 1997;104(6):898-900.

270. Apple DJ, Whiteside SB, Riddle HK, et al. Complications of foldable IOLs: A study of explants and eyes obtained postmortem. *ASCRS.* Boston, MA: 1997;288:73.

271. Apple DJ. How we can stamp out posterior capsular opacification? *Review of Ophthalmol.* 1997;10:170-171.

272. Ram J, Wesendahl TA, Auffarth GU, Apple DJ. Evaluation of phacoemulsification techniques; insitu fracture vs. phaco chop. *J Cataract Refract Surg.* 1998;24(11):1464-1468.

273. Lim SJ, Kang SJ, Kim HB, Apple DJ. Ideal size of an intraocular lens for capsular bag fixation. *J Cataract Refract Surg.* 1998;24:297-402.

274. Lim SJ, Kang SJ, Kim HB, et al. Analysis of zonular-free zone and lens size in relation to axial length of eye with age. *J Cataract Refract Surg.* 1998;24:390-396.

275. Kent DG, Peng Q, Isaacs RT, et al. Mini-haptics to improve capsular fixation of plate-haptic silicone intraocular lenses (Part II). *Eur J Cataract Refract Surg.* 1998;24:666-671.

276. Peng Q, Hennig A, Vasavada AR, Apple DJ. Posterior capsular plaque, a common complication of cataract surgery in the Developing World: Pathogenesis and clinical significance. *Am J Ophthalmol.* 1998;125:621-626.

277. Apple DJ. Harold Ridley: A golden anniversary celebration and a golden age. Editorial. *Arch Ophthalmol.* 1999;117(6):827.

278. Assia EI, Blumenthal M, Apple DJ. Effect of expandable full-size intraocular lenses on lens centration and capsule opacification in rabbits. *J Cataract Refract Surg.* 1999;25:347-356.

279. Apple DJ, Peng Q, Ram J. The fiftieth anniversary of the intraocular lens and a quiet revolution. Editorial. *Ophthalmology.* 1999;106(10):1-2.

280. Newland TJ, McDermott ML, Eliott D, et al. Experimental Neodymium:YAG laser damage to acrylic, PMMA, and silicone intraocular lens materials. *J Cataract Refract Surg.* 1999;25:72-76.

281. Visessook N, Peng Q, Apple DJ, Gerl R, Guindi A. Pathological examination of an explanted phakic posterior chamber intraocular lens. *J Cataract Refract Surg.* 1999;25(2):216-222.

282. Whiteside SB, Apple DJ, Peng Q, Isaacs RT, Guindi A. Fixation elements on plate IOLs. Large positioning holes to improve security of capsular fixation (Part III). *Ophthalmology.* 1998;105:837-842.

283. James ER, Solomon KD, Kent DG, Apple DJ, Peng Q, Whiteside S. *Cytokine production after photorefractive keratectomy and laser in situ keratomileusis.* (In Press)

284. Ram J, Apple DJ, Peng Q, et al. Update on fixation of rigid and foldable posterior chamber intraocular lenses (IOLs). Part I. Elimination of decentration to achieve precise optical correction and visual rehabilitation. *Ophthalmology.* 1999;106:883-890.

285. Ram J, Apple DJ, Peng Q, et al. Update on fixation of rigid and foldable posterior chamber intraocular lenses (IOLs). Part II. Choosing the correct IOL designs to help eradicate posterior capsule opacification. *Ophthalmology.* 1999;106:891-900.

286. Apple DJ, Peng Q, Visessook N, Werner L, Pandey SK, Escobar-Gomez, M, et al. Surgical prevention of posterior capsule opacification. Part I. How are we progressing in eliminating this complication of cataract surgery? *J Cataract Refract Surg.* 2000;26:180-187.

287. Peng Q, Apple DJ, Visessook N, Werner L, Pandey SK, Escobar-Gomez M, et al. Surgical prevention of posterior capsule opacification. Part II. Enhancement of cortical clean up by increased emphasis and focus on the hydrodissection procedure. *J Cataract Refract Surg.* 2000;26:188-197.

288. Peng Q, Visessook N, Apple DJ, Pandey SK, Werner L, Escobar-Gomez M, et al. Surgical prevention of posterior capsule opacification. Part III. The IOL barrier effect functions as a second line of defense. *J Cataract Refract Surg.* 2000;26:198-213.

289. Apple DJ, Peng Q, Visessook N, et al. Comparison of Nd:YAG posterior capsulotomy rates of rigid and foldable intraocular lenses. An analysis of 4599 eyes with PC IOLs obtained postmortem accessioned between January 1988 and January 1999. *Ophthalmology.* 2000. [In Press]

290. Visessook N, Apple DJ, Peng Q, et al. Soemmering's ring formation evaluation in a series of 4599 eyes with PC IOLs obtained postmortem. An assay of IOL biocompatibility. *Ophthalmology.* 2000. [In Press]

291. Werner L, Pandey SK, Escobar-Gomez M, Visessook N, Peng Q, Apple DJ. Anterior capsule opacification: A histopathological study comparing different IOL styles. *Ophthalmology.* 2000; 107:463-471.

292. Pandey SK, Ram J, Jain AK, Singh U, Gupta A, Apple DJ. Surgical management of complete hyperplastic persistent pupillary membrane. *J Ped Ophthalmol Strabismus.* 1999; 36:221-223.

293. Apple DJ. Phaco Chop. Reply to Letter to the Editor (1). *J Cataract Refract Surg.* 1999. [In Press]

294. Gayton JL, Apple DJ, Peng Q, et al. Interlenticular opacification: A clinicopathological correlation of a new complication of piggyback posterior chamber intraocular lenses. *J Cataract Refract Surg.* 2000; 26:330-336.

295. Werner LP, Shugar JK, Apple DJ , Pandey SK, Escobar-Gomez M, et al. Opacification of piggyback IOLs. Analysis of an amorphous material between the lenses. *J Cataract Refract Surg.* 2000. [In Press]

296. Pandey SK, Werner L, Escobar-Gomez M, Roig-Melo EA, Apple DJ. Dye-enhanced cataract surgery. Part I. Anterior capsule staining for capsulorhexis in advanced/white cataracts: A comparative laboratory study using human eyes obtained postmortem. *J Cataract Refract Surg.* 2000. [In Press]

297. Werner L, Pandey SK, Escobar-Gomez M, Hoddinott DSM, Apple DJ. Dye-enhanced cataract surgery. Part II. An experimental study to learn and perform critical steps of phacoemulsification in human eyes obtained postmortem. *J Cataract Refract Surg.* 2000. [In Press]

298. Pandey SK, Werner L, Escobar-Gomez M, Werner LP, Apple DJ. Dye-enhanced cataract surgery. Part III. Staining of the posterior capsule to learn and perform posterior continuous curvilinear capsulorhexis. *J Cataract Refract Surg.* 2000. [In Press]

299. Linnola RJ, Werner L, Pandey SK, Escobar-Gomez M, Znoyko SL, Apple DJ. Adhesion of fibronectin, vitronectin, laminin, and collagen type IV to intraocular lens materials in human autopsy eyes. Part I. Histological sections. *J Cataract Refract Surg.* 1999.

300. Linnola RJ, Werner L, Pandey SK, Escobar-Gomez M, Znoyko SL, Apple DJ. Adhesion of fibronectin, vitronectin, laminin and collagen type IV to intraocular lens material in human autopsy eyes. Part II. Explanted IOLs. *J Cataract Refract Surg.* 1999.

301. Pandey SK, Ram J, Werner L, Brar GS, Jain AK, Gupta A, Apple DJ. Visual results and postoperative complications of capsular bag versus sulcus fixation of posterior chamber intraocular lenses for traumatic cataract in children. *J Cataract Refract Surg.* 1999; 25:1576-1584.

302. Pandey SK, Werner L, Escobar-Gomez M, Visessook N, Peng Q, Apple DJ. Creating cataracts of varying hardness to practice extracapsular cataract extraction and phacoemulsification. *J Cataract Refract Surg.* 2000. [In press]

303. Pandey SK, Werner L, Vasavada AR, Apple DJ. Induction of cataracts of varying degrees of hardness in human eyes obtained postmortem for cataract surgeon training. *Am J Ophthalmol.* 2000. [In press]

304. Ram J, Pandey SK, Werner L, Brar GS, Singh R, Chaudhary KP, Gupta A, Apple DJ. Posterior capsule opacification after cataract surgery and in-the-bag fixation of intraocular lenses: A comparative study between PMMA, silicone and acrylic lenses. *J Cataract Refract Surg.* 2000. [In press]

305. Pandey SK, Ram J, Werner L, Gupta A, Apple DJ. Persistent pupillary membrane (Letter to the Editor). *Br J Ophthalmol.* 2000. [In press]

306. Tyson FC, Pandey SK, Werner L, Apple DJ, McIntyre D, Peng Q. Optical topography: A new method of IOL property analysis. *Invest Ophthalmol Vis Sci.* 1999;40:S298.

307. Peng Q, Pandey SK, Escobar-Gomez M, Apple DJ. The reduction of posterior capsule opacification. *Invest Ophthalmol Vis Sci.* 1999; 40:S295.

308. Pandey SK, Werner L, Apple DJ, Escobar-Gomez M, Visessook N, Peng, Q, et al. Topographical analysis of foldable IOLs: A useful technique for evaluation of IOL surfaces. In: Pasricha JK, ed. *Proceedings of AIOS Congress.* Chennai, India, 2000. [In press]

309. Apple DJ, Peng Q. Harold Ridley Knighted. (Letter to the Editor) *Ophthalmology.* 2000;107:412-413.

310. Apple DJ. Letter to the Editor. *Surv Ophthalmology.* 2000. [In Press]

311. Snellingen T, Shrestha JK, Hug F, Husain R, Koirala S, Rao GN, Pokhrel RP, Kolstad A, Upadhyay MP, Apple DJ, et al. The South Asian cataract management study: Complications, vision outcomes, and corneal endothelial cell loss in a randomized multicenter clinical trial comparing intracapsular cataract extraction with and without anterior chamber intraocular lens implantation. *Ophthalmology.* 2000;107(2):231-240.

312. Wesendahl TA, Hunold W, Auffarth GU, Apple DJ. Kontaktbereich von kunstlinse und hinterkapsel. Systematische untersuchung unterschiedlicher kaptikparameter. *Ophthalmologe.* 1994;91:680-684.

313. Werner L, Apple DJ, Escobar-Gomez M, Ohrstrom A, Crayford BB, Bianchi R, Pandey SK. Postoperative deposition of calcium on the surfaces of Hydroview intraocular lenses. *Ophthalmology.* 2000. [In press]

Index

BUILD Your Library

This book and many others on numerous different topics are available from SLACK Incorporated. For further information or a copy of our latest catalog, contact us at:

**Professional Book Division
SLACK Incorporated
6900 Grove Road
Thorofare, NJ 08086 USA
Telephone: 1-856-848-1000
1-800-257-8290
Fax: 1-856-853-5991
E-mail: orders@slackinc.com
www.slackbooks.com**

We accept most major credit cards and checks or money orders in US dollars drawn on a US bank. Most orders are shipped within 72 hours.

Contact us for information on recent releases, forthcoming titles, and bestsellers. If you have a comment about this title or see a need for a new book, direct your correspondence to the Editorial Director at the above address.

Thank you for your interest and we hope you found this work beneficial.